Psychiatry as a Human Science

Contemporary Psychoanalytic Studies
18

Contemporary Psychoanalytic Studies (*CPS*) is an international scholarly book series devoted to all aspects of psychoanalytic inquiry in theoretical, philosophical, applied, and clinical psychoanalysis. Its aims are broadly academic, interdisciplinary, and pluralistic, emphasizing secularism and tolerance across the psychoanalytic domain. CPS aims to promote open and inclusive dialogue among the humanities and the social-behavioral sciences including such disciplines as philosophy, anthropology, history, literature, religion, cultural studies, sociology, feminism, gender studies, political thought, moral psychology, art, drama, and film, biography, law, economics, biology, and cognitive-neuroscience.

Psychiatry as a Human Science

Phenomenological, Hermeneutical and Lacanian Perspectives

Antoine Mooij

Translation
Peter van Nieuwkoop

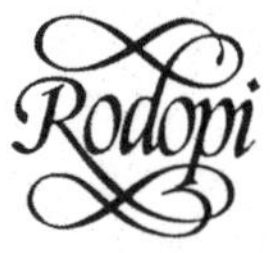

Amsterdam - New York, NY 2012

This book is a greatly revised edition of:
“De psychische realiteit”. Published by Boom, Amsterdam, 2006 (3rd edition)

Translated from the Dutch by Peter van Nieuwkoop

Cover illustration: Marcel Schellekens, Jar on kelim, etch 55x50 cm, 2000.

Cover Design: Studio Pollmann

The paper on which this book is printed meets the requirements of “ISO 9706:1994, Information and documentation - Paper for documents - Requirements for permanence”.

ISBN: 978-90-420-3596-6
E-Book ISBN: 978-94-012-0871-0

Printed in the Netherlands

Contents

Acknowledgements

The present book offers a translation as well as a thorough reworking and substantial extension of the 2006 edition of *De psychische realiteit. Psychiatrie als geesteswetenschap*, which saw its first publication in 1988. In the course of the revision process, comments and suggestions from readers and users were integrated. As a result, the book has reached a state of virtual completion, fully justifying publication in the English language.

I would like to thank Boom Publishers, Amsterdam, for kindly giving their permission to carry out this undertaking. The present book includes a number of text fragments which, in a slightly different form, were published in A. Mooij, *Intentionality, Desire, Responsibility. A Study in Phenomenology, Psychoanalysis and Law* (Brill Publishers, Leiden & Boston, 2010), more specifically, pages 62-68, 69-73, and 192-195. I would also like to thank Brill Publishers for giving their permission.

I am very grateful to Jon Mills for his willingness to include this book in the series 'Contemporary Psychoanalytic Studies'. I would like to thank Petra Kaas (Amstelveen) for her assistance with text and literature reference processing and Wieneke Matthijsse (Willem Pompe Institute for Criminal Law and Criminology, University of Utrecht) for her highly detailed attention to text layout and typography and for her assistance with compiling the Index. A special word of thanks goes to Peter van Nieuwkoop, Anytext Translations, for his careful and meticulous translation of these texts. Effectively, this book also carries his signature.

Antoine Mooij

No longer in a merely physical universe, man lives in a symbolic universe. [...] No longer can man confront reality immediately; he cannot see it, as it were, face to face.

E. Cassirer, *An Essay on Man*, p. 25

[...] the fashioning of the signifier and the introduction of a gap or a hole in the real is identical.

It creates a void and thereby introduces the possibility of filling it. Emptiness and fullness are introduced into a world that by itself knows not of them. It is on the basis of this fabricated signifier, this vase, that emptiness and fullness as such enter the world [...].

J. Lacan, *The Ethics of Psychoanalysis*, p. 150 and 149

Introduction

Looking back on the past two centuries of psychiatry, we cannot but conclude that modern psychiatry is truly flourishing in the 21st century. The various developments within psychiatry (biological psychiatry neurosciences) have largely defined the scientific status it holds today. And yet something was lost in the process as well.

In retrospect, we find that psychiatry has always had a keen eye for underlying biological aspects of mental disorders, while also considering a case in its individuality – adding new dimensions to diagnostics, keeping an open mind to anthropological issues. In addition to having a medical and natural-scientific orientation, its scope was also hermeneutical. Psychiatry has been conceived as being part of both the natural sciences and the humanities. Today this orientation appears to have been jettisoned: in the psychiatric field, little or no attention is paid to experience, to life history, to meaning and signification – in other words, to the psychic reality.

Perhaps we should argue it is just as well that such questions are no longer being asked, considering that they cannot be answered with the degree of certainty that has become the standard within the medical discourse. And yet we could also say that the traditional opposition between the natural-scientific and hermeneutical approaches is no longer valid. Anything requiring scientific validation needs to conform to the methodology of exact sciences and may therefore include meaningful connections and hermeneutical elements as well, both of which are processed in a natural-scientific way. As a third and final point, it appears that 21st-century psychiatry, despite its undisputed accomplishments, has fallen victim to one-sidedness, neglecting as it does the hermeneutical perspective.

Valid objections might be raised to the first two approaches. The first option will lead to an unnecessary reduction of the disciplinary field. Narrowing down the scientific effort to what the exact sciences can process, excluding issues of hermeneutical and reflexive nature, is not an inevitable scientific requirement but a deliberate metascientific choice. The second approach, with its plea for 'unitarian science', disregards the actual scientific landscape we see today, with its multitude of scientific efforts and its acknowledgment, in the very least, of a dichotomy. The third option holds that psychiatry shows undue neglect for the hermeneutical perspective, conceived in a broad sense.

Yet, this unilateral approach is in fact far from being accidental. Indeed, the medical discourse, when applied to modern psychiatry, was built precisely on the elimination of subjectivity. This introduces the need for an additional approach – the hermeneutical approach, in its broadest sense. An all-encompassing synthesis is not yet forthcoming, as major conceptual barriers need to be overcome first – nor is this expected to happen any time soon, if ever. In the meantime it has become essential that the legacy of the hermeneutical approach is not forgotten and that conceptual space is provided for the sake of revision. This sums up the fundamental thesis of the present book.

Its purpose is twofold: first of all, to offer a description, outlining the hermeneutical perspective and its scope, also taking into account the natural-scientific perspective. The second purpose, however, is even more ambitious: an attempt at indicating how a hermeneutical approach, also in this day and age, can add significance, while meeting scientific standards. Yet, the opposition between the natural-scientific and the hermeneutical perspective turns out to be a complex one, as it involves three types of distinctions: a conceptual, an ontological and a methodological one. The first aspect reflects the conceptual differences in use, while addressing physical reality and the psychic reality: the 'logical space of physical objects' (the 'realm of law') and the 'the logical space of reasons' (Sellars, 1956/1997). The ontological aspect concerns the nature of, and the relationship between, both spheres of reality: the mind-body issue. The methodological aspect is about the way both two basic conceptual schemes are put in scientific practice: empiricism and hermeneutics. Lastly, there is the historical point of view.

This results in the following structure. Chapter One outlines the nature of medical thought as the application of natural-scientific methodology on the medical discourse. Unable to take account of the variety of aspects of the psychic, this methodology leaves a space to be filled by psychiatry. Chapter Two describes how psychiatry (in the 19th and 20th centuries) conquered the space created by the medical discourse. In this process, we recognise a pendulum movement, with the hermeneutical and natural-scientific movements dominating alternately and the natural-scientific approach winning out in the end. Both chapters represent a historical point of view.

Chapter Three introduces the concept of psychic reality and describes how the relationship between the psychic and physical reality may be envisioned: the ontological aspect of the divide. It has meanwhile developed into a central philosophical theme, given the predominant position of the biological line of thought, which is also essential to any practice that strives to give psychic reality its rightful place. Rejecting monistic views, a dual approach is embraced. Reality should not be made identical with external reality, as it is not reducible to mere physical reality but also refers to psychic reality.

Chapters Four and Five are devoted to conceptual and methodological challenges. Chapter Four outlines the nature of the medical, natural-scientific approach within modern psychiatry, its conceptual scheme, and the obstacles it encounters, despite its achievements: the medical discourse in psychiatry. From this point on, the largely descriptive and critical approach in Part I gives way to a more argumentative approach in Part II, in order to explore the actual possibility of a new alternative.

Chapter Five develops the conceptual and methodological aspects of this complementary alternative. Central to this approach is hermeneutics – the discipline of interpretation relative to experience, speech and action – which falls into three types: hermeneutics of the signification (Dilthey), of the situation (Gadamer), and of the signifier (Lacan). A case will be presented for bringing these three different lines of thought together under the single heading of hermeneutics, which may look like a surprising effort. Following on these three types of hermeneutical methodologies, a distinction is made between three types of hermeneutical psychodiagnostics: descriptive (Jaspers), relational and structural (Lacan).

After presenting a partially historical overview of the psychic, Chapter Six introduces a twofold distinction between the spheres of emotion and ratio (passion and reason) on the one hand, and of conscious versus unconscious on the other. Referring to the notion of intentionality, phenomenology (in the sense of early Husserl) is also taken into account as an element of the field of hermeneutics, while belonging to the hermeneutics of the signification.

With regard to psychic reality three levels are distinguished: intentionality, being in the world, and the language dependence of human existence. These three levels are enabled and supported by what, following Lacan and Cassirer, may be referred to as the symbolic function. Lacan's (1966/2002) psychoanalytic theory of the symbolic order and the philosophy of the symbolic forms of the (Neo-Kantian) philosopher Ernst Cassirer (1929/1994b; 1953-1957) are brought together, notwithstanding their mutual differences. Both consider man as a living being that is able to symbolise reality from within a symbolic order or symbolic forms, while being stamped by language itself. Man is to be conceived as an *animal symbolicum* (Cassirer), fallen prey to language (Lacan). The difference between the two lies in the fact that the essence of the symbolic function (according to Cassirer) may disclose the real, while (according to Lacan) its essence rather puts the real at a distance. For a more technical-philosophical justification of the rapprochement between phenomenology and hermeneutics, as well as between Lacan, Husserl and Cassirer, reference can be made to A. Mooij, *Intentionality, Desire and Responsibility. A Study in Phenomenology, Psychoanalysis and Law* (2010, pp. 19-36, 93-166, 277-320). The emphasis in the present book, *Psychiatry as a Human Science*, is on the basic idea and its applicability on psychopathology.

Chapter Seven offers an outline of a phenomenological, hermeneutical and Lacanian-inspired psychopathology, based on the three levels of psychic reality. Use is made of the categorization employed within traditional psychopathology distinguishing three types of mental disorder (neurosis, personality disorder, psychosis). These types of disorder are reinterpreted as psychopathological structures, each of which have three subtypes referred to as subject positions. These psychopathological structures are interpreted as a product of the symbolic function, one that may be intact (in the case of neurosis), deficient (personality disorder) or altogether ineffective (psychosis). The basic idea is that the process of symbolization discloses its value where it no longer operates unhindered (Cassirer), with psychopathology offering crucial examples of impediments (Lacan). This perspective enables understanding of the very nature of the various psychopathological structures. On the other side, psychopathology turns out to be of great value to the understanding of the workings of the symbolic function.

Chapter Eight stresses the importance of the life history to the coming about of these psychopathological structures and subject positions, while contributing to the development of a corresponding type of psychodiagnostics: life-historical diagnostics. The psychopathological structures and related subject positions are again illustrated, now from the viewpoint of the life history. Together, the Chapters Five, Six, Seven and Eight constitute a – tentative – attempt at synthesising modern phenomenological, hermeneutical and Lacanian perspectives, putting these into perspective as well as adding clinical significance.

To complete this book, the Epilogue offers a brief outline of the nature of the correlation between the two types of psychiatry distinguished here – natural-scientific psychiatry and hermeneutical psychiatry – and two different lines of thoughts. While both have their validity, to some extent they are also mutually exclusive and cannot be merged into a single elegant conceptual synthesis, while both of them are needed in practice. Still, the effect is positive rather than negative. Particularly in view of its long tradition, it is obvious why medical science was able to spawn psychiatry, burdening it with a double nature that will continue to have a defining influence. In retrospect, it also becomes clear why the psychic – the psychic reality – represents a dimension that is essential for psychiatry and must not be neglected. Only then will psychiatry become a truly human-oriented science. This view is reflected in the title itself: *Psychiatry as a Human Science.*

It is founded in a specific, hermeneutical conception of man, namely that of an intentional living being, which engages in a shared world and is dependent on language, as is confirmed by the subtitle: *Phenomenological, Hermeneutical and Lacanian Perspectives.* These perspectives, pivotal as they are for 'an essay on man', constitute an essential part of any viable, comprehensive philosophical anthropology, insofar as they can be applied to the practice of human sciences. In line with this point of view, this book also aims to contribute to a philosophical anthropology made concrete.

PART I

One

The Medical Discourse

The Exclusion of Psychic Reality

Psychiatry and its core discipline, psychopathology, both have intimate ties with medical science. Psychiatry is a specialty taught at medical schools whose impact, despite its essentially limited basis, is remarkably broad. Within the vast field of mental health care, its medical background serves to effectively legitimise any practice labelled as 'mental health care'. Thus, its sphere of action extends well beyond the medical field. If we wish to explore the relationship between psychiatry and medical science, or the medical characteristics of psychiatry, first we shall need to identify the nature of medical science itself. An attempt will be made to establish whether a coherent 'medical' type of observation, thought, reasoning and action exists at all. Which raises the question: is medical science – both today and in the past – actually underpinned by a coherent conception or vision?

This question, which itself inquires into the foundations of the medical field, transcends medical science and is therefore not medical in nature. Originating in what may be termed the philosophy of medicine, it does not constitute an inquiry in a narrowed-down historical sense either. Nonetheless, it should be the objective of any scientific discipline's philosophy to inquire into its own origins, following two paths: the nature of the scope of reality addressed by this science, and the way this science deals with its scope of reality, respectively.

Two quite opposite stances may be adopted here. The first considers medicine – both today and in the past – to be a conglomerate of disparate subjects. In this view, medicine or medical science is little more than a cluster of isolated topics, bound together at best by biology as a common denominator on the one hand, and by psychology on the other. Yet they lack any real degree of unity, the inevitable conclusion being that medical science merely has a derived status (Shaffer, 1975). This view would turn out to be the undoing of medical science as a coherent discipline.

We should ask ourselves whether this position is tenable – if perhaps we can find a way after all to structure this multitude of themes, indeed even bring about some degree of unity. For example, we may argue that medicine does include fundamental disciplines (like physiology and anatomy) in addition to clinical sciences (like internal medicine and surgery), but that the specific nature of medicine is reflected in the convergence of those disciplines in medical practice, i.e., in the interaction between doctor and patient. Theory and practice combined could define the objective, which is found in the spheres of health promotion and curative care, respectively (Pellegrino and Thomasma, 1981, p. 26). Following Aristotle, medicine might be conceived as one of the so-called productive sciences – sciences that actually produce something, in this case physical and mental well-being.

Yet either position fails to plead its case convincingly. Medicine is more than a hotchpotch of disciplines that have a raison d'être found well outside the medical realm itself. In fact, it is governed by a unifying principle that addresses health and disease, remedying disorders. From this perspective, medicine could in fact be interpreted as a 'productive science'. However, where the former vision lacks ambition, this vision is rather over-aspiring. In the medical field, the definition of 'health', rather than describing physical and mental well-being, in a Platonic sense (Kenny, 1969), is commonly narrowed down to a purely somatic view. It is also doubtful whether the doctor/patient encounter actually merits the pivotal position it has been allocated here. In the following we shall argue that medical science – by necessity – strives to minimise, or even abstain from doctor-patient interaction, because that is precisely the reason why this discipline rose to fame in the first place. How exactly would we describe the nature of the encounter between patient and medical science?

The Scientific Quality of Medical Science

A more or less uniform pattern emerges, with an individual taking the initiative (except in the case of public health monitoring). It is this individual who comes forward with a complaint, a request or a desire: "I'm suffering from chest pain", "Doctor, can you give me something for my sore throat?", "I'd give anything for just one day without a headache", and so forth.

In a decisive step, medical science, rather than accept it as a problem defined by an individual or subject, transforms it into a disease symptom. This demonstrates the inadequacy of the first position, but also of the second. Contrary to what is expressed in the first position, the medical project is bound together by a central notion. This unity, however, is not forged by the doctor/patient interaction, but by the concept of 'disease', disease being an underlying, essentially somatic event exposed by the symptom. Thus, 'chest pain' may be a symptom of a heart condition, but also of a stomach ulcer. It turns symptom and disease into mutually linked concepts, with a corresponding diagnostics serving to solidify a more or less abstract disease concept. The history of medical science has witnessed a variety of disease concepts and their corresponding diagnostics: humoral pathology, which centred on the mutual relationship between the various bodily fluids; the pathological-anatomical disease concept, which gives prominence to organ damage; and the aetiological approach, focusing on invasive agents (e.g., harmful substances and germs), etcetera.

The transformation from complaint to symptom is crucial in this respect. It is what brought medical science into being, exercising an effect that is both positive and negative: the complaint ceases to be regarded as a subjective condition (the negative effect), instead becoming an objectifiable symptom of a yet hidden status (the positive effect). In one fell swoop, the complaining party is transformed into a carrier (of a disease), with medicine assuming the role of an empirical science extrapolating the outcomes of its investigations to other carriers of a similar disease in an objectifying manner.

Although doubt has been cast on the scientific quality of medical science, they lack any degree of credibility. Indeed, its procedures rigorously conform to the methodology of the exact, natural sciences. Like any other truly exact natural science, medicine gathers its data from experience. What exactly is the character of those data, and of the 'path of experience'? Today, it is commonly believed that a number of required stages can be distinguished, which in practice will be applied with some degree of licence.

Scientific research of this character will be based on observation, which does not necessarily imply that these observations lack focus. Through focused observation, the medical field strives to gain insight into a status by verifying expectations that have been developed based on a particular theory or conceptual point of view. As a next step, an attempt is made to satisfactorily address any issues that may have arisen in the process. Subsequently, a hypothesis or assumption is developed that may take the form of a law or a law-like statement ('correlations'). An assumption will not become a true hypothesis until the necessary conditions have been formulated that may either corroborate or refute it. As a further step, it will be ascertained whether the projected outcomes actually occur. Depending on the outcome, the hypothesis will have been confirmed until disproven, or refuted in its current form. In the latter case, an alternative assumption needs to be developed to resolve the fundamental issue, or the conclusion should be that the issue was misformulated. Any corroboration will have a provisional nature – there is always the risk that other predictions will fail and that the hypothesis will be refuted at a later stage, requiring adjustment. A refuted hypothesis, it has been argued, will be more relevant to the progress of scientific research than any confirmation, because verification inevitably has a provisional nature, while falsification brings finality (Popper, 1959/1968). Refutation will cause the hypothesis to be either rejected altogether or to be modified, and will consequently bring growth and progress of knowledge (Popper, 1972). The scientific construct will find its provisional conclusion in the development of concepts and theories that offer a coherent explanation of the findings. As such theories and concepts will fan new practical research efforts, scientific research apparently incorporates a cyclic element. Therefore, maintaining a clear-cut distinction between observing facts (using an 'observational language') and the construction of theories (based on a 'theoretical language') is no longer warranted.[1] In a similar way, the analytic-synthetic distinction no longer holds sway (Quine, 1953/1961, pp. 20-46).

Medical research would fit eminently within the framework of this type of philosophy of science. Then again, we do recognise a divergence between fundamental medical research on the one hand and practical diagnostics on the other, which is caused by a difference in emphasis. Fundamental medical research, seeking explanatory theories, will look upward, along the path leading from observation to theory. For example, in the days of Pasteur only 'essential fever' was known. Later, a distinction between various infectious diseases was introduced, with the concept of infection itself expressing a law or law-like pattern ('correlation'): in specific conditions, contamination by a particular germ is associated with a specified set of symptoms. Now, this generalised concept can be explained by a theory utilizing the concepts of immunity and virulence. Here, the emphasis is on a path leading upwards, from

[1] This model was proposed by post-positivist authors, first by Hanson (1958) and Popper (1959/1968). The latter formulates the theoretical dependence of experience as a programme (1959/1968), p. 107: "Observations are interpretations in the light of theories"; and p. 423: "We are theorizing all the time, even when we make the most trivial statements".

data to theory, with the theory offering an explanation for the data and the established empirical laws. This process is in line with the mainstream of today's philosophy of science.

In medical diagnostics, we would expect to see a different picture, because its aim is not to establish laws or law-like patterns ('correlations'). However, also in this field, medical science remains well within the methodological confines of the exact sciences. In medical diagnostics, the emphasis is not on the 'inductive path' leading upwards, but on the 'deductive, downward path', from the theoretical level down to that of experience. Within the context of today's diagnostic systems, factual data are collected, based on which a hypothesis or diagnosis is formulated and predictions are made that result from this hypothesis or diagnosis, reflecting a specific theory. As a final step, the predictions made are validated. This describes the process of differential diagnostics, in which a range of possible diagnoses are tested individually, each of which is either confirmed or (temporarily) rejected.

An example may illustrate this. If a person suddenly develops a pain in the left arm and a constricted feeling in the chest, an acute myocardial infarction would be the most obvious hypothesis or diagnosis. The theory of the aetiology of a myocardial infarction tells us that the ECG will show specific abnormalities, and that after a certain time period haemochemical changes in the enzyme spectrum can also be identified. Finally, perfusion defects and tissue loss can be visualised. When establishing whether such abnormalities actually occur, a positive outcome will confirm the diagnosis, whereas negative findings will rule it out.

In its pursuit to establish laws or law-like patterns ('correlations'), it follows an upward path, while the medical diagnostics being derived from a well-established diagnostic system – like the International Classification of Diseases (ICD) – leads down. Still, they do have one feature in common: their investigation invariably springs from a dominant notion and is cast in a more or less well-defined theoretical framework. Within the current philosophy of exact sciences, the primacy of theories and of conceptual structures has been generally acknowledged, albeit that there is still disagreement on the status of its theoretical concepts, among other things. Do they merely offer a convenient summary, do they perhaps constitute an empirical construct, or even carry an element of 'reality'? Pragmatism (Putnam, 1974), constructive empiricism (Van Fraassen, 1980), realism (Popper, 1972) and pluralism (Kuhn, 1970; Latour, 1987) offer competing views.[2] Yet they all acknowledge the importance of theoretical constructs.

From a scientific-historical perspective, it would be interesting – as it would once again underscore the harmonious relationship between medical science and the methodology of the exact sciences – to corroborate that medical science did acknowledge the relevance of theoretical concepts and constructs at a point in time when the philosophy of science itself was not yet up to the challenge; methodologists still adopted an inductivist approach, understating the value of theories or conceptual structures.[3]

Science as a Symbolic Form

Meanwhile, the priority of concepts, theoretical construction, is deeply rooted in the very idea of science. It was the Neo-Kantian philosopher Cassirer who in the first half of the twentieth century anticipated these more recent developments of the philosophy of science (Friedman, 2000). He felt that science in its modern form does not offer a mirror of nature, a sheer reflection of brutal reality, of the real (Rorty, 1979). On the contrary, it generates a theory-dependent scientific world view – including the 'scientific image of man' (Sellars, 1963) – disregarding aspects of the real which cannot be integrated in its conceptual scheme. Science is not a film, a mirror, of the real – the real itself is appropriated by science and its symbolic means. Just as any form of symbolisation, any symbolic form, scientific symbolisation is never complete, is always 'one-sided' and leaves a remainder, a residue, to be symbolised by other types of discourse. According to this line of thought, man, in order to be able to access reality, relies on symbolic systems: the symbolic form of language and language-dependent cultural systems as well as the symbolic form of science, both of which transform reality – the real existing outside man – into a language-dependent life world and into a scientific image of the world, respectively.[4]

---

[2] This issue is particularly relevant to the field of natural sciences: do electrons, quarks, superstrings, etcetera, actually 'exist'? It is also relevant to the field of psychiatry, be it at a much lower and less abstract level: does schizophrenia actually 'exist'?

[3] See Claude Bernard, *Introduction à l'étude de la médecine expérimentale*, 1865.

[4] Cassirer, (1944/1966, p. 25): "No longer can man confront reality immediately; he cannot see it, as it were, face to face. He has so enveloped himself in linguistic forms, in artistic images, in mythical symbols or religious rites that he cannot see or know anything except by interposition of this artificial medium".

Later, this view on symbolisation was to be embraced by the French structuralists (Jacobson, Lévi-Strauss), finding its most prominent expression in Lacan's theory of the symbolic order.[5] Indeed, structuralism rooted in classical French epistemology (Koyré) runs parallel to Cassirer's Neo-Kantian philosophy, both of which are drawing a sharp line between experience and the formalisation in science (Granger, 1967, pp. 7-22).

So there is a fundamental difference between the symbolisation inherent to language *and* symbolisation inherent to natural science, in the scientific discourse. Language offers a content-wise conceptualisation or symbolisation of the real, constituting a life world and its specific categories dependent on language – the concept of man as 'man-in-the-world' (Sellars, 1963, p. 6-8). Science on the other hand refrains from the content-wise conceptualization inherent to the life world, refrains from the description of everyday reality, offered by ordinary language. It presents a process of formalisation in which phenomena are analysed in formal elements, those which are present or absent (+/-) without any direct relation with the fullness of lived experience, allowing to be functionalized (if $p \rightarrow q$). Therefore, formalization and functionalization go hand in hand. In a final step, laws and law-like patterns can be established. H_20 for water; if heated it will be boiled at 100^0. A, B, Rh+/- for blood; if mixed, it will not/coagulate (Zwart, 1998). A whole range of reality can be explained scientifically just by using these formal symbols. In this process of formal symbolisation, of formal representation, formal concepts – idealizations (Husserl, 1953/1970), pure meanings (Cassirer, 1929/1994) and master signifiers (Lacan, 1991/2007) – not derived from lived experience but constituting scientific experience – play a pivotal role.[6]

Defining Medical Science

It is hardly surprising that traditionally medical science should have focused on the priority of a theoretical framework, a conceptual scheme,

---

5 Lacan (2002, p. 209): "It is the world of words that creates the world of things – things which at first run together in the *hic and nunc* of the all in the process of becoming – by giving it concrete being to their essence, and its ubiquity to what has always been [...]".

6 An essential difference between Lacan and Cassirer lies in the fact that, with time, Lacan put more and more emphasis on the real as both a barrier and an impossibility, while Cassirer, in line with Neo-Kantianism, choose reality to coincide with its symbolic being processed (Mooij, 2010, pp. 7-10, 153-156). See Chapter Six.

a master signifier, even before the philosophy of science was inclined to do so. For the very reason that its main driver is a central, direction-giving concept: the concept of disease. For all the historical diversity of the various concepts of disease – pathological-anatomical, bacteriological, endocrinological – they have one feature in common. Medical science formalizes the phenomena that make up its own domain, supervised by its fundamental concepts and signifiers, excluding anything that does not fit its conceptual scheme. Following the concept of disease, phenomena of lived experience are selected and transformed into formal symptoms, which are then combined into disease profiles and subordinated to a standard. Indeed, disease refers to health, a normative concept.

Exactly what kind of normativity is at stake here? Overall, two types of normativity may be distinguished (Frankena, 1963). First, a set of rules adopted by a society or culture. A person speaking a particularly language will have to adhere to its rules if he wants to be understood: you cannot join in a game unless you follow its rules. Rather than being universal, such rules will be valid only within a given culture – they were selected, in a sense. Any person wishing to be part of a culture will have to abide by its inherent set of rules. As a result of this element of 'bondage', this type of normativity may be referred to as 'deontological', a term that is used ethically neutral within this context. The second type of normativity is focused not on culture but on nature, more specifically, on a sense of purposivity that is supposed to be inherent in nature, particularly living nature. Most likely, purposivity characterises all living beings whose efforts may, for example, be geared towards survival. This second, 'purposive' or 'functional' type of normativity may be described as teleological (Taylor, 1964, pp. 3-53).

Based on the foregoing, we might conclude that the concept of disease and health adopted by medical science, from a normative point of view, is a teleological one, where the 'telos' or purpose may of course be defined in a variety of ways. It can be done on a modest scale, as in cases where the teleological norm is supposed to be the attainment of a baseline state in physiological or chemical settings, or by maintaining an equilibrium. Alternatively, more ambitiously, the norm might include adaptation of an organism to its environment. Yet, in each case, we recognise a narrowed-down, somatic health concept, as opposed to the broad Platonic-Aristotelian concept of mental and physical well-being. It is this narrowed-down concept that enables medical science to manifest itself as a technical science which, based on generalised knowledge, is able to restore a natural state of balance by technical means.

This constitutes a basic definition of medical science. Medical science, being a symptom-oriented discipline, a 'symptomatology', may develop into a natural science that conforms to rigid standards. Through the concept of disease and health, its symptomatology will introduce a normative and more specifically functional or teleological moment. As a result, the pattern of medical science is both symptomatological and teleological in nature.

THE LIFESPAN OF MEDICAL SCIENCE

Medical science manifests itself at the moment of transformation from complaint to symptom – in specific curative-medical settings (doctor's surgery, laboratory or hospital), in disease prevention efforts, but also in daily conversation, whenever disease- or health-related topics are brought up. The crumbling authority of religious or world-philosophical traditions sparked fresh interest in fact-oriented sciences such as the medical field, which gained prominence as a result.

Its omnipresence and major impact on today's society are the result of a rich and well-established tradition. Medical science itself predates 19th-century medicine based on pathological anatomy, and even the dissection-oriented anatomical approach of the 16th century. The first tentative steps towards medical science may be traced back to the late 5th and early 4th centuries BC, with the advent of early Hippocratic medicine in Greece.[7] Surprisingly, even though Hippocratic medicine was not dissection-based, this turned out to be the very reason why it earned itself a scientific status. Once this type of medicine develops from a craft – a visually oriented barber-surgery – into a study of internal diseases, it becomes a 'science', in today's terms, because of the fact that the body is not invaded. Indeed, its non-invasive character prompts the formulation of theories describing processes occurring inside the body, while theoretical development is controlled by experience. We might say that early Hippocratic medicine acknowledges the difference between experience and theory in that they are mutually dependent, as a result of which medicine ceases to be a hands-on craft, while also failing to

---

[7] The early Greek setting of the medical course follows Clavreul (1978), a Lacanian psychiatrist. Despite the Greek origins of the medical discourse, not all later types of medicine conform to this model. For a discussion of Hippocratic medicine see Magner (2005, pp. 93-98).

provide a speculative type of philosophy of nature (Mansfeld, 1973, pp. 13-14, 28; Popper, 1969).

Nonetheless, there was still ample opportunity for the traditional view of the body as an animated entity to be sustained. For example, Plato opposed the reductionist view of health as a purely somatic concept, as it limited what he envisioned: the well-being of body and mind as a whole. This Platonic – or even Platonic-Aristotelian – more or less holistic view of an animated corporeality took root and for a long time dominated the mainstream of thought (Porter, 1996, pp. 90-93).[8]

Within this historical development, we see a whole new figure emerge, with the first explorations of the human body in the 14th century: the internal is externalised and the unseen becomes visible. It constituted a crucial step when, for the first time in Western history, the mediaeval physician Mundinus opened up the bodies of convicted criminals. While Mundinus only saw what was supposed to be there based on Galen's traditional views, he did not see – obviously could not see – what was really inside this body. It took the best part of two and a half centuries for a new conceptual frame to emerge, with the publication of Vesalius' *De Humani Corporis Fabrica,* in 1543.[9] This landmark publication would pave the way for today's modern medical science. In a strong sense, according to Cassirer (1943), Vesalius created empirical descriptive anatomy as the core discipline of biology and medicine. Visualising what was invisible made the distance between the manifest symptom and the obscure disease increasingly smaller. The mechanistic conception of the body gave birth to notions such as 'fabric' (Vesalius' anatomy) and 'pump' (Harvey's physiology).

A new phase may be identified when, in the late 18th century and early 19th century, the relationship between the clinic and pathological anatomy becomes more and more intimate, resulting in a shift of function of the clinic itself.[10] Formerly a place where established knowledge is taught, it finds itself transformed into a hotbed for new discoveries

---

[8] Plato, Charmides, 156d-157b. Lain-Entralgo (1970, pp. 108-139) emphasised that early medicine centred on dialogue, and that it was Plato who wished to reintroduce this element, contrary to the prevailing beliefs of his contemporaries.

[9] This process is described by the phenomenologist Van den Berg (1959/1965, pp. 30-74, 171-193).

[10] The purpose of this list of keywords is not to refer to a 'history of medicine' as a history of great names. Essentially, its aim is to refer to a history of ideas (Lovejoy, 1936/1964, pp. 3-24), i.e., how a number of variations led to the realisation of one central concept: the externalisation of the internal.

through direct observation of the body, both outside and inside, for example, using instruments like a stethoscope or speculum, visualising the inner workings of a body that is still alive, rather than the anatomy of a corpse.[11]

The broad range of imaging technologies available to today's medical science – e.g., anatomy, radiology, endoscopy, ultrasound and MRI – demonstrates that the original distinction between symptom and disease becomes blurred, but also that this tendency cannot be effective unless set against the background offered by this initial distinction. Opening the body, in addition to exposing the invisible, will externalise the internal. The microcosm that is the body's interior begins to resemble the macrocosm of the physical environment, while the parallel process of mechanization of the world picture is extended to include the human body (Dijksterhuis, 1986).

Evidently, it took some time for a movement that introduced revolutionary new elements and – considering the new technologies introduced by today's medical science – is still far from its completion, to be accepted and integrated. For example, after the first incision by Mundinus, two centuries would elapse before Vesalius, in the 16th century, followed up on it. This venture has always been met with some degree of reserve, which explains why an alternative to this mechanization trend developed, taking the form of a Platonic-Aristotelian view of the body as an animated corporeality, one that was particularly favoured in the days of Romantic medicine. This countermovement has a long history as well, but still this does not detract from the fact that today's medical science, in its turn, is a branch sprung forth from an ancient trunk, and that mechanistic and visualising trends continue to be based on a symptomatological approach.

The Medical Discourse

In view of the long and well-established tradition of medical science it would be appropriate to speak of a 'discourse' rather than a 'model'. In the latter case, we may think in terms of design, modification or rejection

---

[11] This is the central thesis proposed by Foucault (1963/1994). The 'medical gaze' therefore differs from the practice of observation in the medicine of the Greek, which leaves the body uninvaded. The rise of the pathological-anatomical conception of disease may be dated between 1761, when Morgagni published his *De sedibus et causis morborum*, and 1858, when Virchow's *Die Cellular Pathologie* was published.

(Black, 1962). However, the licence of design inherent in this concept does not offer an acceptable match for the history of medical science.[12] The term 'discourse' suggests that medical science reflects a development in Western thought – particularly in modernity – that is tied to a variety of fundamental positions which cannot be ignored and span many generations.

The relative supremacy of a discourse should not be interpreted chronologically, but as a principle. More than being a precursor to the establishment of future facts, it underlies the process of ascertaining facts that fall within the scope of the discourse. It was not until a mechanistic conception of reality began to find currency that Harvey, back in the 17th century, was able to recognise the flow of blood as a circulation system, with the heart as its pump. Only when a view including its concepts and signifiers finds acceptance can phenomena be interpreted within the context of this view: a particular discourse, or a variety of this discourse, enables well-described perception and conceptualization. In addition to this positive effect, a discourse also has a negative effect, in that it closes the door to a different type of perception and conceptualization. Any form of discourse offers a symbolisation of the real, by constituting its specific form of reality, disregarding and excluding what fails to match its form of conceptualisation. While creating opportunities for reasoning and acting, it eliminates opportunities for reasoning and acting differently.

This applies to the medical discourse as well. In a positive sense, the medical discourse is expressed in the transformation from complaint tot symptom, while allowing medical science to develop in a objectifying manner towards reality and constituting the human body as an object, as a merely physical reality. The negative effect would be that the suffering subject is transformed into a carrier or substrate of a disease, excluding him or her as a person with a psychic reality. By the symbolic construction of medical reality medical science does exclude subjectivity or the psychic reality, because this exclusion actually constitutes the reverse of the process of transformation from complaint to symptom.[13] As a result, entities such as the 'subjectivity of the patient' or the 'doctor-

---

[12] The concept of 'discourse', in the broad yet formal sense indicated, played a key role in French philosophy, insofar as it was influenced by Foucault (1969/ 1989) and Lacan (1991/2007). More or less related but more limited in scope is the notion of '*priority of paradigms*' developed by Kuhn (1970, pp. 43-52).

[13] See also Clavreul (1978), who was inspired by Lacan's theory of discourse.

patient relationship' – odd though it may sound – have no place within medical science. It is a remainder, a leftover, instituted by the symbolization of the medical discourse.

PRACTICE AS AN ALTERNATIVE PATH WITHIN MEDICINE

And still, anyone who positions himself outside medical science and is willing to listen to the patient's story, will find that the complaint, more than being a symptom of a physical substrate, actually has meaning, by expressing a question, request or desire: for example, the desire to see the doctor fail and to come out triumphantly as a patient, the disease still intact. Obviously, the complaint can be interpreted within a variety of personal contexts (family, work and such) and may be a manifestation of a disturbed or disrupted communication.

Like medical science was built formally on the exclusion of subjectivity, of the psychic reality, the medical practitioner has always been aware of the subjective dimension, of the historicity of existence and of the significance that should be attributed to disrupted relationships. Undoubtedly, he will have made an effort to take these factors into account, yet without being able to include this dimension into the discourse.

In the 20th century, tentative attempts were made to integrate this approach into the theoretical domain. We may recognise efforts to retain certain aspects of traditional views of human nature as an 'animated body', or an 'embodied self' (Clark, 1997; Varela, 2002). Already established was a psychosomatic approach that identified how a complaint or disease may reflect certain issues originating in life history and psychic reality (Alexander, 1950; Boss, 1954). The direction that anthropological medicine took, particularly during the 1950s (in Europe), focused on integrating specifically human aspects falling outside the scope of natural-scientific concepts, into a widened concept of disease and medical practice (Von Weizsäcker, 1940/1973). We witnessed the arrival of so-called integral medicine, which aimed at taking somatic, psychological and social factors into account. Building on this approach, the 1970s saw the emergence of the biopsychosocial model (Engel, 1980; White, 2004). A more recent development is so-called family medicine, which has a keen eye for the involvement of family factors in conditions with a merely somatic presentation. Some endeavours reached back to the countermovement that had manifested itself earlier – as in Romantic medicine – reflecting a revival of the Platonic-Aristotelian view of an animated corporeality.

Most of these attempts were not particularly successful, and future efforts may suffer the same fate, although not necessarily. However, it is hard to see how any such attempt could ever succeed, because they would inevitably affect the nature of the medical discourse. Apart from having a well-established tradition, medical science is firmly embedded in the mechanizing trends that define the dominant Western mode of thought, which, since Descartes, Galileï and Kant, has come to see nature as one great single mechanism. Today its position, rooted in this mode of thought, is quite strong – perhaps even stronger than ever before – as is exemplified by recent spectacular advances (in the field of surgical techniques, antibiotics and chemotherapies, genetics, and advanced imaging technologies such as MRI). Pleas for more efficient and yet improved health care underline the unchallenged status of medical science. In its present form, however, it is driven by the assumption that disease is mostly or chiefly a mechanical or primarily biological event that affects people randomly, well removed from our psychic reality, history or personal relationships.

In his interactions with patients, the medical practitioner is aware of this alternative path, which defines disease as a meaningful entity, a way of suffering, rather than merely as a mechanical fact (Hanson and Callahan, 1999; Cassell, 2004; Rosenberg, 2007). Yet, medical science finds itself incapable of integrating this point of view, and the field of medicine, a conjunction of medical science and medical practice, now appears to be built on a disjunction: because the constitute each other's exclusion, medical science and medical practice are more or less at odds. And still, its effect is positive rather than negative: it is the very driver of success in medical science and, ultimately, of its major impact on society and its members. What was excluded by science, however, will return in practice. Still, this return fails to affect the autonomous status of the medical discourse, it seems. Thus, medicine has a dual foundation, with one pillar, rooted in science, excluding the psychic reality, while the other, rooted in practice, integrates it without being able to offer an adequate theory.

The void both left *and* created by the medical discourse has partly been filled by psychiatry which, being a medical discipline, is focused on offering a theory of psychic reality. Modern psychiatry, however, emerged as an extension of the medical discourse, which explains why, like medicine, it is characterised by a fundamental dichotomy. Its history will be discussed in the next chapter.

Two

The History of Hermeneutical Psychiatry

The history of care for the mentally ill and thoughts on mental disorders go back to the beginning of mankind (Porter, 1996). As regards the date of birth of modern psychiatry there is common agreement, however, as it coincides with the period of the French Revolution: in the year 1792, Philippe Pinel, in an effort to promote dedicated treatment of mentally disabled people, literally unchained a group of asylum patients. This led, in the early years of the 19th century, to the founding of the first psychiatric institutions. The underlying notion was that an environment of discipline and tranquillity would have a healing effect. From that moment onwards, modern psychiatry – originated from nursing and care settings rather than from academia – would go on to establish itself in the world of science. It purposefully positioned itself outside medical science, which in the same period was allying itself with university clinics in a bid to give its actions a natural-scientific basis (as was pointed out in Chapter One). Its consequences would be twofold. Little though could be accomplished in practice, the objectives of psychiatry were not essentially scientific, but practical or even therapeutic in nature. Its emphasis – another consequence – was on the psychological approach to the patient. This approach, described at the time as '*traitement moral*' or '*moral treatment*' resonated strongly throughout Europe. Important were Tuke in Great Britain and Guislain in Belgium.

Early Institutional Psychiatry

In the early days of institutional psychiatry, ideas on mental disorders still had strong religious overtones. Mental illnesses were associated with the religious concept of sin as well as with guilt. In addition, man was conceived as a single mental and bodily unit, while mental illness was assigned a position somewhere in the polarity between freedom and lack of freedom. Thus, a religious approach was supplemented with an anthropologically informed view.

Within this religious-anthropological field, 'Psychics' were head-to-head with 'Physics'. We should be careful not to misinterpret these two concepts (Verwey, 1980, pp. 6-55). The early 19th-century struggle between Psychics and Physics was nothing like today's definition of the word. Ancient views of nature still held sway, a far cry from the modern concept developed by natural sciences. Both 'Psychics' and 'Physics' still shared these ancient views, which held that nature appears as a natural force or power (*physis*) of genesis and decay. Rooted in the Platonic-Aristotelian tradition, this concept of nature effectively separated contemporary psychiatry from a world view that increasingly became dominated by the natural-scientific approach.

So how did 'Psychics' and 'Physics' relate within the Platonic-Aristotelian tradition? Plato regarded the soul as being superior to the body, as an autonomous entity, still leaving room for a limited degree of unity between body and soul. The Platonic concept was embraced by the Psychics. A protagonist of this Platonic line, Heinroth felt that the body may be the carrier of the soul, but that the soul actually owns the body.[1] In other words, he describes a cohesion between body and soul, while attributing a superior position to the latter. This superior and ultimately autonomous position of the soul will make it possible for a *Seelenstörung* – a defect of the soul itself – to develop. It is the very reason why the champions of this doctrine are referred to as 'Psychics'.

The 'Physics' (Jacobi, Nasse), by contrast, adopted an Aristotelian approach. Certainly, Aristotle chained the soul – as the form of life or as its defining principle – more firmly to the body than did Plato. The soul defines life, either as a form or as an essence. Because the soul functions as a life form or life-giving principle, it can never be imperfect in itself – only the matter in which the soul expresses itself can be flawed. Therefore, any disorder originating from the soul will not compatible with this view, and a mental disorder will always be organic in nature. This explains why the followers of this doctrine are called 'Physics'.[2]

Despite their diverging views, both Psychics and Physics shared a common fundamental view, viz., that of man as an animated body or an embodied soul. Arguably, it was the – partially – religious background of institutional psychiatry that caused the Platonic-Aristotelian view of

---

[1] Heinroth (1823, p. 75): "Der Leib enthält die Seele, ist der Träger der Seele, wie alles äussere der Träger des Inneren ist. Der Leib gehört der Seele an: aber die Seele nicht dem Leibe, denn alles Innere ist als das ursprüngliche auch das höhere".

[2] Wyrsch (1956, p. 30), after offering a quotation fromThomas of Aquino, summarizes it as follows: "In unserem Sprachgebrauch auf Deutsch und in einem Wort gesagt: es gibt nur organische Psychosen".

man to take hold beyond the realm of the natural and medical sciences, which gained ground at a steady pace.

THE EARLY MEDICAL DISCOURSE IN PSYCHIATRY

The situation changes dramatically with the emergence of academic psychiatry in parallel with institutional psychiatry, a development that is associated with the increasing practical significance attributed to psychiatry: the desire to include psychiatry in medical training, in order to provide new doctors with some practical knowledge of the field. And so *Universitätspsychiatrie* (Psychiatry in university clinic) emerged next to *Anstaltspsychiatrie* (Psychiatry in mental hospitals) – adding small-sized university clinics to the existing large-scale institutions (Jaspers, 1913/1997, p. 846). It would bring a profound change to the cultural landscape.

Griesinger

Obviously, academic psychiatry gravitated towards natural scientific medicine, causing this brand of psychiatry to be performed in a mental setting that was fundamentally different from institutional psychiatry. As a result, the religion-inspired Platonic-Aristotelian mode of thought gave way to the scientific approach of medical science or the medical discourse. This revolutionary institutional and discursive transformation is associated with Griesinger.

Man, no longer conceived as an embodied soul in a Platonic-Aristotelian sense, now became the physical-chemical-mechanical entity, a theme of natural science. This historic break is marked by Griesinger's work 'Pathology and Therapy of Mental Illnesses for Physicians and Students', published in 1845. Griesinger proceeded from a differentiated naturalism conceiving mental functioning as a symptom of matter to which, however, it can never be fully reduced (Verwey, 2004, pp. 27-34). In light of this, it would be useful to investigate mental functions as a function of the brain, while conceiving mental illnesses as the product of a brain disorder. Thus, Griesinger laid the foundations for 19th-century biological psychiatry, as is exemplified by his famous thesis that mental illnesses are diseases of the brain. He postulates that mental diseases will always reflect some kind of brain disorder.[3] Thus, psychopathological phenomena would be symptoms of some underlying somatic event. In line with the medical discourse, psychiatry was able to develop as a natural science. In this respect, it is hardly relevant whether Griesinger's choice for naturalism was dogmatic or hypothetical in nature. Indeed, the difference in scope between dogma and hypothesis will not detract from the impact of this endeavour (Jaspers, 1913/1997, p. 459). What is implied is a symptomatic existence of the mind in relationship to nature – an interpretation pursued more fervently by Griesinger's followers than in his own efforts. Griesinger adopted a more restrained position in that he renounced any radical type of reductionism that fully reduces the mental to the material aspect, as it allowed him to also take mental factors into account (Griesinger, 1843/1964, pp. 168-172).

This nuance was lost, however, in the further development of biological psychiatry which, in line with contemporary beliefs, favoured an even more radical reductionism. However, these far-reaching ambitions also widened the gap between the ambitions of biological psychiatry and its accomplishments. Then again, there were a number of breakthrough events at the time, such as the discovery of speech-regulating brain centres (Broca and Wernicke) which for the first time in history could be visualised using newly developed staining techniques. Nonetheless, insights into the various brain functions were still limited. Eventually, this programme failed to live up to its promise – a promise that could never be substantiated anyway with the technical means available at the time.

Moreover, the need was felt for a less dogmatic, more 'empirical' approach. The spirit of the times changed, and materialistic reductionism began to lose some of its sheen. The fact that biological psychiatrists were notorious for their callous approach to patients certainly did not help. A new paradigm was needed: clinical psychiatry.

---

[3] Griesinger (1845/1964, p. 1): "Welches Organ muss also überall und immer nothwendig erkrankt sein, wo Irresein vorhanden ist? Die Antwort auf diese Frage ist die erste Voraussetzung der ganzen Psychiatrie. Zeigen uns physiologische und pathologische Tatsachen, dass dieses Organ nur das Gehirn sein kann, so haben wir vor Allem in die psychischen Krankheiten jedesmahl Erkrankungen des Gehirns zu erkennen".

Kräpelin

The idea was that it would be beneficial for psychiatric patients to be examined more empirically, particularly with regard to the course of their disorder. Kräpelin (1856-1926) is the true champion of this approach. His textbook, which was published in a number of editions in the late 19th and early 20th centuries, earned him the title of Father of Clinical Psychiatry. We might say that Kräpelin succeeded in bridging the gap between institutional psychiatry, with its penchant for clinical description, and the neuropathological orientation of academic psychiatry. Admittedly, the approach he adopted did put academic psychiatry on a pedestal.

He intended to create order in the multitude of disorders identified at the time. He even made it his quest, testimony to which are the constantly changing classifications introduced in the various editions of his textbook. He felt that rather than the momentary state of mental dysfunctioning, it was the course of a disease that would offer conclusive evidence as to its nature. It was Kräpelin who gave the 'careful description' the scientific status which it lacked in biological psychiatry. In doing so, he perhaps did not create clinical psychiatry, but he certainly gave it scientific legitimacy.[4]

Two of the distinctions he made have retained their currency to this very day. The first one concerns the distinction between endogenous and exogenous causality (from the inside or the outside) of a mental disorder, regardless of its precise definition. The second distinction is that between 'affective' and 'non-affective' psychoses, for which he coined the phrases 'manisch-depressives Irresein' (manic-depressive psychosis) and 'Dementia praecox' (dementia praecox), respectively (now referred to as bipolar disorder and schizophrenia). In doing so, he created some kind of basic order which has never lost its validity as a classifying principle. His efforts met with a lot of resistance at the time, and later as well. His basic assumption was that, like somatic medicine, psychiatry would include a range of autonomous diseases rather than comparatively non-specific 'modes of reaction'. Thus, he turned psychiatry into disease-based or *nosological* psychiatry.

---

[4] France also boasted a rich tradition in the field of psychopathology, with people like B.-A. Morel (the concept of degeneration), P. Sérieux and J. Capgras, V. Magnan, J. Cotard.

At the heart of *nosological* psychiatry was the disease unit concept. Despite the broadening envisioned and accomplished by Kräpelin in his nosological approach, this concept was as much in accordance with the medical discourse as was neurological psychiatry. This is caused by the nosological line of thought itself. A mental disorder constitutes a psychiatric disease if it is characterised by the simultaneous finding of an identical present condition, course of the disorder, final condition, cause, and organic substrate. A nosological diagnosis should be considered as a 'logical product' of its constituting partial diagnoses regarding presentation, substrate, cause and course of the disorder. In fact, a nosological diagnosis presupposes a law-like (nomological) relationship. If one or more conditions (to which one or more partial diagnoses refer) have been met, it follows that other conditions (to which other partial diagnoses refer) have been met as well. As a result, a nosological diagnosis will express a law-like relationship, and so we would be justified in describing a *nosological* diagnosis as a *nomological* proposition. It makes the nosological diagnostics congruous with natural-scientific and medical-scientific methodology, which also strives to identify causal, nomological relationships.

It also renders the nosological project quite vulnerable. If one partial diagnosis has been rejected or remains unconfirmed, it follows that the nosological diagnosis, as a 'logical product' of its partial diagnoses, should not be made. Moreover, inductive logic – a branch of logic which deals with probability values – holds that the probability of the nosological diagnosis as a 'logical product' would at best be equal to the smallest probability value of one of its partial diagnoses. Consequently, the standards imposed by the logical structure of the nosological diagnosis would be exacting to the point where such a diagnosis can no longer be made (although this was not realised at the time). Thus, any extreme interpretation of symptomatology within psychiatry will eventually lead to its own downfall, following principles taken from the methodology of the exact (natural) sciences – the very principles that nosology, as a partner of the medical discourse, strives to uphold.

Kräpelin's view was essentially medical-scientific – formal as well as content-wise – as we may conclude from his rejection of the doctrine of psychic causality of mental disorders, or 'psychogenesis'. It may not have been a rejection per se, but he certainly qualified this possibility by criticising "the popular opinion that regards the development of mental disorders from misinterpretations or mood swings as a matter of course".[5] The central concept becomes 'endogeny' – the cause of a mental disorder 'lies within'. With Kräpelin, its scope varies and its precise meaning changes, depending on whether it refers to hereditary traits, general physical constitution or an idiopathy. The concept deals with the elimination of environmental factors, particularly those of mental or interactional nature.

Again we recognise a tendency to consider a mental disorder – and thus psychic reality – as a symptom of an underlying process, much like Griesinger had done in his biological interpretation of psychiatry, rather than as an autonomous event. At the heart of this lies the fact that nosology aligns itself with the medical discourse, both in its methodology and in its content. Once again, however, this effort was bound to fail at the time, because an exclusion of the psychic reality, as dictated by the medical discourse, will upset the balance within the psychiatric field.

THE ALTERNATIVE PATH IN PSYCHIATRY: UNTIL 1950

Psychiatry adopted a systematic approach to the 'alternative path' – which includes rather than excludes psychic reality – much more so than somatic medicine, or psychiatry did or was able to do in its early years. It also attempted to account for this at a theoretical level, by following two lines of inquiry. The first line is that of psychoanalysis, which emerged, and also found currency, outside academia. The second line remained embedded in the university clinic, whilst attempting to broaden its scope. Two stages may be distinguished. Overall, the first stage refers to the pre-World War II period, the second stage to the period that followed.

In the following, both aspects of this 'second line' will be discussed in accordance with this chapter's objective: the history of hermeneutical psychiatry – 'hermeneutical' in a broad sense. This objective is limited and does not include a comprehensive history of psychiatry, as this would have required a different approach. This limitation offers another advantage, namely that it highlights a part of psychiatry's history that is less well-known today. Moreover, we shall briefly outline a number of figures that will be brought up in more detail later in the book.

---

[5] Kräpelin (1909, p. 120). The four bulky volumes of this 8th edition can be seen as the highlight within Kräpelin's development. It constituted an attempt to refute objections raised against previous versions. See also: Bercherie (1980, pp. 139-153; 220-232).

Freud and Psychoanalysis

Freud (1856-1939) was not a product of institutional psychiatry, but originated from an academic background in the neurological field causing him, by extension, to be shaped by the neurological private practice. Finding himself confronted with cases that defied any neurological explanation, he attempted to clarify symptoms by proceeding from a person's experience and life history (Ellenberger, 1970). Freud's approach may well have been inspired by "the popular opinion that regards the development of mental disorders from misinterpretations or mood swings as a matter of course". The popular opinion or common sense interprets behaviour as an expression of needs, intentions, expectations and representations. Freud extended this interpretation by adding that mental states may constitute an unnoticeable or unconscious process. As a result, rather than simply following the popular opinion, he enlarged this concept, prompted by the need to treat the symptoms in addition to explaining them. This need was reinforced by the fact that he worked as an independent practitioner and not at an asylum or university clinic, environments that demanded little in that respect.

Thus, psychoanalysis was shaped on the basis of milder 'neurotic' disorders – hysteria, compulsive neurosis, phobia – that would not lead to the patient being sectioned (Freud 1909/1955a; 1909/1955b). Essential in this respect was the construct of a new treatment modality where the patient was encouraged to speak freely, with the psychoanalyst listening with 'free floating attention'. Freud effectively distanced himself from the medical discourse, which was focused on identifying symptoms of an underlying disease process by consistent diagnostic questioning. In doing so, Freud did not focus on symptomatology – instead, he set out to define the implicit message of a complaint, or its expressive value, proceeding from the notion that acknowledging the hidden message would remove the need for obscuring it, causing the phenomenon to recede. A person losing her voice after 'failing to say either yes or no' in a situation where it really mattered to speak up, may have lost her voice for the very reason that she 'could not say either yes or no', thereby manoeuvring herself out of an awkward situation. Insight into the conflict would cause the symptom itself to disappear. Fundamental in this respect is the notion of an unconscious driven by conflict, with insight into the nature of these conflicts serving as a remedy. Essentially, he reached back to the ancient notion that people may suffer from ignorance, and that truth – fighting ignorance and active oblivion – is a healer. It was the ancient Greek notion of 'Know thyself' that, since the Age of Enlightenment, has survived in a different guise, in modern philosophy, redefined as a presupposition that man can and should liberate himself from mental fetters.[6] By thus stressing the significance of self-reflection, he strayed beyond the boundaries of natural-scientific psychiatry, where mental disorders are supposed to be a consequence of natural processes, in a materialistic sense. This constituted an unequivocal paradigm shift.

In yet another field Freud distanced himself from natural-scientific psychiatry, a second leading thought being that a mental disorder was the product of a life history or the sum of a person's experiences and actions throughout his or her lifetime. Once again, we recognise a concept inspired by the popular opinion, which again was extended in the sense that the focus was on childhood upbringing and on the affective ties existing within the family. Its concept of sexuality was quite broad, including the whole of binding relationships but without relinquishing its original, more limited definition, thus turning it into psychosexuality (Freud, 1905/1953b). The significance of life history, of 'psychogenesis' and therefore of self-reflection, widened the gap with the naturalistic tendencies of contemporary psychiatry, which was dominated by the notion of 'endogeny'.

Freud's world-picture, however, was also informed by medical science, and he always kept a deep respect for his teacher Von Brücke, who was a professor of physiology (Jones, 1953/1981, p. 39). Von Brücke, Helmholtz and Du Bois-Raymond championed a mechanical-scientific explanation of the world. Their view of nature was one that could be the theme of life sciences. Freud discovered – or rather, rediscovered – the significance of psychic reality, developing a method of empirical investigation. However, he then chose to add a theoretical surfeit of physicality, describing it as a 'psychic apparatus' using electric, hydraulic and energetic concepts that only served to undermine it (Freud, 1950/1966; Habermas, 1968, pp. 300-331).

This masquerade proved rather futile. Guided by Kräpelin, contemporary psychiatry continued to frown upon Freud's ideas. This rejection was partly due to the shift of field envisioned by psychoanalysis: the shift from the 'major psychiatry' of psychotic disorders (requiring

---

[6] The motto featured in *Die Traumdeutung*, 'The Interpretation of Dreams', is an unmistakable pointer. Freud (1900/1953a), p. ix: "Flectere si neqeo superos, acheronta movebo".

sectioning) to the 'minor psychiatry' of what was then referred to as 'neurotic issues'. At a deeper level, it rejected the interpretative approach and metaphysical roots of psychoanalysis. In the eyes of contemporary psychiatrists, psychoanalysis meant retreating to a pre-scientific stage from the scientific realm they wished to gain a foothold in.

Jaspers: Descriptive and Understanding Psychology

The aim of the second line of enquiry was to broaden the field of psychiatry. This effort took place within the clinic itself, affecting the traditional domain of psychiatry. Within this context, Jaspers' 1913 publication *Allgemeine Psychopathologie* can be considered a milestone. Although Jaspers had little affinity with psychoanalysis as such, his theoretical conceptualization had much in common with Freud's. Jaspers' (1883-1969) thinking had been shaped by university psychiatric training, which was firmly positioned within the medical discourse tradition. While Freud, in his theoretical construct, attempted to combine an interpretative and natural-scientific approach into one single system, Jaspers went to great lengths in order to keep the two separate. Moreover, he attempted to give his interpretative approach a theoretical basis by embracing the theory of humanities developed by Schleiermacher en Dilthey in the 19th century. In doing so, he introduced – and rigorously enforced – a stark dualism between psychic phenomena on the one hand and natural elements on the other.

Phenomenology. Initially, Jaspers intends to describe the patient's unique experiences, a process he describes by coining the phrase 'phenomenology': "it (sc. phenomenology) *gives a concrete description* of the psychic states which patients actually experience and *presents* them *for observation*. It reviews the interrelations of these, *delineates* them as sharply as possible, differentiates them and creates a suitable terminology" (Jaspers, 1959/1997, p. 55). In Jaspers' phenomenology, the emphasis is on describing the patient's inner experiences, in order to identify phenomena that can be associated with one's own experiences, being enlargements, reductions or combinations of such experiences as well as experiences that the investigator is unable to relate to. Familiar though we may be with feelings of anxiety and compulsion, compulsive phenomena in a obsessive-compulsive disorder will be more intense or of a different variety. The investigator may even find himself unable to relate to certain negative symptoms – e.g., the feeling of ceased personal activity.

Although Jaspers' intention is to describe subjective and unique experiences, looking for generalization he does not wish to limit himself to descriptions of individual experiences alone. Yet he shows remarkable restraint in that respect. For example, he writes: "Close contemplation of *an individual case* often teaches us of phenomena common to countless others" (Jaspers, 1959/1997, p. 56). The word 'often' is typical of Jaspers. It reflects his prudent approach, whilst indicating that in his view a scientifically developed overall concepts can never be carved in stone. That is precisely why he objected to both contemporary psychoanalysis and phenomenology as favoured by Husserl. Indeed, in his conception of phenomenology, Husserl attempted to define the essence of phenomena: the phenomenon of perception, of memory, of hallucination (Walker, 1994). Jaspers considered this overambitious and quite unacceptable. He chose instead, from a Kantian perspective, to emphasise the perspectival and consequently limited nature of human knowledge (Walker, 1995). So great was his resentment of overall conceptions that he even imagined such conceptions where there were none. For this reason, the more restrictive term 'descriptive psychology' would be more appropriate with regard to Jaspers' views than 'phenomenology'. Indeed, thanks to Husserl, phenomenology has become associated with definitions of essence.

As a result, on the one hand Jaspers contributed significantly to the development of psychiatric or psychopathological research, while on the other he never went – or aspired to go – beyond contributing to single phenomena, 'Einzelphänomene'. Still, his was a significant contribution, and Jaspers' pioneering work has done a lot to enrich the field of psychopathology. Moreover, it brought a shift in emphasis to the inner experience into the sphere of psychiatric practice. It invited the psychiatrist to try and connect with the patient's situation, thus legitimising an individualised approach in which empathy and sympathy became firmly established.

Understanding. As a next step, Jaspers intended to offer an explanation for the experiences described. The explanatory process is assigned to 'understanding' (*Verstehen*) or, should that prove no longer possible, to a causal explanation in its more restricted sense (*Erklären*). Again, Jaspers succeeded in introducing a now well established distinction, for which reason he is regarded as one of the founding fathers of 20th-century psychiatry (Schwarz and Wiggens, 2004). The following has become a household phrase in this respect (Jaspers, 1959/1997, p. 301): "1. We sink ourselves into the psychic situation and *understand genetically by empathy* how one psychic event emerges from another. 2. We find by repeated experience that a number of phenomena are regularly linked together, and on this basis *we explain*". The distinction is fundamental, and ignoring it has been – and still is – the cause of much confusion within the world of psychiatry.

Yet, Jaspers' elaboration of this distinction is far from being flawless. In his interpretation, meaningful connections (between loss and grief) are derived from a generalised sense of self-evidence rather than reflecting actual experience. Jaspers only managed to represent them as *Idealtype* (as defined by Max Weber) or as ideal-typical models or search schemes that do not have to occur in reality but only function as pointers in the world of psychic reality. This limitation was brought about by Jaspers' conviction that there was only one type of knowledge rooted in experience: the natural scientific type, phenomenology or descriptive psychology only being descriptive, from his point of view. In his conception of psychopathology, the psychological domain did not align with the natural-scientific sphere. A distinctly different view was held by Kronfeld (1920), who valued – from his Neo-Kantian perspective – the unique, intrinsic, significance of the psychological ('autological') method to psychiatry in relation to the natural-scientific ('heterological') much more explicitly than Jaspers was inclined to do. Ultimately, Jaspers regarded natural science and medical science as the only 'true sciences', and never quite succeeded in integrating the humanities in his thinking. Having said this, Jaspers did succeed anyhow in pushing the boundaries by introducing a descriptive and 'verstehende' type of psychology.

In doing so, he broadened the psychopathological concept, which led to the emergence of the influential 'Heidelberger Schule', but also proved quite successful in a broader context. The efforts of the Heidelberger Schule led to a broadening of the view on man within the psychiatric field, by validating life's 'inner side' (experience) as well as its history (historicity).[7]

[7] Although he did not belong to the Heidelberger Schule, Kretschmer deserves special mention, in that he contributed significantly to the broadening of psychiatric diagnostics ('multidimensional diagnostics'). A first step towards this effort was offered by *Der sensitive Beziehungswahn*, published in 1927/1950.

Phenomenology and Binswanger

The issues raised by Jaspers were elaborated further by Binswanger (1881-1966). Some of his earlier publications can be seen as a discussion with Jaspers, influenced by Husserl.

Phenomenology. Binswanger agreed with Jaspers in that he regarded empathy and sympathy with others as a prerequisite, yet disagreed in the sense that he did not want to limit himself to single phenomena, instead preferring to conceive these phenomena as expressions of a person as a whole. In doing so, he distanced himself from Jaspers, who focused on subjective experience. Binswanger intended to reach more deeply, starting from experience and probing down to the person expressed through it. This is where the specifically phenomenological aspect lies. Ultimately, the phenomenology developed by Husserl does not deal with experience itself, but with the intentional connection between an I (-pole) and an object (-pole) within the context of this experience. That which an perception focuses on – its object – may differ from the object of memory in its presentation. In parallel, its relationship with the 'I' is also different. According to this line of thought, the description of a hallucination – an objectless perception – would not suffice in itself, because it fails to include the person hallucinating. Seen from this perspective, there are no 'hallucinations': there is an 'I', a person, who is hallucinating and who engages in an intentional relationship with his 'objects' (of perception, hallucination, and such). Engaging a person's perspective or, more generally: that of intentionality, will cause a descriptive psychology to change into a phenomenology which, as was mentioned before, strives to capture the intentional relationship (Binswanger (1922/1965a, pp. 271-272).

Understanding. Binswanger (1955, pp. 67-81) also further developed the issue of understanding, unlike Jaspers, by emphasising the aspect of experience, in his article 'Erfahren, Verstehen, Deuten in der Psychoanalyse'. We may argue that his aim was to escape the unyielding alternative that holds that knowledge either derives from a scientific, 'nomological' experience, or manifests itself in 'logical' or ideal-typical connections made explicit. As a third option, removed from this alternative, he identified the experience of expression as a quintessential mode of experience. It proved a fortunate choice, considering the absence of both a logical and a nomological relationship between the expression itself and what is expressed. Rather, the relationship does exist in an inner, internal way. However, his elaboration of this premise left much to be desired. We can hardly blame Binswanger. Indeed, it required a great deal of energy to develop a satisfactory concept, with the Anglo-Saxon philosophy of the latter half of the 20th century developed by Wittgenstein (1958/1963) and Von Wright (1971) – rendering a particularly significant contribution to improving our insights (see Chapter Five). Here the concept of internal relationship or relationship of expression comes into its own, a concept that is fundamentally different from any external relationship that would merely reflect an incidental or causal connection.

Considering that the concept of understanding is referring to factual experience, the opposition between understanding and explaining is played out differently as compared to Jaspers. Indeed, understanding, unlike Jaspers, doesn't refer to a supra-temporal or ideal-typical, more or less logical type of relationship – but to the life history expressed in life events. Essentially, this much more fluid conception of understanding will qualify the 'understandable' and 'non-understandable' opposition as defined by Jaspers, which also functioned as an demarcation criterion between 'endogenous psychoses' (that cannot be related to) and 'non-endogenous psychoses' (that can be related to).

In addition, the meaning of causal explanation becomes broader and is actually changed: no longer restricted to natural-scientific or somatic explanations, it is now extended to 'life-functional' connections, including bodily and mental functions, in their dysfunctionality, if any. The diagnostically relevant question would not be whether a disorder is mentally or somatically determined, but whether it has a life-historical or a life-functional connection.

In this respect, Binswanger (1947, pp. 50-74) stood in his article 'Lebensfunktion und innere Lebensgeschichte' in a different tradition than did Jaspers, or the tradition that Freud believed to be part of. His conception of nature and life did not originate in natural sciences, but in a Platonic-Aristotelian tradition, as becomes evident from his notion of 'life function', which does not agree with any mechanistic interpretation of nature. While Freud and Jaspers stayed close to the medical discourse, adding a type of discourse that included the psychic – with Freud adopting the somewhat ambiguous approach of a *discours mixte* (Ricœur, 1965/1970) and Jaspers favouring a strict methodological distinction – Binswanger stood in the Platonic-Aristotelian tradition.

Philosophy of Life and Psychopathology

The alternative concept of nature was even more manifest in a different line of psychopathological thinking, one that turned out to be just as influential: psychopathology based on the philosophy of life. Contemporary philosophy of life was also driven by a criticism of a mechanistic view of life. In France this movement was represented by Bergson, among others, and also in Germany it found wide acceptance. A naturalistic conception of nature was met with a broader conception of nature, bringing the need for the system of life-defining categories to be extended beyond the realms of physics and chemistry. In France, Minkowski (1927/1997) made an attempt to develop a concept of schizophrenia, particularly schizophrenic autism, based on Bergson's philosophy of life ('*perte de contact vital avec la réalité*'). In Germany, Straus and Von Gebsattel, also working from a life's philosophical perspective, developed a conception of depressive disorders, i.e., of melancholy, with special emphasis on the disturbances of internal time (Straus, 1928/1963; Von Gebsattel, 1954, pp. 1-18). Depression would then be conceived as a stagnation of the essentially (or perceived) forward-moving motion of time, barring the melancholic's access to the future and leaving him trapped in the past. Also outside psychopathology, in neurology and general medicine, philosophy of life left its marks, invariably as part of an effort to overcome the limitations of a mechanical-physical explanation of life (Straus, 1935; Goldstein, 1934).

During this period, up until the Second World War, as well as being influenced by the contemporary philosophy of life, psychopathology as a whole opened up to a more philosophical line of thought. One of the reasons is the abstract, 'philosophical' nature of the concepts employed, viz., endogeny and fundamental disorder. Endogeny could have one of several meanings: it could refer to a presumed genetic disposition, to an unknown somatogenesis, to a mental constitution, to an aetiology lacking a connection to life history (without a demonstrable psychogenesis). The following central meaning emerged: independent onset, autonomous course and non-understandability. Yet this central meaning failed to obscure its speculative background.

The second theme constituted a supposed fundamental disturbance to which psychotic phenomena of endogenous psychosis could be reduced, which might pinpoint the specific nature of these psychoses to distinguish it from psychogenetically determined psychoses. For example, Bleuler (1857-1939) substituted the concept of schizophrenia for that of *dementia praecox*, while extending it by qualifying its unfavourable prognosis (that Kräpelin had associated this disorder with). He positioned the fundamental disorder within an *Assoziationslockerung*, while others spoke of 'psychic ataxia', or a mismatch between mental faculties. In France, the concept of '*automatisme mental*' (Clérambault) had found currency to describe this fundamental disturbance or, more specifically, the initial, prodromal, symptoms of a psychosis which also form its nucleus. To the patient, these phenomena – voices that are meaningless – appear to come wholly from outside and cannot be controlled, as a result of which he secondarily develops a delusion intended to give 'meaning' to these meaningless phenomena, emerging from 'brutal reality'.[8]

Although these fundamental disturbances were often associated with a presupposed organic disorder, their definition tended to take a psychological or philosophical form rather than a physiological one. Ultimately, the notion of a fundamental disturbance (*Grundstörung*) concerns the ultimate basis of the diverse nature of psychotic phenomena.

THE ALTERNATIVE PATH IN PSYCHIATRY: AFTER 1950

In every domain, the Second World War constituted a juncture in history, and hermeneutical science was no exception. After the war, however, when life had returned to normal, its continuity proved virtually unbroken.[9] A contributory factor was that, for obvious reasons, biological lines of thought had become tainted, and would take a long time finding reinstatement. Moreover, the war experience had brought a qualification of the significance of 'endogeny', now that people had witnessed the impact of traumas, life experience and life history, seeing it reflected in patients. The need for reaching back to a phenomenological hermeneutical tradition, which after all represented a humanity ideal, was strongly felt.

---

[8] Lacan has been strongly influenced, with respect to his conception of psychosis, by the notion of 'automatisme mental' of Clérambault (Lacan, 1981/1993; Grigg, 2008, p. 11).

[9] Its leading members were H.W. Gruhle, K. Schneider, H. Tellenbach, W. von Baeyer and W. Janzarik, W. Bräutigam. The school has existed until the 1990s.

'Verstehende' Psychopathology

This humanity ideal featured strongly in the rebirth and rise of the Heidelberger Schule after the war. The 1950s and 60s were important decades, seeing the publication of work done privately during the war period. Some had based their work on Jasper's modest premises, while other efforts proved more ambitious.

Tellenbach (1961/1983) described the melancholic character type *Typus melancholicus*, which is partly characterised by self-limitation and may underlie melancholy in its traditional interpretation. Going further than Jaspers, he attempted to record key moments within this structure. He distinguished the 'symptom', in its clinical-psychiatric meaning, from the 'phenomenon' in a phenomenological sense, which needs to describe the characteristic and essential elements of the state of affairs. He argued in favour of the significance of the concept of 'endogeny', enlarging it by separating it from somatogenesis, thereby giving it the meaning of 'thrownness', in the sense of Heidegger: *Dasein* is thrown in the world being nature itself. (Tellenbach, 1961/1983, p. 42)

K. Schneider (1959/1980), by contrast, stayed close to Jaspers' intentions. He identified criteria based on which schizophrenia could be diagnosed with a high degree of certainty. These were so-called first-rank symptoms (including advanced types of hallucination and the controversial concept of delusional perception). This effectively limited the concept of schizophrenia while also refining its diagnostics. The sharp contrast we see with Jaspers between non-understandable and understandable psychopathological disorders, between endogenous and non-endogenous psychosis or, between the so-called 'process' and 'development', still echoed strongly.

The scope of phenomenology was extended. In the 1950s, Conrad (1958/1987) more or less rounded off the field of descriptive phenomenology, more particularly with respect to the field of delusions in schizophrenia, as the most extreme psychotic condition. He felt that schizophrenic delusions originated in a manner of perception that tends towards 'apophenia' (epiphany), with patients experiencing events happening around them as being particularly significant to them. This is evidence that the patient assumes a particular vantage point in relation to the world, which he describes as 'Ptolemaeic': the patient finds himself frozen in a passive central position within the world, unable to change perspective.

Work was also done in the field of delusional disorders, or paranoid psychosis, within the so-called *verstehende Anthropologie* developed by Zutt (1953/1963b; 1957). This orientation chose a specific anthropology as its point of departure, rather than an ingenuous experience, and was therefore not part of the phenomenological movement. A central notion within this line of thought was that human existence was tied to hierarchies, the so-called *Daseinsordnungen* (e.g., the societal hierarchy and the hierarchy of housing), which offer some degree of protection. The disruption caused by a delusion as part of a delusional disorder is less profound than the Ptolemaeic world perception associated with schizophrenia, where we see a complete reversal of the balance of human existence. Yet, as part of the decay of the existential order, the resulting delimitation may trigger delusional episodes (Kulenkampff, 1955). The protective shield offered by limitation disappears, causing the person to feel pursued by an omnipotent other and exposed to unlimited scrutiny. This does not necessarily explain the delusion itself, but merely interprets it from a specific (in this case) anthropological perspective.

Binswanger's Daseinsanalyse

In Binswanger's later period, the anthropological aspect becomes more prominent. Building on the *Daseinsanalyse,* it is elaborated and refined. This elaboration is strongly indebted to Heidegger's philosophy, to whose work Binswanger added his own personal interpretation. The project of the Daseinsanalyse actually predates World War II (1931-32/2000), but it did flourish after the war. Abandoning the objective to describe a person as an unique individual, it sets out to offer a description of a person's world or his fundamental world design – the frame of reference that will allow something to be interpreted as something (Frie, 2003, pp. 142-145). A world design of a particular person that is based on continuity – to mention the famous example of *Absatzphobie* – will cause a sudden event to be experienced as traumatic, which is of course more likely to occur with a person whose world design is susceptible to bursts and fragmentation (Binswanger 1947, pp. 204-207). In this case, 'continuity' becomes the central category based on which the world, in all its aspects of time, space and intersubjectivity, is constructed and experienced. 'Continuity' is, in the case of the *Absatzphobie* the basic category, the *existential apriori* of its world design, its being-in-the-world (Needleman, 1975, pp. 31, 70-72, 112).

This interpretation does not 'explain' nor does it wish to explain, because the *Daseinsanalyse* merely intends to offer a comprehensive description. Many of his cases became famous: Ellen West, Lola Voss, Jürg Zünd, and Suzanne Urban (Binswanger, 1957). These cases are still a fruitful source of inspiration, adding a deeper descriptive level to psychopathology. Yet, obviously such a description cannot be neutral, and is actually derived from the categorical system of Heidegger. It articulates the forms in which experience of a patient takes place, not the content of the experience itself (Binswanger, 1947, pp. 204-207). The emphasis on the formal aspects brings out its close relationship with traditional psychopathology which, after all, focuses on the form rather than the content of a psychopathological phenomenon.

Within the *Daseinsanalyse*, the assumption of a biological or endogenous determination of psychiatric disorders would not pose a problem. A biological or endogenous determination of mental disorders, for example melancholy, would be wholly compatible with the *Daseinsanalyse*, as it merely offers a description and not an (causal) explanation. This made Binswanger's *Daseinsanalyse* perfectly acceptable within traditional German clinical psychopathology, whereas it met with some criticism in France, where the psychoanalytical, psychodynamic orientation was dominant (Ebtinger, 1986; Giudicelli, 1996, p. 101-102). Nevertheless Binswanger, through his Heidegger-inspired *Daseinsanalyse*, was determined to counter the reductive effects of standard psychopathology by highlighting a more profound dimension of psychopathological phenomena than classical psychopathology was willing to acknowledge.

Heidegger, however, rejected this source and believed Binswanger to have misinterpreted him – he even criticized Binswanger's famous description of the *Absatzphobie* (Heidegger, 1987, pp. 254-258). His criticism was both justified and not justified. Binswanger tried to offer an 'empirical' description of specific world-designs, where Heidegger developed a formal analysis of any world design as such. In other words, while Binswanger provides a variety of *Daseinsanalyses,* Heidegger offers one single *Daseinsanalytik*, valid for every *Dasein*. Heidegger and Binswanger are each involved in different projects, a philosophical and a empirical project, respectively. In that sense Heidegger's criticism is not justified. However, Heidegger's inquiry goes further than merely designing a philosophical anthropology. His frame of reference would not be able to cover an all-encompassing anthropology anyway. A curtailed type of 'anthropology' is sufficient in his case, because essentially it does not focus on a philosophical anthropology as such, but on a fundamental ontology, on the 'Question of Being'.[10] Binswanger tended to downplay this distinction, so in that sense Heidegger's complaint is justified.

There is yet another issue. Implicit in Binswanger's *Daseinsanalyse* is a strong normative component that finds expression in the qualification of world designs as being aberrant or abnormal (Holzhey-Kunz, 1994, pp. 25-27). It has been argued that schizophrenic world designs are essentially private designs, whereas all melancholically driven ways of being-in-the-world are more or less similar, a conclusion that would also apply to mania (Tatossian, 1979). A person with schizophrenia will be 'schizophrenic' in his own individual way, whereas the melancholic has 'everyone's' depression. Whichever the case may be, any aberrant life form – in a unique or generalised sense – will meet its own standards and can therefore be regarded as a specific world design. Subsequently, this specific design can be qualified as a disruption of a general human life-form, or as a disruption of the interplay of structural moments within a human life, respectively. Effectively, this introduces a normative-anthropological conception of the nature of man.

Yet, contrary to what Binswanger believed, the normativity of his *Daseinsanalyse* cannot be inferred from Heidegger's *Daseinsanalytik*. Heidegger offers a system of existential categories (*existentiales*) based on which all human phenomena should – and could – be described. It is precisely the formal nature of Heidegger's analysis that precludes the introduction of a content-related normativity.[11] Of course, this does not detract from the intrinsic value of Binswanger's contributions to psychopathology.

---

[10] For a criticism of Binswanger see Heidegger (1987, pp. 236-242). He also speaks of a 'productive misunderstanding' (1987, p. 151). Binswanger saw fit to complement Heidegger's analysis, which would culminate in a central position of 'care', with the concept of 'love'. See Binswanger (1942/1953). In Heidegger's case, the category (or rather: existentiale) of 'care' does not concern any concrete type of care, but a highly formal relationship, in order for the concrete phenomenon of love to be included. Heidegger does have a point, but so does Binswanger. Later, Heidegger's treatment of intersubjectivity – Being-with – would be met with increasing criticism and was considered inadequate. See Levinas (1961/1969). We might say that it is precisely what Binswanger's concept of love refers to. Seen in this light, Binswanger's (implied) criticism of Heidegger was more appropriate than Heidegger would have cared to admit.

[11] The highly normative level of Binswanger's work is pointed out by Holzhey-Kunz (1994, pp. 25-27).

Ultimately, Binswanger took it even a step further from 1960 onwards. He shifted his focus from Heidegger back to Husserl – not the early Husserl, proposing a descriptive phenomenology, but the 'transcendental' Husserl. A new, final step was made. Refusing to limit himself to a categorical and normative description of actual worlds of singular patients, Binswanger went on to describe the constitution of a world as such (in mania, melancholy and delusion) from a general ('transcendental') consciousness (in a Husserlian fashion) that is, or would be, presupposed to any actual consciousness of a world. Rather than look into the content of world designs (of mania and schizophrenia) he explores the constitution of a world design as such within the framework of a general, transcendental, consciousness (Binswanger, 1960, 1965b). This approach, however, met with little acclaim, no doubt a result of the predominantly consciousness-philosophical issues associated with it.[12]

Phenomenological-Anthropological Psychiatry

In order to elaborate the transcendental motive, however, there is no imperative need to relate it to a transcendental consciousness, in line with the later Binswanger. We may establish a link with human existence itself. It is noteworthy that such a kind of inquiry into human existence would actually transcend Binswanger's *Daseinsanalyse.* Despite his heavy use of philosophical jargon, Binswanger's *Daseinsanalyse* first and foremost intended to present an empirical hermeneutics of the various life designs. An inquiry into the very origin of a world design or life style will have ramifications going well beyond Binswanger's conception of *Daseinsanalyse.* Rather than detail an actual life's path, a transcendental inquiry should describe an instance or principle that shapes a concrete life design. Whenever someone experiences and designs his own life as being worthless, the question poses itself what entity actually shaped this life design. On the one hand, it needs to be removed from the design process – to the degree where it actually is the

---

[12] The Daseinsanalyse has actually been followed up through the work of M. Boss, who sought connection with Heidegger, particularly with his later work. A discussion of both positions (Binswanger and Boss) can be found in Holzhey-Kunz (1994, pp. 17-79). The impact of Binswanger's work turned out to be considerably greater than that of Boss' ideas.

designing entity – while on the other hand it can only be known from the life design itself.

In the 1970s, Blankenburg (1971) raised this issue and elaborated it, building on Heidegger's work, much like Binswanger had done in his *Daseinsanalyse*, but in a different way. Contrary to Binswanger he does not explore the contours of a life design, but looks into the conditions that would enable a specific (type of) being-in-the-world. In fact, he examines the conditions of possibility for a symptomless type of schizophrenia – a type of being-in-the-world that he defines as characterized by a loss of natural self-evidence, of common sense convictions, a loss of the sense of familiarity: *Der Verlust der natürlichen Selbstverständlichkeit.* He reduces it to changes in the relationship unto the world, in temporalisation, and in I-forming. Blankenburg's project has borne fruit, proving an inspiration to numerous scholars exploring the symptomless type of schizophrenia (Kimura, 1982; Mishara, 2001; Stanghellini, 2004; 2007; Sass, 2001; Sass and Parnas, 2001; 2007).[13]

Psychoanalysis as a Broadening of Understanding

Where the Heidelberger Schule, the *Daseinsanalyse* and phenomenological-anthropological psychiatry concentrated their efforts on deepening the phenomenological description, psychoanalysis focused on broadening the field of understanding. As was outlined before, psychoanalysis has had its own early history outside of the university, going on to expand rapidly worldwide. Simultaneously, its clinical relevance has become increasingly convincing (Fenichel, 1945). From the 1960s it sprouted a more explicitly 'hermeneutical' brand of psychoanalysis, renouncing Freud's mingling of a 'language of meaning' and a 'language of forces' in Ricœur's (1965/1970) terminology, preferring the 'language of meaning' (Gill, 1983; Klein, 1976; Schafer, 1976; 1983). Its framework became less ambitious, more 'empirical', one might say. With time, psychoanalysis limited its scope to finding meanings, motives, purposes of action, aspects that can be investigated as part of the clinical practice of treatment and diagnostics, abandoning Freud's drive-defence model, which nevertheless still found support (Hartmann, 1964; Brenner, 1980). Kohut's 'self-psychology' (1971) criticised the classical drive-defence model, by introducing a fourth agency alongside Freud's structural

[13] For an exhaustive bibliography with regard to phenomenological psychopathology from 1970 onwards see Charbonneau (2010).

model (ego-id-superego). Yet one may argue that Kohut remains within the frame of intra-psychic theories and does not cross the border of interpersonal theories (Mills, 2000).

Crucial in this development were the theory and practice of interpersonal psychoanalysis, which emphasised the importance of interpersonal connectedness, defining the human being as the total of his relations, reducing drives and an internal, unconscious world to a very limited role (Sullivan, 1953). Next, the object-relational approach came into being – a somewhat misleading term, considering that the psychoanalytical term 'object' in this context does refer to a person or subject (and not to a partial object). The object-relational approach deals with relationships of a person with another person, which may be the actual person (Fairbairn, 1952; Winnicott, 1971/1980; Greenberg and Mitchell, 1983) but also may be of an imagined nature (Melanie Klein). Here, the conceptual framework has also been broadened. The highly influential theories of Bion (1970/1986) deepened its conceptual framework, turning it into a new paradigm. Less speculative and more pragmatic are the intersubjective or relational theories, emerging in the 1980s (Atwood and Stolorow, 1984; Stolorow, Atwood and Orange, 2002). These emphasize the 'irreducible subjectivity of the analyst', the importance of co-construction of meaning and the mutuality in the psychoanalytical process over the role of the unconscious and its interpretation (Renik, 1998). The object-relational and the intersubjective theories taken together may be considered to occupy the space left between the interpersonalists on the one hand and the classical drive/ defence model on the other (Thompson, 2005).

Equally important is the attachment theory – build on the seminal work of Bowlby (1969). It states that the emergence of an inner (*mind*) in a child requires for the child to be first met by another who owns an inner himself. Consequently, primacy lies with the other in the genesis of subjectivity – not until the other attributes states of mind to the child will the child be capable of internalising these mental states itself, in order for a process of subjectification to develop. Thus, the attachment theory, at least in its psychoanalytical form, describes the emergence of subjectivity and the capacity to experience in relation to one's environment (Fonagy and Target, 1996a and b; Fonagy et al. 2002).

Finally, there is yet another line of psychoanalysis, one which aims to offer a global anthropological reinterpretation of traditional psychoanalytical findings. Seminal to this theory is the precept that the meaning of expressions is not primarily based on conscious (or unconscious) intentions, but also and particularly on governing patterns of language and culture with an intersubjective and transsubjective validity: the symbolic order. One should bear in mind that these expressions do not originate solely in actual governing patterns within a current linguistic and cultural system, but also in those of a seemingly defunct past: the early childhood and the parental history. Here we do find a 'primacy of the Other' – in the sense of intersubjectivity (of the relational theories) and in the sense of the environment (of the attachment-theory). We also find a 'primacy of Otherness' (an intersubjectivity being rooted into a linguistic and cultural structure, into the symbolic order). This line of psychoanalysis, developed by Lacan, defines human existence – a result of subjecting oneself to the symbolic order – as being characterised by an internal split, by an inherent lack (Lacan, 1966/2002).

Definition of the Alternative Path within Psychiatry

Psychiatry set out to develop a theory for psychic reality, which after all had been excluded by the medical discourse. Its initial efforts were Platonic-Aristotelian in nature and did not involve a medical scientific approach. After the early stages of biological psychiatry as developed by Griesinger and others, and following from the criticism raised against Kräpelin's traditional clinical psychiatry, an alternative path emerged: psychiatry as a human science. This approach, it turned out, alternately reaffirmed or undermined the validity of the biological (or endogenous) determination of a disorder type. Overall, however, the need was felt to distance oneself from what was regarded as a reductionist approach. Jaspers kept both paths well separate, yet showed restraint in his elaboration of the second path. Later, his work was extended through the description of the mental disorder (the descriptive phenomenology of the Heidelberger Schule and the *Daseinsanalyse*), while the concept of psychogenesis was broadened from a psychoanalytical angle. Thus, psychiatry bade farewell to a singular type of symptomatological scheme, which held that a mental disorder would merely be a symptom of a dysfunctional substrate. Psychiatry was also practised in a 'hermeneutical' fashion, to the extent where hermeneutics reflect the theory and practice of interpretative description (of behaviour, experience and life events).

Gradually, a different type of disease scheme emerged, which was predominantly hermeneutical rather than symptomatological in nature. Its underlying concept was that all experiences and behaviours, including aberrant ones, are meaningful – 'meaning and signification' referring to standards and rules that define this meaning and signification, which would also apply to abnormal behaviour and experiences. At a certain level, all our experiences and actions are guided by standards and rules. Both implicitly and explicitly, hermeneutics refers to these standards – in phenomenology, with regard to the hallucination, the anthropological description of a manic world design, to a halted development from a psychoanalytical point of view. For example, in describing a hallucination as an objectless perception, and a delusion as an incorrigible aberration, psychiatry draws on perception schemes and thinking patterns that are imposed in a normative fashion. The standard referred to does not reflect a normal condition present in physical nature and fails to correspond with the dysfunctions of the medical discourse. It is a type of standard that a person is 'supposed to' live by if we wish speak of a human type of perception or thought. These standards are neither physiological nor teleological in nature – their 'supposed to' aspect makes them deontological (see Chapter One). Like we need to adhere to the rules of a language in order to be intelligible, we also need to obey the prevailing rules of perception and interpretation in order to be understood. Obviously, this type of 'supposed to' does not carry an element of moral rejectability or punishability. Rather, these standards refer to general human boundaries in respect of perception and thought.

The Medical Discourse in Psychiatry: the Next Phase

Throughout its history, even in the 20th century, psychiatry has set great store by the biological aspects of a disorder, as is indicated by its adoption of 'endogeny' as a key concept. Hereditary, constitutional and physical causes were supposed to play a major part in the aetiology of a mental disorder. In the latter half of the last century, this approach grew into a dominant force. This chapter deals with hermeneutical psychiatry, not with the history of psychiatry, and an in-depth historical description would be out of place here. Still, we should mention a few relevant points, in view of the significance of the mutual relationship between the hermeneutical and natural-scientific approaches.

The discovery of the efficacy of psychoactive drugs (antipsychotics, antidepressants, anxiolytics), from the 1950s onwards, changed the face of psychiatric practice, but also influenced the theoretical concepts of psychiatry. Psychology, in the form of clinical and experimental psychology, had made its appearance in the field. It influenced psychiatric practice (behavioural therapy) as well as commonly held views on disorders. We witnessed a strong rise of (behavioural) genetics. Imaging techniques gave a powerful boost to concepts of localisation, and the field of biological psychiatry has seen tremendous advances. The lack that characterised the initial phase of biological psychiatry – insufficient knowledge about the intricate workings of the brain – which only hastened its decay at the time, is gradually being filled by contributions from the field of neuroscience (Andreasen, 1984; 2001).

In fact, the rise of biological psychiatry is so spectacular that it appears to have effectively obliterated its hermeneutical tradition. Indeed, it brought ideas that are striking similar to the naturalistic trends that dominated the late 19th and early 20th centuries. Although the neuroscientific domain covers a wide range of ideas, naturalism still prevails. Traditional medical discourse tends to conceive a mental disorder as a direct consequence of a disturbed cerebral structure, where the finding of a brain abnormality would suffice to explain the psychiatric disorder in its entirety. This constitutes the fulfilment of the promise made by Griesinger's superseded brand of biological psychiatry. Increasingly, psychiatry has been manifesting itself in the traditional sense of the medical discourse (Guze, 1989).

Moreover, newly developed classification systems filled the existing gaps in diagnostics with established facts. DSM-III, DSM-IV en DSM-5 earned psychiatry new respect as a science, facilitating scientific research. Part of the nosological project had to be abandoned, because pathological units could no longer be assumed apriori. However, another part was retained, on account of the fact that establishing diseases in the traditional sense of disease units was the ultimate objective. Within the DSM-III/IV/5 classifications, a hidden system is at work that highlights the biological origin of the disorders.

Also, we recognise a desubjectifying tendency because, for the sake of repeatability, efforts are made to achieve a maximum of unequivocality of terms as well as a predominantly behaviour-oriented approach to identifying symptoms and traits (Hell, 2003; Zarifian, 2005). This will result in a fragmented and externalised world of experience. This finding will not detract from the values of these systems, as it merely points out its reverse side, and thus its scope. Each in their own individual way, these new classifying systems fulfil the inherent promise of Kräpelin's approach.

And thus modern psychiatry, both through its biological orientation and classifying systems, is carrying on the tradition of the medical discourse. Mental disorders are now regarded as a symptom of a brain dysfunction, which psychiatry presents itself as a 'symptomatology' investigating correlations between behaviour and brain dysfunctions. Centred on biology, its standards, despite their social component, are essentially biological and are referring to a natural function (Wakefield, 1992). It lies embedded in the thesis that the mental disorder is fundamentally a disease of the brain, and that today's psychiatrist is a brain specialist. The medical discourse in psychiatry manifests itself, also in its modern guise, as a symptomatology that is normatively associated with a biological or, more specifically, teleological set of standards.

CONCLUSION

The path of the medical discourse, which in today's psychiatry is represented by biological psychiatry, is characterised by a symptomatology that is accompanied by biological standardisation, like the path of hermeneutical psychiatry is characterised by a hermeneutical deontology. It demonstrates that the path of the medical discourse and the alternative path are similar formally and are different content-wise. They are similar in the sense that they are both descriptive and normative, each in their own way. They are different to the degree that the alternative path within psychiatry enabled the integration of the psychic, whereas the first path was biased towards its exclusion. This is what turns the hermeneutical psychiatry into the necessary complement of the medical discourse within psychiatry.

Thus, the hermeneutical and the natural-scientific perspectives appear to belong to the same system, even though they exclude each other conceptually: meaning is of a different order than a natural fact. A person doing scientific research will exclude any alternative approach for the duration of this research. The effects of this 'dualism' are less dramatic than is sometimes believed. It merely means that both perspectives and their derivative forms cannot be adopted simultaneously, only in parallel or sequentially (Bracken and Thomas, 2005). Also, they summon each other 'performatively' or in the act itself, as the movement of abstraction will leave enough space for that which is abstracted. Moreover, they are historically interconnected, because of the alternation between the hermeneutical discourse and the natural-scientific discourse, and because the natural-scientific discourse (within the medical field and later also within psychiatry itself) creates the void to be filled by the hermeneutical discourse. Also in practice they are complementary. Within a treatment and a diagnostic setting, either perspective may be chosen, in order to prevent the threat of a unilateral approach (Phillips, 2004).

The next three chapters will discuss the inquiry into the precise nature of their relationship in more detail. First of all, the focus will be on the ontological issue of defining the relationship between body and mind. Next, the more conceptual and scientific-theoretical issue concerning the boundaries of a natural-scientific approach and the possibilities of a hermeneutical approach will be addressed.

Three

The Relationship between the Psychic and Physical Reality

The previous chapter demonstrated that the biological turn taken by psychiatry triggered an intensive enquiry into the relationship between body and mind. The solution to this issue seems to be biased in a particular direction, driven by a strong urge to reduce mental functions to mere brain processes and, by extension, to define mental disorders as the product of a brain dysfunction. The rationale offered is as follows: "Once the brain disorder has been identified, the psychiatric disorder has thus been explained". This effectively reduces the psychic in general and a mental disorder in particular to a derived status, to a mere symptom of a substrate-level disorder. Increasingly, psychiatry has been manifesting itself in the traditional sense of the medical discourse.

This creates the need for this position, with all its various nuances, to be analysed and its plausibility to be examined. In view of the overwhelming complexity of this issue and the scope of this chapter, it can be addressed only in the most general of terms. As a next step, we shall try to establish whether – even now – there may be possibilities to define a position that would add significance to the concept of psychic reality.

THE BASIC ALTERNATIVE

Significant beyond psychiatry and its core discipline, psychopathology, the relationship between body and mind has long been the object of much philosophical debate (Rentsch, 1980). In this regard, many stances may be adopted, and have been. Repeatedly we came across the concept of an animated body or an embodied soul, reflecting the ancient teachings of Plato and Aristotle. Plato regards the soul as being superior to and independent of the body. Although some degree of cohesion is assumed, the emphasis is on separation, the overall approach being dualistic. Aristotle's views, by contrast, have strong monistic overtones: Aristotle conceives the soul as a life form or defining principle, and form as being one with the material aspect.

Dualism and monism, or dualistic and monistic accents, are not tied to the concept of animated body – quite the contrary in fact. Indeed, it was the anti-Platonic-Aristotelian tendency of the 17th- and 18th-century Classical Modern line of thought that intensified and absolutised the opposition between body and mind. Where, by and large, reality came to be conceived as a single great mechanism, a mechanistic interpretation of man was still met with hesitation. It led Descartes to conceive man as being composed of two substances: a spatial or physical substance, and a mental substance. This explicitly dualistic approach would earn him much criticism from later philosophers. On the one hand, this dualism is essential with Descartes, in the sense that he gave free reign to the then unfolding process of mechanisation of the world picture, while simultaneously creating a safe haven for both man and man's will, in order for man to remove himself from the mechanistic and deterministic consequences of the natural-scientific project. We might even say that any brand of philosophy that strives to retain the unique qualities of man – as expressed in the concepts of autonomy (Kant) or intentionality (Husserl), freedom (Sartre) or action as opposed to event (Wittgenstein) – will rely on some form of duality. Yet, the dualistic approach does raise the issue of the relationship between the two entities, regardless of the terms in which this dualism has been written. Descartes' solution took the form of an interaction between the entities of body and mind, which he localised in the pineal gland. The obvious inconvenience of this solution makes it clear that the enquiry into the relationship between two heterogeneous entities is bound to put the dualistic approach in an awkward position.

A monistic or, more specifically, materialistic theory circumvents this problem, as it denies either of the two entities or attributes a derived status to one or the other. Where the Classical Modern line of thought favoured a view of reality as a single great mechanism, their obvious choice was to repudiate any form of mental substance or instance, which sprouted a host of materialistic conceptions.

It is hardly surprising that both basic positions – monistic and dualistic – should be reflected in psychiatry. The materialistic view of the pathogenesis of mental disorders proved dominant. This was to be expected, in light of the strong presence of the natural-scientific approach, the medical discourse, in the psychiatric domain. Then again, clinical practice is often based on a dual scheme, also referring to the autonomous significance of the individual experience – of the psychic reality, in other words. Thus, this issue has both practical and theoretical significance, considering that any answer to this problem will determine the scope and extent of any action taken.

THREE LEVELS OF PSYCHIC REALITY: INTENTIONALITY, WORLD, LANGUAGE AND THE LACK

How does the issue of the psychic reality manifest itself in psychiatry? The patient will formulate a complaint, explaining that he feels inhibited or anxious. He or she does something that is experienced as strange or unsettling. In this sense, a complaint refers to a subject of action and experience, in a broad sense.

Indeed, any type of action or experience will refer to a subject. Perceiving is not the same as receiving a stimulus ('I feel anxious, I am in pain, I experience feelings of lust'). In fact, perception or any form of experience is endowed with a 'subjective' or 'qualitative' aspect. It may take a variety of forms such as pain experience ('I am in pain') or colour experience ('this particular red').[1] The same will apply to actions: human action presupposes subjectivity being involved. It makes the differences between 'my arm being moved' and 'moving one's arm'. Any experience or action will refer to a subjective quality, a subject.

Moreover, the person acting does 'something' and does it in a particular way (carefully, recklessly); a person perceiving will perceive 'something', doing it in a particular way (seeing, hearing). This 'directedness towards an object' in acting and experiencing is called intentionality ('aboutness'). It comes in various modes. Man is able to imagine, to remember, to fantasize, to hallucinate, to have delusions and so on. Thus, action and experience are informed by subjectivity as well as by intentionality. The emphasis, at this initial level, is on the 'subject pole' – the subject as a source of object focus.

Experience and action are both forms of subjective, intentional involvement, but there is more to it. A person acting will act within a field of action. A person who perceives, performs a function while building a field of perception that holds the 'objects' perceived, in the broadest sense of the word (things in space and time, as well the relationship among other). We are not only subjective and intentional beings but we are also in a world that encompasses us. This constitutes

[1] Searle (2002), p. 26: "Conscious states by definition ar inner, qualitative, subjective states of awareness or sentience". The term 'qualia' has found currency to describe a qualitative state.

the second level of psychic reality, next to that of subjectivity and intentionality: the world. The emphasis here is on the 'object-pole'; the world that we both find and design.[2] This world will be affected by the subjectivity of the person involved, yet this subjectivity is also reflected in the objectness of this person's world: a small world limited by fear, a world in which the other is powerful or dependent, etcetera.

A third level of psychic reality concerns the possibility of reflection, which retrogradely affects both the first and second levels. Each intentional insight ("I feel threatened") is potentially accompanied by a reflexive insight ("Am I actually being threatened, perhaps I'm just imagining things"). Each trait of this world can be questioned reflexively, by asking 'Is it really so?' It can well be maintained that the capacity to reflect is rooted in man's language capacity. Indeed, language mediates between the 'subject pole' and the 'object pole' by offering the universality of the concept while bringing an unprecedented broadening of experience, as it introduces a host of complex connections, such as negativity or denial, as well as a range of logic modalities – possibility, impossibility, necessity.[3] A language user, a subject subordinate to language is eminently capable of distancing itself from both a surrounding reality and itself. Such a human subject may think: "Is it actually real what I'm seeing there; what I feel inside, is that a genuine feeling; could it be that there is something else going on here", etcetera. A human subject is capable of distancing itself from the surrounding reality, with subjective and intentional consciousness developing into reflective consciousness.[4]

These three levels are interconnected. The pole of subjectivity/intentionality constitutes the foundation that enables the more complex 'finding/designing a world' (the object-pole), while reflection retroactively affects the preceding levels, like linguistic framing is informing them.

---

[2] Perhaps these two levels of the psychic (of subjectivity/intentionality and of being in the world) can be attributed to animals as well – to the higher primates at least (consciousness and species-specific *Umwelt*) – although the inaccessibility of animal consciousness will probably keep this a controversial issue.

[3] Sellars would deny the thesis (1956/1997, § 31), "that there is any awareness of logical space prior to, or independent of, the acquisition of a language".

[4] Habermas writes (2008, p. 173): "Conscious participation in the symbolically structured 'space of reasons', jointly inhabited by linguistically socialized minds, is reflected in the accompanying performative sense of freedom".

MONISTIC POSITIONS: MATERIALISM AND FUNCTIONALISM

Now that we have reached a – provisional – definition of the psychic, we may start considering its relationship towards the physical. We need to look at the physical, because when examining the psychic, we are bound to come up against limits. A person may both help and offend another person, but he cannot simultaneously raise and lower the same arm. In addition to such fundamental limits, there are also truly physical limits. A human cannot run 50 kilometres or simply choose to stop breathing. This concerns the biological aspects of human existence. These biological aspects have become major objects of study, to which the expansive growth of physiology, pharmacology and the modern neurosciences bears testimony.

Thus, the question of the relationship between the psychic and the physical is begged. How exactly do they relate? To find out, we need to look more broadly at the monistic and dualistic positions distinguished above. We cannot hope to do more than define its boundaries, the body-mind issue being the object of an extensive and highly technical debate, but also because the issue possibly falls outside the order of 'solvable' problems, probably because of its overambitious nature.

The position of monism, taking the form of materialism, is strong. It is based on the notion that any reality is material and that psychic phenomena, produced by intentionality, can be reduced to non-mental, physical terms. The dominant position of the natural sciences explains why this view is strongly favoured today. Central to this idea is the concept of a causal closure of physics. Based on this concept, it would be inconceivable for a gap to occur within natural causality. If a mental element, e.g., a wilful decision, were to be an autonomous and causal factor, the physical reality would cease to be closed and become exposed to encroachment from another, non-physical sphere, showing gaps. This would invalidate a purely physical theory of physical phenomena, an outcome which of course would be quite undesirable. Consequently, several attempts have been made to overcome this problem, which were invariably aimed at eliminating non-physical (mental or psychic) factors.

Behaviourism constituted the first and best-known effort, with the British philosopher G. Ryle (1949/1966), in the post-World War II years, as its foremost protagonist. Behaviourism rejects the anthropological dualism which holds that two entities, a mental and a physical entity, would be involved in a mutual interaction. Ryle used the intriguing expression 'ghost in the machine'. The dualism of a 'ghost in the machine' will lead to a number of hard-to-accept consequences ensuing from an open rather than a closed reality, while also being rooted in a misconception. Psychological terms describing notions such as intelligence or mood relate to a hierarchy in behaviour rather than to mental conditions. A person's intelligence refers to the procedure or organisation of actual behaviour, not to intrapsychic thought processes. In Ryle's view, psychological terminology is not about the mental course of events but about behavioural dispositions. Mental conditions, of an either cognitive or affective nature, are conceived as tendencies or dispositions towards a specific behaviour.

Since the 1950s, the *identity theory* has championed yet another strategy, one that comes in different flavours. The underlying principle of the identity theory is as follows: It distinguishes three languages, viz., the language of behaviour, the language of neurophysiological processes and the language of introspection. Each of these three languages would offer a unique description of the same reality. A common example would be Venus as either the Morning Star or the Evening Star. Although their descriptions and significations differ, they both refer to one and the same reality: that of Venus. Continuing the analogy, the various languages – of behaviour, of neurophysiology and of experience – would result in different descriptions, each referring to a single identical reality, which may or may not be material in nature (Feigl, 1958).

Explicit materialism has no such limitations. Likewise, it covers a number of different flavours. First, consciousness or the mental may be conceived as an additional, supervening quality of matter that has a particular condition, like water can be liquid or solid (Davidson, 1980, pp. 207-225). A more radical type is represented by materialistic reductionism, which posits the identity of the psychic and the physical (Smart, 1963). Here, pain would be identical to the stimulation of specific nerves. The most radical approach is that of the eliminative materialism, which strives to rule out any mental terms relating to subjective experience or intentional attitudes. This view disqualifies psychological terminology ('folk psychology') as an incorrect form of speech that requires elimination, because reality can only be attributed to its underlying neuronal networks or structures (Churchland, 1984). With this type of elimination, nothing is lost – it merely intends to correct a fundamental fallacy. The very opposite of materialism is represented by a line of research that is not in any way based on any form of materialism, yet essentially it produces a similar outcome in that it denies the unique nature of the psychic, viz., functionalism.

Functionalism as a movement came to the fore in the 1970s. Its point of departure is an argument raised in order to refute or challenge the materialistic basic position – the identity of an experience involving a particular condition or stimulus. This is contrasted with the fact that sensory experiences, e.g., pain, can be produced in a number of ways and by a variety of systemic conditions. This multiplicity would invalidate putting the mental on an equal footing with the physical: if a similar mental phenomenon can be produced physically in different ways, the possibility of equalization is effectively eliminated. Developing this argument, the functionalist will put any relationship with the cerebral substrate on hold, focusing on the function of cognition, which may manifest itself in the desire to avoid pain.

These considerations will lead to a type of functionalism, a functional conception of the mind, that expressed itself particularly in the form of cognitivism. It conceived the mind – up to a point at least – as a digital computer programme using customised software, running on hardware which is the brain (Putnam, 1975; Fodor, 2000). It effectively sheds the link between the mind and a specific function of the brain, thus paving the way for an enquiry into the mind independently of the brain, as well as for imitating or simulating it through computational programmes. Moreover, the mind was stripped of its intentional subjective and experience-related qualities – a point that is essential within the context of the present review. The mind was defined as a computer programme which eliminates intentional states and subjective experiences, while reducing semantic, sense-giving, relations to formal, syntactic ones (Searle, 2002, pp. 203-225).

This view does not rule out consciousness entirely, but uses the limited conception of a 'psychological consciousness' or 'access consciousness'. This type of consciousness relates to consciousness contents, e.g., cognitions, which may be accessible by consciousness but are merely processed as a 'unit of information' by an information-processing, computational system. Within the framework of 'psychological consciousness', the individual in question has a visual perception or cognition, but without actually experiencing it in a sense-giving ('semantic') way. It has been excluded from subjective and intentional experience or awareness. Apparently, the psychological consciousness leaves a gap, to be filled by the 'phenomenal' or 'subjective' consciousness. This is what we recognised in the description of the psychic reality: "I am in pain, I see a tree, I am thinking". The emphasis with regard to subjective consciousness is not on the sheer presence of a representation of an object, but on the subjective focus on an object, on subjective experience. Here, intentionality goes hand in hand with subjectivity.

CRITICISM OF THESE MONISTIC POSITIONS

Can intentionality (intentional involvement) and subjectivity (the accompanying subjective experience) actually be reduced to a material as well as a functional event? The themes of intentionality and subjectivity should be discussed separately.

Intentionality. First, we have intentionality, which is addressed differently by materialism (or physicalism) and functionalism, respectively. Is the perspective of intentionality fully reducible to the perspective of a (physicalistically rewritten) third person? The presumption would be that, once again, the language describing the psychic can be reduced to the language that describes the physical. However, we seem to be up against an impregnable conceptual barrier (Sellars, 1956/1997). A language dealing with physical entities, in addition to logical constants (expressions such as: not, and, or), will only hold expressions to describe physical conditions ('natural facts'). This language differs fundamentally from a type of language that also deals with intentional entities ('epistemic facts'). More than logical constants and expressions to describe physical conditions, it contains expressions to describe intentional involvement: intentional attitudes, subjective positions – in fact, the intentional ingredients of the psychic reality. In other words, this language contains an additional category of expressions.

The presence of such a category means that the logical structure of this language differs from that of the language type mentioned earlier. The truth conditions for its propositions will differ. For example, a proposition from the physical language may take the following form: "The case is that the sun is shining" – this phrase would imply, if true, that the sun is shining. A proposition from the intentional language on the other hand, might be: "He imagines that the sun is shining", or "He believes (hopes, hallucinates) that the sun is shining". If true, this phrase – uttering a 'propositional attitude' – does not necessarily imply that the sun is shining. We can and should maintain that either language cannot be reduced to the other, if only because of a fundamental difference in formal-logical structure (Davidson, 1980, pp. 207-225).

The view of functionalism will also be addressed. Like intentional phenomena cannot be reduced to physical events – according to materialistic views – the concept of intentionality cannot be reconciled with that of a computational process based solely on formal principles either, a claim which represents the functionalistic tenet. The famous thought experiment of Searle's Chinese room (a type of computer) demonstrates that a person who is capable of adhering to formal, syntactic rules, does not necessarily grasp its underlying meanings: semantic rules (which control intentionality) cannot be reduced to any set of syntactic rules that would determine mutual relationships between the various terms (Searle, 2002, pp. 16-17).

Qualia. Reducing or eliminating the intentional aspect – in a physicalistic or functionalistic way – is a problem, but so is the elimination of the subjective, qualitative aspect of psychic reality. This is the second theme, next to intentionality, to be discussed. Traditionally, this problem has been cast into the form of a question: "What is it to be like a bat?" (Nagel, 1974). This subjective or qualitative aspect of experience does not refer to the species-specific world of a particular type of organism, nor to the way an object is presented. In fact, it relates to the quality of experience itself. The experience can be non-intentional, like there can be non-intentional feelings (e.g., pain, listlessness): it makes experience merely qualitative, non-intentional. Next and most commonly, experience can be both qualitative and intentional, without the qualitative aspect itself being intentional, whilst bestowing the quality of subjectiveness upon intentional phenomena (e.g., colour experience). Visual, auditory perceptions, as well as dreams, experiences, and desires each have their own unique qualitative aspect. Therefore, the qualitative aspect of experience is not reducible to the mere presence of a representation, or to an intentional relationship (Reynaert, 2002). To the extent that the language of intentionality cannot be reduced to a physicalistic language, this would also apply to the language which encompasses the qualitative aspect of experience.

In summary, there is a fallacy in attributing a quality – the intentional and qualitative aspect of experience of a person as a whole – to the physical domain, being merely a part of the whole: the 'mereological fallacy'. The attributing of these aspects would only make senses when referring to a whole, e.g. the sphere of the person (Bennett and Hacker, 2003). Despite the perfect feasibility of the materialistic or functionalistic premise, many feel that a consistently materialistic or functionalistic view of consciousness, including a complete reduction of the mental to the physical, would not be possible (Nagel, 1986; McDowell, 1994; Sellars, 1956/1997; Searle, 2004). An *explanatory gap* will always remain.

A particularly unique position is taken by *epiphenomenalism*. Recognising irreducibility, it does not grant any explanatory power to consciousness, to self-awareness, or to the experience of freedom of will. It merely affects the existence of these intuitions as an evolutionary by-product, lacking any degree of impact on behaviour. Their existence is not denied, but these intuitions exist only as an illusion produced by the cerebral structure. It is this illusion that leads people to believe their behaviour is being dictated by experiences and thought, that they can actually reflect and have freedom of will (Wegner, 2002). Any feeling of pain is merely an echo, a side-effect, occurring well after the body has responded. This view seems to have found currency in psychiatric practice, if we assume that mood disorders are merely the result of a neurotransmitter system disorder. It would mean that psychic experiences are no more than a side-effect of events occurring at a substrate level.

It will serve to explain an external aetiology. According to this theorem, man is exposed to external influences, for example toxic agents (aetiological factors) that produce a change of condition in the cerebrum (pathogenesis), which in its turn produces disturbed experience and behaviour, which behaviour may then serve as a harmful agent triggering a new string of events. This view, although recognising the psychic factor, does reduce it to the status of a mere side-effect.

Dual Positions: Dual Aspect Theory and Interactionism

By contrast, the dualistic positions do acknowledge the unique quality of the psychic reality. They challenge the sovereignty of the naturalistic and physicalistic discourse, making a strong case in the sense that they are based on the intuition of people that their experience matters. The weakness of naturalism – the subordinate position of this intuition – is turned into a strength. Defining their relationship, however, here turns out to be the real problem.

The most prudent type of dualism is the *dual aspect theory*. It is based on the notion that the mental and the physical are two aspects of the same substance, both being inseparable and irreducible (Nagel, 1986, pp. 19, 18-32, 40-49). It represents a venerable tradition going back to Spinoza and Schopenhauer. In a practical sense, it offers the advantage that psychic factors can be taken into consideration without any restraint. Again, this theory met with acclaim in both the psychiatric and neurological fields (Damasio, 2003). Drawbacks include its highly metaphysical character and ultimately weak explanatory power. How are we supposed to imagine the relationship between these two domains of reality? Stating that reality always has two aspects is describing the problem rather than offering a full-fledged solution.

The *theory of interaction* takes up a more explicit position, recognising body and mind as disparate entities, each with their own autonomy. The somatic is supposed to exercise an effect on the psychic, and vice versa. The neurophysiologist Eccles and the philosopher Popper both championed this view (Popper and Eccles, 1977) in combination with Poppers 'theory of the three worlds': the physical world (world 1), the mental world (world 2) and the world of meanings (world 3). We find that this dualistic interactionism has also been embraced by general psychiatry. This is exemplified by the concept of a 'circle of anxiety': An external stimulus is perceived, producing the thought: "Danger". In turn, this thought will bring feelings of anxiety and, consequently, physiological changes and physical symptoms (which will then be perceived), etcetera (Hell, 2003, p. 162). A similar depression model may be described: Impaired activity, negative self-esteem, overcompensation of such, stress, physiological changes, physical symptoms, impaired activity, and so forth. This view offers the advantage of offering a bidirectional approach to causality rather than a unidirectional one. A stimulus will produce a thought, a thought will trigger a physiological response.

A major obstacle would be that it is hard to imagine a mutual influence between the mental and the physical. Then there is the law of energy conservation, which poses a difficulty. Although it is argued that the amount of physical energy required to produce a psychical change is minimal and negligible – being 'vanishing small' – within the context of the overall energy condition of the body, this does sound like an argument of convenience (Popper and Eccles, 1977, p. 545).

Yet the enquiry itself raises some fundamental objections, which also apply to non-interactionist and monistic explanations of a supposed causal relationship between the mental and the physical. Indeed, they are based on two premises, the first being that a direct correlation exists between mental and physical processes. It presupposes that the psychic can be analysed atomically in a similar way as perhaps the physical. Unless this condition is fulfilled, such a correlation cannot be established or even imagined. However, this atomistic approach – if physiologically practicable – would constitute an artifice at the psychic level, and would to all intents and purposes be unfeasible. The artifice lies in the fact that the experience involves a complex process of various modes of thought and perception, all of them presupposing intentionality, rather than a set of isolated thoughts and emotions. Even if, in retrospect, certain aspects may be isolated, they can never be separated from the overall subjective position.

Yet, artifice may not be the overriding objection, but the real problem is that this type of atomism simply does not work: thoughts – assuming that there would be a point in isolating them – are not available objects that can be found or constructed. After all, thought and feelings are intentional – they refer to something or are focused – as opposed to physical entities, which lack this quality. Consider the distinction between a psychical and a physical language mentioned earlier, which demonstrated that psychical language holds expressions describing intentional relationships (thinking, imagining) that physical language lacks. The intentional object of, for example, a thought, cannot be fixed in any way, because a thought may hold a number of contents at the same time. Thinking of a table, I may think of this particular table, but also of other tables that I may have seen in the past or will see at some point in the future. Implicitly I am thinking about the essence of a table, which allows me think of this table as 'a table'. Its intentional quality will cause a thought to break up into a variety of thought fragments, without any possibility of stopping this fragmentation at an atomistic level. Or, in more concise terms: consciousness and consciousness contents do not constitute an 'event' that can be correlated causally to another 'event' (Cassirer, 1923/1994a, pp. 27-52). Consciousness is a 'holistic' concept and psychic functioning is 'holistic' as well. The 'contents' of consciousness presuppose the 'formal structure' of consciousness as a whole.[5] This implies that, assuming that any atomistic approach to the psychic would be impossible, likewise a supposed correlative relationship between the psychic and the somatic – atomistically speaking – cannot exist either.

AN ALTERNATIVE CONCEPTION

Consequently, it is pointless to speak of a causal relationship existing between the psychic and the physical in general. Are we perhaps

[5] Cassirer writes (1923/1994a), p. 37: "In all diesen Verhältnissen [...] zeigt sich derselbe Grundcharakter des Bewusstseins, dass das Ganze hier nicht erst aus den Teilen gewonnen wird, sondern dass jede Setzung eines Teiles die Setzung des Ganzen [...] seiner allgemeinen Struktur und Form nach bereits in sich schliest".

witnessing a case of confusion between categories? Most likely. Fundamentally, the concept of 'cause' serves to structure a sphere of reality, determined as it is by causality. Introducing the principle of causality adds a structure to 'the real' resulting in the sphere of causality that is defined by causal relationships. Within this sphere of reality, events are supposed to take place based on mechanisms of cause and effect. Therein also lies its limitation. If the category of 'causality' serves to structure one sphere of reality, this category cannot be used as a structuring principle among different spheres of reality.

This issue might be equated with the relationship between land and property. A piece of land may be my or someone else's property, but the terms 'land' and 'property' cannot be used interchangeably, as they originate from different fields of meaning. Likewise, the presence of land cannot be the cause of me or anyone else owning it. Indeed, ownership is defined by the prevailing title to this land, and therefore not by physical reality – it is defined by the social reality of legal ownership of this property. The 'language of ownership', to coin a phrase, can never be reduced to 'language of land' (Hart, 1948-1949). The two languages hold different concepts or categories, and there is no point in using a category from one language to describe the relationship between both languages and their corresponding spheres of reality. Nonetheless, the presence of land does constitute a prerequisite for the fact – contended or not – that this piece of land belongs to a particular person. If there is no land, no physical entity, then there can be no property – this is self-evident.[6]

Returning to the psychic and the physical, we may argue that the physical represents the land or the prerequisite for the psychic to exist, and that, e.g., a disorder of cerebral regulating systems would be the prerequisite for disorders to occur at the level of action or meaning. Still this is not enough to warrant the statement that one actually causes the other. Fulfilling a necessary prerequisite – the presence of a substrate – does not necessarily make it a sufficient prerequisite. A phenomenon or set of phenomena may cause another phenomenon if it constitutes more than just a necessary prerequisite for the phenomenon to be explained, and actually includes a sufficient prerequisite. The tendency to speak in

---

[6] This mode of thought seems to be in line with the notion of the bio-psychosocial model (Engel, 1980), bearing in mind that the conditionality thesis imposes a categorical divide between the biotic on the one hand and the psychosocial (which is taken as a whole) on the other.

terms of necessary and sufficient prerequisites is even misleading in this case, in the sense that this terminology is consistent *within* a particular sphere of reality, rendering it unfit to support a hierarchy *between* spheres of reality. Considering the difference in level between the two spheres of reality, we cannot hope to offer more than a general statement that the substrate fulfils a 'preconditioning' function in relation to the sphere of meaning. Alternatively, the term 'relationship of foundation' (Merleau-Ponty, 1945/1962, p. 394) may be used, because the substrate does provide the foundation for actions and experiences to occur. Like property can never be described adequately in terms of land, an adequate description of actions and experiences in terms of substrate cannot be offered. Thus, what is described in terms of substrate, cannot 'cause' that which is described in terms of actions or experiences. There exists a fundamental difference between the two.[7] This will preclude any degree of causal relationship to be assumed between singular phenomena from either sphere, or types of phenomena between collective ones. The phenomena will differ: having an experience is essentially different from a sense being stimulated, like an intentional action differs essentially from a body movement (Wittgenstein, 1958/1963, § 621). What it does is prevent a causal relationship to be assumed between types of phenomena from the two spheres or between singular phenomena.

Explanation

Moreover, psychic reality is determined not only by subjectivity/intentionality, but also by being in a world or a situation and, in the final analysis, by language and culture in a structural way, which also makes reflection possible. The meaning of, for example, an action is established as a result of a subjective intention but also by attributing meaning from a shared situation as well as by the connotations offered by language. In addition to the individual intention, there is the element of signification offered by a person's social environment. The same applies to knowledge and emotion: they are shaped by experience, but also by situation and culture. Thus, the inner world (of man) is profoundly affected by the outside cultural world. To put it in Hegelian terms: The 'subjective mind' of man is most profoundly informed by the 'objective

---

[7] The view outlined here is close to Searle's in the sense that an ontological difference applies between the physical and the mental, while, contrary to Searle, no causal dependence in respect of the physical is assumed. See Searle (2002, pp. 7-60).

mind' of culture.[8] This will only widen the gap between the spheres of reality, of intentionality, and of causality.

Yet an intimate, deep relationship does exist between the two – one, however, that cannot be causal, because the range of action of causality is limited to the sphere of causality, unable to control the relationship between the two spheres. There must be some form of correlation between the two based on which correlative connections can be investigated and determined: a stimulus of the retina will be accompanied by a visual perception, a stimulus of the tympanum, will lead to an auditory perception. These are the themes of (neuro)psychology and some branches of modern neuroscience. There is yet a deeper aspect to this relationship – in the sense that physical factors may be able to underlie psychic phenomena without actually explaining them. Thus, the biological substrate can be regarded as the foundation enabling both actions and experiences to happen, while eluding an adequate description in terms of this substrate. We may study the biological conditions of perceptions, of actions, of anxiety, of mood swings, bonding behaviour, etcetera. Anxiety, it seems, is mediated by two distinct cerebral pathways, while the reflexive function may be partly dependent on prefrontal cortical areas, and a disorder of this area may limit the level of reflection (LeDoux, 1996, pp. 225-266). The biological base functions as a boundary or delimiter for psychic dispositions.

Yet these conditions merely constitute the basis for psychic functions, which is also determined by other factors. It seems that biochemical and electrochemical factors are conditionally part of a much more complex structure that is defined by experience as well as by situative and cultural elements. Still, this takes away nothing from their significance. The condition of the body and the brain supports psychic functioning and influences experience, making actual signification wholly dependent on biological conditions. However, signification is also dependent on the external situation, cultural standards, linguistic phrasing, and on how the individual sees himself and his situation – the capacity to reflect. This is where a divergence may occur.

Anyone who takes an interest in how specific and actual behaviour is determined, as in psychotherapy, will not focus first and foremost on the biological foundations of psychological dispositions, because these are presupposed. Also, a person looking into the biological foundations of

---

[8] It is also the fundamental theme of hermeneutics of the signifier, which was elaborated by Lacan. See Chapter Five and Six.

dispositions, as in neurophysiology, might ignore actual aspects of meaning, even though they may help identify actual pathological and non-pathological actions and experiences. Here we would be dealing with research into the biological underpinnings of the delicate structure of psychological existence (Damasio, 1995; Kandel, 1999; LeDoux, 1996; Panksepp, 1998).

We recognise both an 'upward' and a 'downward' trend. An example of the former would be the perception of a physical process of dehydration as part of a subjective experience of thirst, which triggers an action (drinking). The latter could be exemplified by the fact that anyone who drinks too much alcohol will develop an addiction as accompanied by a higher physical alcohol tolerance. As a result, the body will need more and more alcohol in order to have a similar experience, to reach the same level of pleasure. Thus, the physical sphere enables both experience and action, with the action affecting the level of the physical body. The relative weight of the relevant factors from these two spheres may work out differently, depending on the situation: sometimes the emphasis will be on the biological substrate, sometimes on meaningful connections, sometimes on both.

It may well turn out that the influence of the physical component is considerable. The presumed relationship of conditionality does not imply any kind of separation. The psychic reality is established through 'collaboration' with the brain and body as a whole. This high-level collaboration goes well beyond that of a marginal condition (Waldenfels, 2004, pp. 142-154). The condition of the body and the state of the brain determine the experience, so we can truthfully speak of biological conditions of concrete given meanings. For example, the presence of elevated cortisol levels will cause a person to see the world differently than at lower levels, while systemic oxytocin levels co-determine bonding behaviour. However, a major limitation applies here. Indeed, no explanation is offered for the possibility of signification per se, which is presupposed with this type of empirical research into correlative relationships. We should actually ask ourselves whether a 'biology of meaning-giving' is possible at all – a much more ambitious project than merely investigating the 'biological conditions of concrete given meanings' – which is a fruitful enterprise anyway.

ULTIMATELY A PROBLEM WITHOUT ANY SOLUTION

Does the thesis of conditionality actually put paid to the problem of the relationship between the psychic and the physical? So far we have offered an explanation why the answer may be yes, but any solution will be partial. Still unanswered is the question of the leap between what lacks meaning (the electrochemical processes) and what does have meaning. To describe this we may use the word 'emergence', although this does not really provide a solution in itself. We are still left with the problem of the 'mental effect', the fact that consciousness exists and that we perceive something. Another problem is that of 'mental causation', or the possibility that actions such as bodily movements are also informed by thoughts and experiences – the explanatory gap remains. This gap may well be tied to an insurmountable problem. It may prove too much of a stretch to imagine what the brain, the organ of imagination and representation, actually does. Trying to imagine one's own process of imagination and representation would be tantamount to leaping over one's own shadow.

A solution may not be forthcoming, and so we should limit ourselves to simply identifying a state that eludes further enquiry. Most likely there is no point either in wondering why stimulation of the eye by light of a particular wavelength results in the visual perception of 'red', while another wavelength will lead to the perception of 'violet' – these are simply given facts. Indeed, the fact that stimulation of a sense produces a particular perception (a visual or auditory perception) may also be regarded as a given fact. The reverse also applies: the experience that a particular thought will lead to a particular action is another given that is no more intriguing than the fact that stimulating a sense will produce an experience. These correlations can be explored by neuropsychology and other neurosciences: so called 'easy problems'. How exactly this stimulation produces an experience, is quite another matter: the 'hard problem' (Chalmers, 1996, p. xii). Inspired by the scientific picture of the world, it may be tempting to offer a neuroscientific explanation for this question as well: The way brain processes 'produce' experience or are accompanied by inner life and consciousness. The relationship between body and mind may ultimately elude us (McGinn, 1999). After a long life of thought and research, the physiologist and psychologist F.J.J. Buytendijk (1965, p. 77) wrote:

> Even the most general and evident experience, something that takes effect through its meaning, is beyond our imagination. And yet this is the very hallmark of any perception, action, expression or symbol (word gesture).

Ultimately, we are dealing with the question whether a complete explanation of man can be offered based on 'things' or natural processes, or only up to a point (Habermas, 1988, p. 443).

A major bonus of this view of conditionality is its negligible ideological content, while it also lacks any form of materialism, which is often ideologically charged and militant in nature. And thirdly, it avoids autonomisation of the psychic reality and psychosocial sphere. This offers a pragmatic advantage, because the recognition of the disparity of two distinct modes of thought or languages games (of natural events, and of experience and action) will enable an ingenuous enquiry into events to be initiated in both spheres and from both perspectives, in order to identify correlative connections. Also in both the diagnostic practice and general practice the two perspectives can be drawn upon, even switching between them in one diagnostic session. However, this approach will preclude an enforced type of integration between two perspectives and spheres of reality whose overall formats are fundamentally different. This does not prevent the free use, however, of both left and right hands, provided they are *not* bound together in a scheme that rejects the unique character of both perspectives. Perhaps we should consider them both unique in their own right, each with their own separate validity (Mooij, 2010, pp. 93-129).

Also, their designs have a distinct and individual scope, which, however, is not predetermined. One of the 18th-century pioneers of modern physiology, Von Haller, probably had little idea of the range of themes physiology was going to cover later on. Equally, pre-20th-century psychology could never have envisioned the kind of physiologically presented phenomena that were to prove meaningful from a psycho(pathological) point of view. And yet the reverse also applies: much of what appears psychic at first glance, turns out to be biological conditioned.

A Hermeneutics of the Body

The human body constitutes the arena where the two are pitted against each other in battle. On the one hand, the body is the substrate, while on the other it functions as a perceiving and acting body-subject. Medical practice was more or less built on this dichotomy: a person performing a venous puncture will stick a needle in a vessel (a substrate) but also in a person (a subject). It is conceivable, indeed we know for a fact, that the human body, which hitherto has been dominated by the biological approach, can be incorporated much more prominently into the design of meaning than has been done so far.

Psychosomatics

In the past, traditional psychosomatics did some work in this field, using the limited resources available at the time. This movement had its heyday in the 1950s and 1960s, and was strong in Germany (Von Uexküll, 1963), in France (Marty, De M'Uzan, and David, 1963) and the United States (Alexander, 1950), establishing a tradition that has survived even to this very day. Its followers were prone to drawing hasty conclusions, however. For example, a simple interaction model was often employed as a conceptual basis – criticised by Boss (1954, pp. 27-78). In addition, the biphasic model (Mitscherlich, 1967), based on the thesis that the patient will not proceed to somatisation until 'psychisation' has failed, proved highly questionable. Its psychosomatic specificity thesis (Alexander, 1950) is tenuous at best, and is not particularly convincing either when assuming a conditional relationship between substrate and psychic reality.

In order to avoid a simple interactionist approach, the psychogenesis of a somatic disorder may be imagined as an 'instrumentalisation of the body': utilising the body as a means towards solving a psychic problem. This would make the path of somatisation only one path of out of range of possible paths that might be taken (Wyss, 1987). In this way, anorexia could be interpreted as an expression of refusal of the female body. Refusing food will result in the patient retaining a boyish figure (Lang, 2000b, pp. 264-281). Without neglecting other aspects of anorexia nervosa (self-esteem, connection with bipolar disorder or addiction), this may help to visualise the path of somatisation of a mental problem or conflict. From this perspective, the psychosomatic project looks modest, staying safely within the 'well-trodden paths'.

Nevertheless, the concept of 'somatization' remains on a more general level of vital importance, as it refers to an inability to mentalize or, in Lacanian terms to 'symbolize'. This inability may be to some degree equated to the concept of 'alexithymia' (Sifneos, 1973), which is conceived as the incapacity to identify feelings and distinguish between feelings and the bodily sensations of emotional arousal: an inability giving meaning to somatic events, a concept that is derived from the concept of 'pensée opératoire', introduced by the Paris school of psychosomatics (Marty, De M'Uzan, and David, 1963). Lacan integrated this notion in his concept of the 'holophrase', i.e., a sentence consisting of one single word or a cluster of words without intervals ('help'), with the subject being stuck to these expressions ('signifiers') as they mutually solidified, finding himself unable to put these into perspective using other signifiers, to symbolize the event in a dialectical way (Lacan, 1973/1986, p. 237). If conceived in such a way – as an inability to symbolize feelings and bodily sensations – the concept of 'psychosomatic phenomena' remains valid, while excluding specificity-claims way (Guir, 1983, pp. 147-154).

One's Own Body, Embodied Cognition and Embodied Symbolic Order

One's own body. There is yet another approach next to the traditional psychosomatic approach that might be adopted. We might introduce the sphere of meaning and signification at the level of the body, rather than at the level of psychic reality, of individual actions and experiences. This allows the body, monopolised as it is by the physiological or biological approach, to be incorporated into a design of meaning. This will turn the body into a phenomenon of meaning. This is the fundamental concept developed by Merleau-Ponty (1945/1962). Merleau-Ponty argues that the conscious, reflexive and personal relationship between man and the world is limited, representing only a part of its function as a subject ('*moi-sujet*'). In addition, man is already a subject, receptive to, and creator of, meaning at a pre-personal, anonymous and preconscious, i.e., bodily, level. The field of the intentionality of the '*moi-sujet*' is supported and motivated by that of the pre-personal intentionality of the body-subject, the '*corps-sujet*', one's own body: meaning is dependent not only on conscious signification from the sphere of conscious intentionality, but also on the pre-personal signification originating in the sphere of functioning intentionality. The primordial bodily and pre-personal ties with the world will bring a bodily oriented space and time into being, supplying the foundation for a personal, conscious intentionality and its worldly correlates, which in turn are related to the primordial world of the preconscious intentionality, residing in the body (Matthews, 2003; 2006).

This concept of a preconscious intentionality was hardly new within phenomenology, and Merleau-Ponty was not the first to introduce the concept of an 'operative intentionality' that functions pre-reflexively rather than reflexively. In doing so he actually relied on Husserl's view (Waldenfels, 2000, pp. 246-264).[9] With Merleau-Ponty, the body ceases to be a readily available thing and is turned into the actual source of meaning. As such, the body creates meaning, e.g., in a spatial sense: a thing is either near or far away because it is engaged in a meaningful relationship with the body. In this manifestation, the body is no longer an object or thing, present-at-hand in Heidegger's terms, having turned into the very subject of things, or their point of access, attributing meanings and significations to the world of things.[10]

Embodied cognition. Remarkably, within neuroscience itself we witnessed the emergence of a movement representing this very concept. Distancing itself from brain-centred neuroscience, the theory of 'Embodied Embedded Cognition' revolves around the finding that cognition is embodied in the brain, the central nervous and the human body as a whole, while also being literally embedded in the world (Clark, 1997; 2008; Noë, 2009; Varela, 2002). Following on, the organism – brain and body – is regarded as being environmentally focused rather than as an electrochemically closed system (Glas, 2003).

Effectively, the theory distances itself from an (eliminative) materialistic approach of the body-mind issue, while also rejecting (cognitive) functionalism, which conceives cognitions as mental representatives of an external reality, based on their computational or syntactic structure. It counters functionalism by postulating that cognitions are bodily mediated, forming a unity with actions in relation to the world, adding that this world (countering materialism) already

---

[9] Merleau-Ponty (1945/1962, p. 254): "There is, therefore, another subject beneath me, for whom a world exists before I am here, and who marks out my place in it. This captive of natural spirit is my body, not that momentary body which is the instrument of my personal choices and which fastens upon this or that world, but the system of anonymous 'functions' which draw every particular focus in a general project". See also Husserl (1952/1989), section 35-42.

[10] When asked why in *Sein und Zeit* (1927/1962) he made no or little mention of the body, Heidegger (1987, p. 292) replied: "[...] dass das Leibliche das schwierigste ist und dass ich damals eben noch nicht mehr zu sagen wusste". And also (p. 215): "Das Leibliche des Menschen kan nie, grundsätzlich nie als etwas bloss Vorhandenes betrachtet werden, wenn man es sachgemäss betrachten will; wenn ich das Leibliche des Menschen als etwas vorhandenes ansetze, habe ich es zum vorhinein schon als Leib zerstört".

carries meaning at the most fundamental level. Even at the level of physical mediation, the organism endows the environment with the quality of a 'world', as an entity upon which meaning is bestowed. Conceptual weaknesses within this programme are found particularly in the 'upper side' and 'lower side' of mental functioning. The 'upper side' refers to the problems encountered in trying to validate higher 'disembodied' mental functions like thinking and logical reasoning (Bechtel, 2001). At the 'lower side', once again a persistent gap is identified between the physical, meaningless reality of causal relationships and the meaningful world within which the organism operates. Truly striking, however, is the similarity between this view of the body as an entity that shapes itself through direct contact with its environment, and Merleau-Ponty's tenet.

Similarly, champions of this view make frequent reference to Merleau-Ponty (Gallagher, 2005; Dreyfus, 2007). For example, Gallagher (2005) distinguishes a body scheme that controls body movements as well as a body image that defines the perception of the body itself – in inter-subjective interaction. Supporting the mental processes of a conscious intentionality, this embodied self is closely related to Merleau-Ponty's concept of a body-subject, of pre-personal intentionality.

Embodied symbolic order. The body gives meaning, in line with Merleau-Ponty's interpretation, but also takes meaning. Meaning-giving activity is accompanied and preceded by meaning-taking passiveness: Meaning-giving activity of man always takes place within a symbolic world (Cassirer (1944/1966, p. 24/25).[11] Above, the symbolic worlds, symbolic systems – different as these are from animal's *Merknetz* of signals – acquire an objectivity, an objective status, which has a long-lasting and wide-ranging effect (Krois, 2004).

This point was highlighted particularly in the field of Lacanian psychoanalysis. With man being embedded in the symbolic order, symbolization implies limitation, which will become also manifest at a bodily level. Whenever the body becomes part of a cultural or symbolic order, body movement – ranging from digestive to facial and vocal expressions – may be meaningful, but can never assume all meaning. Thus, the meaning-bestowing and signifying body also becomes the signified body. The human body is intertwined with culture, assuming

[11] Cassirer's views did not only stimulate Merleau-Ponty's thinking (Merleau-Ponty, 1945/1962, pp. 122-127) but it may be said that these views offer a supplement to Merleau-Ponty's philosophy as well.

the forms that culture and the symbolic order will impose (Leclaire, 1968, pp. 77-97; Lemoine-Luccioni, 1976; Soler, 2011, pp. 51-54).[12] The body, being embedded in the symbolic order, 'embodies' culture, the symbolic order in its turn. Lacan (1966/2002) writes (p. 6): "As we know, it is in the experience inaugurated by psychoanalysis that we can grasp by what oblique imaginary means the *symbolic* takes hold in even the deepest recesses of the human organism", and (p. 346): "[...] the symptom's signifying structure [...] shows the omnipresence for human beings of the symbolic function stamped on the flesh." The body, the organism is always 'overwritten/overridden' by language (Fink, 1995, p. 12; Verhaeghe, 2001, p. 17). Not only the 'subjective mind' is strongly defined by the 'objective mind' of language and culture, the organism, the 'subjective body', is as well. The body is not only an embodied subject (Merleau-Ponty) or an embodied cognition, but actually offers an embodiment of the symbolic order. This idea constitutes probably one of Lacan's most fruitful and profound insights.

Remarkably, also here – not only in the field of the body-subject, but also with respect to the environmental influence – a connection with neuroscience may be recognised (Kandel, 1999). In this respect, we often see an opposition between a neuroscientific ideology that is often – or sometimes – present, and the actual outcome of neuroscientific research itself (Northoff, 2011). The ideology is that of a rigorously enforced naturalism defined by 'neuronal man' (Changueux and Ricœur, 1998). The outcome will be a different one, involving aspects such as course of life, life history and cultural bias with respect to behaviour (Pommier, 2004).

The notion of subjectivity of the body and the significance of environmental influences combined foster the expansion of the sphere of meaning and signification – through enlarging the 'active' and 'passive' route. The extent to which this sphere will be extended cannot be predicted. It includes all intentional actions but also, to a lesser or greater extent, any ostensibly non-intentional behaviour as well as digestive movements of the organs, the respiratory system and sexual functions. This will lead us to develop a 'hermeneutics of the body', a context that may enable respiratory and digestive or other disorders to be related in a meaningful way. Essential is the insight that this hermeneutically accessible body with its organs is essentially different from the body

[12] Lacan, 2001, p. 418: "[...] le corps, il en (sc. de la passion du signifiant), devient le lieu de l'Autre".

defined by the biological approach. Merleau-Ponty distinguished the 'body-subject' from the 'body as object'. This last, physically and scientifically accessible body is located at a level – in metaphorical spatial terms – below that of the hermeneutically accessible body (Bermúdez, 2005).

Having said this, in the course of the 20th century efforts have been invested in developing the hermeneutics of the human body. The phenomenological movement has always paid a great deal of attention to this topic.[13] Without assuming that anything described in these contributions remains valid, it might be worth investigating what might still be useful, particularly in light of recent neuroscientific developments

Explanation

In the foregoing, a case was made for the thesis of a (at least) two-layered structure of the approach to reality, and effectively of reality itself, rejecting any hybrid form of the two approaches. This would imply that the psychosomatic specificity hypothesis, which assumes a unilinear route – from 'psyche' to 'soma' – would not fit the bill. Then again the reverse is also implied: a rejection of the notion of a sharply defined biochemical specificity of mental disorders, with well-described disorders at a substrate level underlying specific disorders at the level of behaviour or experience. Even the role of a limited number of neuro-transmitter systems in a multitude of mental disorders – as well as the sometimes sweeping effects of psychoactive agents – would argue against this thesis. Also, when imaging techniques identify a stronger activity in a certain brain area compared to other areas, we should bear in mind that this particular activity is tied to the overall brain activity. Moreover, thinking in terms of anatomical localisation of psychic functions yields to conceptualisation in terms of functional inter-connected neuronal circuits. The effort put into the search for a neurological correlate of consciousness (NCC) might better be diverted to a more worthy cause (Searle, 2002, pp. 50-58). Indeed, consciousness, while functioning in a 'holistic' way, may be present 'everywhere' (Cassirer, 1923/1994a, pp. 27-52). Therefore, it is hardly likely that the nucleus of human consciousness which, as a fact or potential, pervades

---

[13] Goldstein(1934); Straus (1935); Von Weiszäcker (1940/1973); Zutt (1938/1963); Gehlen (1966); Plügge (1962); Buytendijk (1965). For a review of these authors see Spiegelberg (1972).

psychic functioning in its entirety – intentionality – could be reduced to one single area of the brain.

Obviously, this qualification of a rigorous attempt at localisation does not imply a rejection of a conditional relationship. Quite the contrary, it underscores it. We may act at a biological level to produce effects at a psychic level, e.g., through psychoactive drugs. Yet this would not be proof of a causal relationship, let alone a unilateral one, in the sense of a necessary and adequate basis. These chemicals produce a change at the substrate level, changing the physical conditions of a personal (and pre-personal) existence. At the level of meaning, the subject finds himself in a position to change his world, either personally or pre-personally, consciously or unconsciously. Psychoactive drugs thus create the conditions required to produce changes at the level of the psyche or the level of meaning.

In view of the conditionality involved, a correlative connection between the psychic and the somatic sphere is feasible and could be explored further. This correlation does not exclude a certain degree of autonomy of either sphere, but this autonomy is presupposed. If denied, this autonomy may trigger a battle between the research projects associated with the respective spheres.

The next two chapters will examine the legitimacy and the conceptual and methodological boundaries of both projects in more detail.

[illegible] ... and [illegible] ... with [illegible].

Four

Empiricism in Psychiatry

Despite the vast gamut of elaborations available today, there is common agreement on the nature of the pursuit of natural science and the scientific disciplines orbiting around it: They all intend to reproduce, describe and explain the experience-based phenomena they investigate, in a bid to answer the question why things happen the way they do. Once an explanation has been offered, it is not deemed scientific until validated by research and framed in theory. This prompted E. Nagel (1961/1971, p. 15) to write in his classic work *The Structure of Science*: "[...] the distinctive aim of the scientific enterprise is to provide systematic and responsible supported explanations".

The type of 'why' question may vary, however: why does a particular object expand when heated, why does the pulse rate increase following blood loss, why does social isolation increase the risk of a suicide attempt, and so on? Based on these examples one may gather that the explanatory approach cannot be separated from the object of explanation. This may be a natural phenomenon or a social event or, at a higher level of abstraction, laws or statistical correlations tied to somatic or social reality, which in turn need to be explained by a general theory. Obviously, natural-scientific psychiatry – biomedical psychiatry – will draw on this scientific view. But what exactly are the basic coordinates of this philosophy of science?

THE NATURAL-SCIENTIFIC EXPLANATION

A specific, formal pattern seems to have emerged. Overall, two conditions need to be met for an explanation to be deemed valid. First, the statements underlying the explanation must be empirical in nature. The aim of this prerequisite is to eliminate speculation: some form of test implication is needed. A statement that cannot be tested is not acceptable. Thus, the criterion of testability separates scientifically acceptable statements from unacceptable ones – it functions as a 'criterion of demarcation' of scientifically meaningful language (Popper, 1959/1968, pp. 34-39, 85). Obviously, the key question is what exactly is meant by 'testable' and what type of experience is 'acceptable' (Kraft, 1960, pp. 27-49). One may adopt either a strict or a lenient position, and both positions have their own drawbacks. An open-minded stance, prepared to embrace psychic factors, is bound to clash with orthodox scientific minds bent on rejecting entities that elude verification, such as inner experience. However, a choice for rigidity may have its pitfalls too.

Testimony to this is the debate that took place between Karl Popper and Rudolph Carnap in the mid-20th century. If we argue, like Carnap did in line with early logical-empiricism, that only statements which are strictly verifiable should be allowed, by extension this would mean that laws of nature are inadmissible, as they cannot verified in a strict sense. A law will take the form of a universal proposition, referring to something that will occur each and every time, although it would be practically impossible to verify each single case. Support by empirical evidence or corroboration would mean little, as a law cannot be verified in a strict sense. However, a law *can* be refuted, or falsified. Popper argues that all it takes is the finding of one instance – the instance that is prohibited by the law, the universal proposition: the finding of one single black swan suffices to refute a universal proposition that states that all swans are white. This debate led to the decline of a rigid type of positivism that distinguishes ruthlessly between observational language and theoretical language, to be superseded by a more liberal interpretation of science.

This extended concept of science highlights the theoretical embedding of laws, and the dominance of theory within observation, where refuting or falsifying laws and theories will bring separation, elimination and, at any rate, correction. The falsifiable quality of theories will offer conclusive evidence about their ultimate scientific quality. Despite the resulting extension of the scientific field with the attributed significance of theories and conceptual structures, the demand of testability is maintained in its strictest sense. Invariably, the implication is represented by external observation: "Here is a black swan" (Popper, 1959/1968. pp. 27-49; Putnam, 1974). Mental conditions, dispositions and competencies can be processed, provided they are fully objectified. This enables a scientific psychology and psychopathology to be developed. However, any subjective attribution of meaning will fall outside the scope of these sciences. Limitation of the range of the experience and the elimination of a more generalised concept of experience still apply. In view of the limitation intended, this approach should be termed empiricist or empirical-analytical rather than empirical, because the latter lacks specificity. It limits the concept of experience to what can be perceived externally, precluding a broader concept of experience.

The second element of an explanation is the prerequisite of predictability. An explanation should indicate why, given certain baseline conditions, a particular event is expected to happen. By extension, we can say something about cases that have not yet happened but may happen at some future moment. Once such cases have been accounted for, an expectation needs to be formulated in order to predict future cases of a similar kind. However, the events or cases predicted must be described with enough accuracy to satisfy the prerequisite of verifiability formulated above. Again, the limitation of the experience comes into play, so also in this respect we may speak of empiricism.

This term is used in its most generalised sense, and should not be conceived as a philosophical brand of empiricism, like the logical-empiricism developed by R. Carnap, its qualification by W.V.O. Quine (1953/1961) or a more recent flavour of constructive empiricism (van Fraassen, 1980). What we actually refer to is a common scientific practice – one that is not directly related to an explicitly philosophical movement – which is guided predominantly by the criteria of testability and predictability.[1]

These criteria – testability and predictability – were developed by C.G. Hempel (1966) into the type of deductive-nomological explanation that became something of a standard. That which is to be explained is referred to as 'explanandum', the explanation as 'explanans'. Thus, the 'explanandum' represents a phenomenon to be explained (an event, coherence of events, etcetera). One of both premises constituting the 'explanans' states the specific conditions in which the phenomenon occurred (p). The other premise formulates a general proposition, a law, that is valid for the set to which the phenomenon to be explained belongs (if p then q). A classic example: iron expands when heated; this is iron and it is heated; it expands. Another example: cardiac output will be increased by vascular dilatation; vascular dilatation occurs; cardiac output is increased. Or: social isolation increases the risk of suicide; social isolation is more pronounced in urban areas. A last example: in

[1] This broad concept of the notion of empiricism leaves unanswered the question regarding the status of theoretical concepts (electron, electromagnetic fields, nosological entities). The may be theoretical constructs, in line with logical-empiricism, or may correspond to reality (from a 'realistic' epistemology).

urban areas a higher risk of suicide is identified. This enables natural sciences, physiology and psychology to exist, in their strictest sense.

The general proposition may cover a law or a law-like statement ('statistical correlation'), as often times we have to make do with lower-order generalisations. This most certainly applies to the field of medical science. Comparing Chapter One, we can distinguish between the level of scientific research where, at an experimental and theoretical level, a general explanation is sought for diseases, as well as the clinical level, in order to reach a diagnosis and to be able to initiate treatment in practice. Both at the theoretical level and the clinical and practical level, limitation to lower-order generalisations will be unavoidable. The explanation implicitly employs a range of laws (kinetic laws, physical laws, chemical laws), as well as specific information taking the form of knowledge about statistical patterns or relative frequencies. The formulation of a natural law will often prove impossible, so one will have to settle for less. And yet, invariably an effort will be made to meet the prerequisites of testability and predictability, as indicated: The prerequisites of the 'covering law model' have to be met. Also medical science turns out to be empiricist both in its practice and in its theory.

THE POSTULATE OF CAUSALITY

Rephrasing the above, we might argue that explanation takes place by describing things and events based on formal and preferably quantitative properties. Consequently, a process of formalisation and quantification is presupposed. *Formalisation* is the introduction of formal terms, in the shape of constants (a, b, c) and variables (x, y, z). *Quantification* goes one step further, as it focuses on 'making countable' – even in cases where that which is to be counted does not yet contain a numeric component (1, 2, 3) – in order to perform measurements or calculations: on natural phenomena, living nature, mental capacities, dispositions, conditions or social phenomena and other kinds of events. As a next step the event can be considered to be something that occurs in specific conditions. This process can be called *functionalisation*: an event is described as occurring in dependence on, in function of, or in correlation with, another event. Therefore, formalization (viz. quantification) and functionalisation go hand in hand. If an event (p), however, represents not only a necessary but also an adequate prerequisite for another event (q) to occur, we can say that p is the cause of q: a mere correlation is turning into a real causal relationship. That means that a causal relationship is of a more fundamental nature, whereas a functional relationship (or a relationship of correlation) merely has a subordinate status. And so it seems that the empiricist scientific approach looking for causal explanations has found its ultimate basis in the postulate of causality.

The introduction of the principle of causality adds a new edge to the prerequisite of predictability. More than representing a formal criterion of scientific research, it expresses a particular conception of nature: the conception that nature (as well as human nature) is predictable and can be defined by laws, with causality being the 'cement of the universe' (Mackie, 1980). Yet, the choice for the term 'postulate' suggests that empiricism does not so much prove this thesis but that only its acceptance will enable evidence to be produced in the sense indicated, while including a variety of phenomena into the 'realm of law' (McDowell, 1994). For example, doubt has been cast on the existence of true universal fundamental laws, with causality being relegated only to low-level causal principles (Cartwright, 1983). Yet, this does not detract from its relevance. In a way, the postulate of causality represents a condition of possibility for natural-scientific knowledge to exist, not being limited to physics, while also including chemistry, biology. This postulate actually turns the natural-scientific undertaking into a project – the empiricist project. Applicability is proof in itself. This does not necessarily mean that the real per se, in itself, is defined by causality, the principle of causal closure. Full acceptance of a deterministic view within natural sciences as well as its dependent disciplines does not imply a deterministic conception of the real, the 'brutal reality of being'.

Essentially, the idea of causal closure of physics is the product of the symbolic system of the natural sciences, with science itself being a specific symbolic form, according to Cassirer (1929/1994b). The idea of causal closure is in actual fact the product of a particular scientific project that allows other projects to be developed as well. Indeed, science in its modern sense does not offer a mirror of nature, a pure reflection of brutal reality, of the real. On the contrary, it is offering a form of symbolisation of the real by generating a theory-dependent scientific reality, in which mathematics and causality play a pivotal role.[2] However, like any form of symbolisation, scientific symbolisation is never

---

[2] Putting 'science' and the 'postulate of causality' on equal footing is not wholly in line with Cassirer: his concept of science includes natural sciences as well as formal sciences (mathematics).

complete, is always 'one-sided' and leaves a remainder, a residue, to be symbolised by other types of discourse.

Therefore, there is a fundamental difference between the symbolisation inherent to language and that to natural science, scientific discourse: between the 'manifest image of man' (i.e. man-in-the-world) and 'the scientific image of man' (Sellars, 1963). Language offers a content-oriented symbolisation of the real, constituting a life world and its specific categories, dependent on linguistic structures: 'the manifest image of man'. Science refrains from this content-wise symbolisation dependent or ordinary language, from the description of lived experience offered by the life world. Science presents a process of formalisation in which phenomena are analysed and formalized while abstracting from the fullness of lived experience. The formalization is essential: 'pure meanings' (Cassirer, 1929/1994b, pp. 329-560), 'idealizations' (Husserl, 1953/1970b, pp. 18-74) or '*mathèmes*', '*petites lettres*' (Lacan, 1991/2007) having a central role. Yet, one has to bear in mind that the reality disclosed by ordinary language – the life world – does not coincide with the real as little as the reality constituted by empiricism, both of these underlying a process of symbolization: the one being more formal (the reality of natural sciences), the other being more content-wise (the reality of the life world) (Granger, 1967, p. 14, 18, 38, 58, 66).

EMPIRICISM IN THE HISTORY OF PSYCHIATRY: NOSOLOGY

The scope of this natural scientific project, however, is quite impressive, as is exemplified by the expansive growth of natural science. Still, the project encompasses more than just the mechanics of natural science or life sciences: it also includes the human body, which is no longer conceived as an animated body, but as a highly complex biomedical unit. This empiricist project firmly took root in the fields of physiology and pharmacology – indeed, in the medical field at large (see Chapter One). It meets the prerequisite of predictability, explaining and predicting as it does the medical-biological phenomena. The prerequisite of testability is fulfilled as well, in the sense that the experience is limited to what can be perceived physically or externally. The body of biology is the physical-chemical body, for which laws of a general or universal nature, or probabilistic laws, law-like statements ('correlations'), can be established in order to design conceptual models and theoretical constructs.

The natural-scientific scheme is not strictly bound to biology and also demonstrates its value in the fields of psychology and psychiatry. For evidence we only have to look at the history of psychology, beginning with W. Wundt and the rise of experimental psychology, in the late 19th century. Another example is the psychiatric field, with the early psychiatry developed by Griesinger, or clinical psychiatry and Kräpelin's pathology (nosology). The nosological approach sets out to identify a law-like relationship between present condition, course of the disease, final condition, aetiology and biological substrate. An example par excellence is *dementia paralytica*, for which the (a) present condition, (b) course of the disease, (c) final condition (d) the cause (*spirochaeta pallida*) and (e) the pathological anatomical substrate were known. Other psychiatric disorders were also supposed to submit to this scheme. Thus, a nosological diagnosis will imply a law-like relationship: if a, then also b (c, d, e), turning a nosological diagnosis into a nomological proposition, and making nosological psychiatry congruous with natural-scientific and biomedical methodologies.

In Chapter Two it was demonstrated, however, that this claim was too ambitious. From a logical viewpoint, it meant that no nosological diagnosis was possible until each single partial diagnosis had been made. Also in practice, the application of the nosological scheme proved to be much more difficult than was believed initially. If we wish to keep the nosological approach, it may be applied as a heuristic principle, in order to be able to identify any of the conjunctions specified. This is how nosology has often served its purpose, while it also functions within the DSM-III/IV/5 line of thought.

The partial retention of the nosological line of thought contributed to the major rise of the biological psychiatry that we witnessed in the latter half of the 20th century (Guze, 1989). Although this was partly due to the advances made in physical technology (imaging techniques) and in chemistry (in-vivo assays), its legitimisation was based on an empiricist conception of psychiatry as a science. This approach consists in the formulation of reductive models, based on the idea that the different levels of explanation (genetic, neural, psychological, social) should be integrated into some kind of unified explanation (Kendler, 2005). However, this may be combined with a reductionistic programme, e.g., that of unified science. It postulates that there is essentially one single science, and the laws of complex wholes can be reduced to the laws of partial objects, and ultimately to the law of elementary particle physics. Yet, the boundaries between formulating reductive models and formulating a reductive ontology may become blurred. Meanwhile, this issue triggered a sophisticated debate, which actually contributed to the raising of psychiatry to a scientific level (Schaffner, 2008). At any rate, the ascendency of biological psychiatry was a major event in the scientification of psychiatry. On the whole, this rise contributed in no small measure to the impressive overall growth of the psychiatric field (Andreasen, 2001).

EMPIRICISM IN PRESENT DAY PSYCHIATRY: DSM III/IV/5

This growth was also dependent on the development of taxonomic systems for the sake of classifying psychiatric disorders, made necessary by the prerequisite of replicability. Essential in this respect was the major step of developing the DSM-III classifying system in the USA: *Diagnostic and Statistical Manual of Mental Disorders* (Third Edition). DSM-III proved of great importance to psychiatry, both as a discipline and in clinical practice.[3] As mentioned before, the design of this taxonomic system owes a great deal to Kräpelin's nosological systems: It can be interpreted as a Neo-Kräpelian project. Moreover, the design of the DSM system was strongly influenced by Hempel (1965), whose empiricist philosophy of science has been mentioned before. It should be obvious, therefore, that this system was embedded in the empiricist tradition.

The introduction of this system put an end to the wide variety of methods employed hitherto in diagnostics. First of all, DSM classification greatly facilitated research, allowing the prerequisite of replicability to be met, while setting up psychiatry to meet empiricist prerequisites. Next, psychiatry could turn its attention to developing as a clinical practice into *Evidence Based Medicine* (EBM). With time, diagnostics became more standardised, while treatment could be controlled based on guidelines and treatment effects investigated using research methods that were completely in line with empiricist principles (Sackett et al. 2000). Only those types of treatment whose effectiveness had been proved based on randomised controlled trials (RCT) were deemed acceptable, an option open to criticism (Slade and Priebe, 2001; Williams and Garner, 2002).

---

[3] American Psychiatric Association, *Diagnostical and Statistical Manual of Mental Disorders: Third Edition*, 1980; *Fourth Edition*, 1994; *Fourth Edition, Text Revision*, 2000; *Fifth Edition*, 2013.

The relative strength of DSM-III (later updated to DSM-IV and later on converted into DSM-5) lies in the importance of operational criteria that apply to each and every class, its emphasis on observable phenomena, as well as in its 'a-theoretical' principles, supposedly eliminating aetiological reference. Classification is based on five axes, the first two being the most important. They comprise clinical disorders (like schizophrenia, paranoid and affective disorders, anxiety disorders) and personality disorders (such as the avoidant type, the borderline type), respectively. The definition of clinical disorders (Axis I) and personality disorders (Axis II) was developed on the basis of point-by-point criteria (of inclusion and exclusion). Speaking in neutral terms of a disorder rather than a disease suggests that any reference to historically evolved pathological concepts would be avoided.

Nonetheless, the supposed a-theoretical principle only covers a limited range of levels, which is meanwhile a well-known fact. The onset of an anxiety disorder is centred around the notion of a panic attack, seen as a purely biological event; primacy is given to a supposed meaningless biological event. A highly complex and detailed classification was developed for mood disorders – well-suited for biological treatment – whereas the delusional disorder is dealt with succinctly. An apparent bias is observed towards underlying biological mechanisms of a psychic disorder. If such mechanisms are not distinct and pharmacological effects of treatment are limited – as in the case of the delusional disorder – interest seems to wane.[4]

Despite the fact that a great deal of ingenuity, clinical experience and consultation went into the positioning of a variety of groups and subgroups, time and again we observe a tendency towards far-reaching operationalisation. This tendency is also reflected in the development of standardised interviews. Common types are the structured interview types SCID-I for Axis I disorders and SCID-II for Axis II disorders (First et al. 1996, 1997).

The classification system (DSM III/IV/5) and the diagnostic medium of the structure interview are not mentioned for the sake of a detailed discussion, but rather to illustrate the prevailing tendency towards operationalisation of concepts, implying a formalisation and functionali-

---

[4] For a criticism of the alleged non-theoretical content, see e.g., Spitzer (1988) and id. (1990); a criticism of inappropriate use of DSM-IV, see Andreasen (2001); for a criticism of the ideological content of the DSM-III/IV line of thought, see Zarifian (1994/1998); major controversies have been recorded in Sadler et al. (1994).

sation of the phenomena. In those cases where the operationalisation of concepts is maximised, the phenomena themselves are formalised as far as possible. e.g., described according to their formal characteristics (duration of condition, e.g., one week, more than six months, less than six months). Formalisation is not an end but a means: its purpose is to investigate whether a relationship of correlation or even a causal relationship exists between the formalised event (a particular type of behaviour) and other formalised factors (of social or biological nature). Yet it *is* important. Only when the empirical content of the concepts has been operationalised adequately, when the events, the phenomena, have been formalised sufficiently, will this research become replicable – the prerequisites of testability and predictability, the basic assumptions of the empiricist approach, will have been met.

Meanwhile a new development has emerged, namely the use of psychometric tools within psychiatry, which is gaining popularity fast. Psychiatry, in its empiricist form, is turning into a measuring science. When applying psychological measurement tools, two types of questions need to be answered: Do these tools produce reliable results? And: do they actually measure what they are supposed to measure? Answering this question allows a critique on the classifying and measuring brand in psychiatry.

A Critique

Reliability and Validity

The first question concerns reliability. Reliability may apply to researchers, to the objects of investigation or to the measurement tool itself. The question would be whether any match identified can be explained by coincidence or not and, if so, to what extent. It may turn out that researchers using the tool did not identify an acceptable match until having received adequate training in using this tool, or that certain patient groups showed a higher match rate than others, or that some components of the measurement tool resulted in a higher match rate than other components. In the last case, the reliability of the tool itself is explored, while an identified relative lack of reliability can lead to the adaptation, further specification, elimination. It turns reliability into a relative concept.

Another issue, one that is tied to the issue of reliability but well distinct nonetheless, is that of validity, which follows from the second question: does a measurement tool actually measure what it is supposed to measure? When rigorously operationalising a concept, at a certain point one may wonder whether the status of operationalisation still matches the original content of this concept. First of all, this problem will occur when developing standards for the operationalisation process, i.e., when validating the measurement tool. A standard may take the form of an expert's judgment. If there is satisfactory agreement between the research outcome established by using the measurement tool (in intelligence, depression or anxiety measurements), and the expert's judgment, the tool may be regarded as being validated. Yardstick, criterion or standard would then be the expert's judgement, while the measurement tool is supposed to 'predict' it: *predictive* validity. Another type of validity concerns the so-called *construct* validity. Further characteristics of the isolated behaviour are investigated, while these characteristics are introduced into the concept, which initially only described the behaviour in a conventional, arbitrary way. The scope of the concept is widened, making this 'isolation' less arbitrary and more strongly justifiable. A third and final type of validity concerns the true *concept* validity. Rather than address the step-by-step extension of a concept, it deals with the question whether a given operationalisation of a given concept will correspond satisfactorily with that particular concept. The question is whether an intelligence test actually measures intelligence, and not some educational adaptation level, or whether a depression scale can truly measure depression. What is needed here is a conceptual analysis of the issue at hand, including answers that touch upon the nature of the phenomenon itself. At any rate, components of the conceptual content need to be described, dealing with factual issues like: "What is depression really?", "What is anxiety really?"

Like reliability, validity is a relative concept (Thorton, 2002). First of all, the value of the commonly used predictive validation is limited, because the criterion or standard – the expert opinion – is established in an arbitrary or conventional fashion. Regarding the construct validity, the tenet is that further investigation should tell us more. At a basic theoretical level, certain diagnostic concepts may have been validated in an acceptable manner, but complex relationships are bound to present difficulties. The third method of validation, conceptual validation, is problematic in its own way, confronting us with the issue of reduction, which is inherent in the empiricist approach. It may be doubted whether the formalised phenomenon and the original phenomenon have much in common.

Empiricism implies reduction and, consequently, a reality in respect of which reduction occurs is presupposed. The psychology of perception abstracts what is phenomenal within perception. Responding to a thesis from psychology of perception, the Dutch psychologist Linschoten, who abandoned phenomenological psychology in favour of experimental, empiricist psychology, wrote the following (Linschoten, 1964, p. 30):

> The equal sign in Weber-Fechner's law (S = k log R) therefore does not necessarily mean that (...) awareness could not be anything else than that which follows the equal sign. Certainly not. (Qualitative) awareness is a different thing altogether, more than just the logarithmic value of stimulus strength multiplied with k. Such an interpretation would be utterly pointless.

Thus, the (empiricist) psychopathology of hallucination abstracts that which is phenomenal within the hallucination. It is here that phenomenology, as eidetic phenomenology, enters the stage, which focuses on exploring essences – to be distinguished from Jaspers' merely descriptive psychology (Sadler, 1992). A current definition of a hallucination is 'object-less perception'. Misjudging its operational character would turn this definition from a purely phenomenological point of view into utter nonsense – of course a hallucination has an object, a *perceptum*. Something is 'heard or seen', and the pretension of reality is never called into question. However, only the patient is privy to this reality and, more essentially, it concerns the patient only, and him alone. That is why hallucinations should not be referred to as perception, but as surrogate perceptions at best. A different type of object will therefore change the perspective on this object, as phenomenology will point out. Moreover, it should be borne in mind that a thing that essentially has a private character differs fundamentally from something that lacks this characteristic. Therefore, it would be a fallacy to speak, in the case of hallucination, of reality or the attribution of reality – reality or worldliness being essentially intersubjective. This example of a hallucination demonstrates that a phenomenological analysis of a phenomenon, i.e., a description of the essence of this phenomenon (including a conceptual analysis of a concept) is actually capable of measuring the distance between this phenomenon and its formalisation, between this concept and its operationalisation. The extent of the measure, of the gap, also reflects the validity (in the third sense) of the operationalisation.

It may be that the researcher or research community overlooks the fact that reduction does take place within scientific research (Thorton,

2004). Yet reduction is inherent in the process of formalising, quantifying, functionalising. Science consists in developing and testing models – reductive models. To give an example (quoted by Linschoten, 1964, p. 33): William James argued that a Beethoven string quartet could be investigated as an instance of scratching cat gut with horsetail hair, and that an exhaustive description based on this perspective would be possible. However, it also allows for a different kind of description, one that is closer to phenomenal reality. That is legitimate, but once again, one has to bear in mind that the phenomenal reality does not coincide with the real as little as the reality constituted by empiricism, underlying both a process of symbolisation as such. All modes of perception and conceptualization are underlying a process of symbolization.

Modes of Conceptualisation

The inquiry into the validity of measurement tools has a counterpart: the inquiry into the nature of conceptualisation. The three types of validity of measurement tools (predictive, constructive or conceptual) are mirrored by three modes of conceptualisation: *nominalistic, constructive, real.* A concept may take effect based solely on agreement, which corresponds to predictive validity. It makes a concept little more than an agreement to group phenomena, and the concept would become a 'name', nothing more. This type of conceptualisation is nominalistic in nature. Alternatively, the concept may gradually gain (empirical) support, making the process of grouping less arbitrary. This describes the constructive mode of conceptualisation. As a third form, the concept is supposed to reflect phenomenal reality per se – be it partially – which is why this type is called 'real'.

At the symptom level, a (partially) real conceptualisation seems to present few obstacles, considering that a link with a more or less controversy-free phenomenology can be established – with perception, with thought, with desire (see the example of the definition of a hallucination and its phenomenology). Conceptualisation with respect to psychiatric disorders, however, is much more problematic. Indeed, it is most *unlikely* that psychiatric disorders described in classification systems would truthfully reflect a disorder occurring in reality. Even the history of modifications within the DSM-III/IV/5 would argue against it. The focus is actually on conventions that – to a smaller or larger degree – found empirical support, which elevated them to the status of a construct. Some constructs have a long history and are firmly established as in the field of dementia (Dillmann, 1990); others will be exposed to dispute from time of time as in the case of the concept of schizophrenia (Blom, 2003). This is not a problem in itself – the problem begins if the status of concepts is misconceived, and a higher level of reality is attributed to them than would be warranted. For instance, from a conventional, arbitrary point of view we may rightfully separate a disorder as an Oppositional Defiant Disorder from the similarly conventional established overall Conduct Disorder. And yet this does not justify referring to these disorders as if they actually exist and would consequently have a more elevated status than a 'name' that may develop into a construct, e.g., a social construct (Hacking, 1999, Church, 2004). Nevertheless, these constructs and classification systems often appear to be given 'naturally', as Hacking (1999, p. 111) mentions: "At the time that each classification was in use, it seemed somewhat inevitable, a perfectly way to classify". These constructs are appearing as real entities (Rosenberg, 2007).

Insight into the precise content of the concept, the (social) construct, is of vital importance. If one wishes to explore independent variables, the characteristics already embedded in the conceptual content need to be excluded first. Proceeding from the notion that psychopathy is characterised by factors such as lack of guilt, lack of empathy, deceit, impulsive action, refusing to take responsibility for one's own behaviour and various types of crimes, there would be no point in investigating whether members from the resulting cohort will display a lack of empathy or engage in acts of deceit. Indeed, such characteristics are part of the concept itself (Hare, 1991). If we argue that satisfying psychopathic criteria in the sense indicated would be a strong predictor of future relapse, this would only be an empirical statement to a very limited extent – in fact, it has a highly tautological content, because 'a high degree of relapse' is more or less part of the concept itself. Obviously, this does not mean that empirical research in respect of a conceptual construct would be pointless – certainly not. Yet it *is* imperative that empirical research refers primarily to *in*dependent variables, not being part of the concept itself. Also in epidemiological research into the prevalence or incidence of a psychic disorder, the dependence of the research outcome on its conceptual point of departure should always be kept in mind, as it strongly qualifies the outcome. In other words, no compromising should take place in the sense of presenting a predominantly non-empirical research as empirical – a scientific attitude is not always assumed.

The comparatively artificial nature of diagnostic distinctions is well illustrated by the classification of personality disorders. DSM-III/IV offers a subdivision (on Axis II) into a number of types (dependent, avoiding, narcissistic, histrionic personality disorder, etcetera), specified in bulleted lists (Millon, 1981). It turns out there is a substantial overlap among the various types distinguished. Particularly the miscellaneous group of Personality Disorders Not Otherwise Specified (NAO), commonly has a remarkably high number of attributions. The presence of such a large miscellaneous group is proof of the comparatively artificial character of this type of overall classification. DSM-5 made an effort to address this problem by cutting down the number of personality disorders and by implementing a more dimensional variety of diagnostics. In turn, this will give rise a to a new problem, in that the boundaries between disturbed and non-disturbed becomes blurred to the extent that it widens the scope of the definition of a disorder substantially. These problems present themselves because essentially only codeable descriptions of traits are supposed to be offered, while this limitation fails to meet the demands of psychodiagnostic practice, which requires a much deeper insight into the underlying personality structure. This results in a particularly complicated system, distinguishing five personality types, five levels of personality functions and six personality traits. This solution is at variance with the initial aim set by the DSM project aimed to offer a convenient system. It reflects the limits of this taxonomic approach, which always tends to expand.

THE CONCEPTS OF DISEASE AND VALUE

The limits that the empiricist approach is bound to run up against, do not actually detract from its significance. On the contrary, its significance remains unchallenged. The DSM system contributed to the emergence of a common language – a language that never existed before – to serve diagnostics as well as scientific research. It is useful to the degree that classes of the system are considered to be of a predominantly descriptive nature and would be regarded as practical tools (Frances, 1995). This would most certainly make them of seminal importance to both epidemiological and biological research. An investigation into the occurrence of psychic disorder and its relationship to social stratification and geographical distribution is of great social relevance. The importance of biological-psychiatric research to the diagnostics, treatment and theoretical development surely does not require any explanation, considering its massive contribution to developing a broad insight into the psychic disorder. Admittedly, not all expectations were fulfilled, and the ever increasing process of system refinement makes it less and less practical as a diagnostic tool. Moreover, the various classes opened up fewer research opportunities than had been hoped (Kupfer, 2002; Kendler and Zachar, 2008). And yet, despite these setbacks, the position of the system has remained strong throughout – hardly surprising, because successful attempts at strengthening the medical discourse have always been welcomed by medical science. It certainly helped to affirm the position of psychiatry as a biological medical science.

The concept of disease is proof of this (APA, 2000, p. xxxi). On the one hand, according to the DSM, it is generic, covering any type of clinically significant mental or behavioural pattern that is clinically relevant and leads to (subjective) distress and (objective) impairment. And yet it only becomes truly relevant once it can be defined as the manifestation of a behavioural, psychological or biological dysfunction. This brings a limitation: for a particular behavioural pattern to be recognised as a disorder, it needs to be linked to a dysfunction. Thus the concept of dysfunction is attributed a key role. Also those who believe the DSM definition to be too sweeping tend to emphasise the functional concept: disease as 'harmful dysfunction' (Wakefield, 1992). In this case, a dysfunction is interpreted as a disorder of a natural mechanism or of an organism. Any specification in terms of a neuronal substrate may be left out (Wakefield, 1992). What *is* essential is the reference to a dysfunction, e.g., a function. Such a functional explanation (in a strong sense, different from the weak sense hitherto used in the pairing of formalisation/functionalisation) is purposive. An organ or a behaviour is only functional if it serves a purpose. Functional, purposive, explanations are teleological in nature, referring as they do to a teleological standard. This will lead us to the very heart of the medical discourse, which is characterised by both a symptomatology (the presence of a concept of disease) and a teleological normativity, as was discussed in Chapter One. Once again, empiricist psychiatry, driven by a teleological concept of disease framed in terms of dysfunction, finds itself firmly rooted in the medical discourse.

And yet what is being masked here is the aspect of value. When exactly is something 'harmful', 'clinically significant' or an 'impairment'? The issue has been raised before by Jaspers (1959/1997, p. 780): "The only single thing in common between events that have been called 'sick' is that a value-judgement is expressed. In some sense, but not always the same sense, 'sick' implies something harmful, unwanted and of an inferior character". That is precisely where the fundamental difference between psychiatry and somatic medicine lies. Rules and values will always come into play when determining if something is adequate, or deviates from the response expected within a particular culture. Rather than a functional, teleological type of standardisation, this reflects a deontological type of standardisation, as was outlined in Chapter Two. In psychiatry, values are very much part of the discourse itself: The psychiatric facts in themselves are charged with meaning (Fulford 2004; Sadler, 2005).

A similar issue is seen in the identification of the ontological status of disorders. According to the Neo-Kräpelian conception of the DSM system, diseases are deemed to exist in reality, while their true nature is to be established through research. However, if the psychiatric facts ("This is inadequate") are also value-based, value predetermined, then the same will apply to any concept of a disorder based on these facts: A disorder becomes a value based 'construct'. Some classes (conduct disorder, oppositional conduct disorder, the ADHD disorder) demonstrate the constructive aspect quite clearly, as was established earlier. However, any set of values is bound to incorporate a cultural bias towards the disorder. For example, from a Western perspective, avoidance behaviour is far more likely to be labelled as a personality disorder than in Oriental cultures. Of course, this does not mean that any disorder would be a myth-like construct (Szasz, 1961) – such a claim could never be substantiated. Yet he notion that psychiatric disorders are occurring actually in reality and need to be investigated merely for their factual content – the 'disease realism' approach – is not tenable (Zacher, 2000).

THE LIMITS OF THE MEDICAL DISCOURSE

It downplays the far more complex nature of psychiatry as compared to medical science, to the medical discourse. To begin with, its concept of disease is different: it includes both a functional-teleological and an evaluative-deontological point of view. Secondly, the status of the concept of disease differs, considering that it is primarily constructionist rather than ontological-realistic in nature. Thirdly, values are also relevant, as they determine the nature of the disorder as well as the therapy selection: psychiatry is partly value-based medicine. This leads to a different practical approach: Essentially, the patient is a discussion partner who, to some extent, can also be held accountable for his or her behaviour. This brings us to the fourth and final point: The medical discourse does not address subjectivity proper. Like medical science, it might have an eye for the subjectivity of the patient, but merely in an objectifying way. It will define the patient as an object suffering from 'distress', 'pain' or 'loss of quality of life to a certain degree'. Likewise, it is aware of the aspect of intentionality and its various manifestations, to the degree that they can be objectified as perception disorders, thought disorders, affective disorders, etcetera.

What is excluded here is the signification from the perspective of the patient himself: What is his attitude towards the symptoms, what is the nature of the signification underlying the symptoms, is there a relationship with the life history? Rather than stress the relationship between the symptoms and the impaired brain function, these questions will focus on the psychic reality. The position of the individual, no longer a mere element within a set, will shift, turning him into a source of signification.

The strategy of excluding meaning, of isolation, formalisation, quantification and functionalisation of phenomena, which is inherent in the medical discourse, will ultimately lead to a causal, mechanistic conception of reality, according to the reductionistic programme (Cartwright, 1999; Thornton, 2004). As a point of departure, it practises what may be termed the 'machine metaphor' – a concrete form and detailed elaboration of the 'mechanisation' of the world image as it has unfolded in modernity, even to include the human body – as was pointed out in Chapter One. Even the contemporary shape of the formulation of biological theories, which speaks in terms of computational processing, biochemical receptors and neurophysiological networks, does not fundamentally affect its orientation towards a machine metaphor. Biochemistry, nuclear physics and electrophysiology have complemented and qualified the mechanisation of the world view, without effectively neutralising it. In this regard, the machine metaphor turned out to be applicable to both nature and the human body, at least to some extent, while leaving some space for a hermeneutics of the body.

This metaphor, this discourse dealing with the confrontation with psychic reality, undoubtedly has its limits, while being perfectly compatible with a variety of disciplines, such as the psychology of mental functioning, behavioural genetics and behavioural medicine. This is clearly manifested by the problems regarding validity, conceptualisation, the concept of disease, the value aspects inherent in the cultural embedding of psychiatric facts. They illustrate most vividly that the project of the medical discourse, which proved so successful in both somatic medicine and psychiatry, is an uneasy match with psychic reality, whose phenomena it is unable to acknowledge fully.

For that reason it would be useful to look into the backgrounds and feasibility of another project – from a scientific-theoretic point of view – one that lacks functionalising and mechanising qualities and is willing to investigate internal relationships between phenomena. The history of hermeneutical psychiatry, in its broadest sense, has proved its viability in the past. Phenomenology, hermeneutics and psychoanalysis have all contributed a great deal to the psychiatric field (see Chapter Two). For the future it may also be a promising path, as it invites psychiatry and psychopathology to adopt a more interpretative and explorative line of inquiry, ultimately leading to a broadening and changing of focus.

PART II

Five

Three Forms of Hermeneutics

In psychiatry, the limitations imposed by the empiricist approach may lead us to explore an alternative approach, taking the psychiatric investigation setting as a starting point. Firstly, psychiatry deals with abnormal behaviour or experience requiring change. In cases where no change is desired by anyone, the behaviour or experience in question will fall outside the psychiatric scope. The desire for change may be expressed by the subject itself, or by someone else (parent, partner, society), through the formulation of a complaint ("I feel down") or an accusation ("He is acting in a compulsive way, he is so confused"). Essential is that the psychic factor conveyed with the complaint and the accusation is not ignored, but is actually taken account of. The problem experienced may involve well-described symptoms (e.g., compulsion, anxiety or dissociation symptoms) or deeply ingrained personality traits (which may reflect character issues or a personality disorder). In such cases, we are faced with a phenomenon removed from what is familiar, or perhaps with a long-standing trait that we may consider odd nonetheless. It proves that anything considered odd or uncommon will only reveal itself against a backdrop of familiarity. This establishes the first connection between the psychiatric investigation setting and an interpretative approach. The issue of interpretation will present itself in any situation in which something is experienced as odd even though it occurs within a familiar framework.

THE SIGNIFICANCE OF HERMENEUTICS TO PSYCHIATRY

The issue of interpretation is particularly relevant to situations in which something is experienced as odd despite occurring within a familiar framework. To interpret means to 'translate'. The learning of interpretation is also referred to as 'hermeneutics', which is derived from the Greek word 'hermeneuein', meaning to translate or interpret (Ineichen, 1991). The need for interpretation will present itself whenever something is not quite clear or is uncommon to some extent. Interpretation is not required in cases where all is clear and obvious. If something is regarded as uncommon, removed from any frame of reference – as perhaps in the case of an non-understandable delusion or a grotesque crime – interpretation will not be possible. Interpretation is played out in polarity of familiarity and strangeness (Gadamer, 1960/1985), p. 262).

The need for interpretation is felt not only in the psychiatric field, but even more so in daily life: human beings are self-interpreting animals (Taylor, 1985a, pp. 45-76). Man lives in a 'space of reasons', while having experience and world-directed thoughts, and manifesting meaningful action, all of them requiring justification and interpretation (Sellars, 1963; 1956/1997). People are creatures of interpretation, constantly assessing their own and other people's behaviour and experience: "He says this, but he may well mean that; why is he acting up like this?" Interpretation finds a unique application in the humanities: in the fields of history, the science of literature, cultural anthropology, law and, to some degree, in psychiatry. What was the significance of a particular political assassination (history)? What is the meaning of the theme of loss within a particular work of poetry (literature)? What is the significance of a particular 20th-century legal text to today's situation (law)? What is the psychopathological background of a particular crime (psychiatry)? Such questions belong to the field of hermeneutics, which deals with the actual process of interpretation ('the praxis of hermeneusis') as well as with selecting a particular type of interpretation ('a type of hermeneutics'), and finally with the principles, possibilities and limitations of interpretation ('philosophical hermeneutics'). What exactly is deemed acceptable as an interpretative procedure will vary widely among the various disciplines. Far from being a foreign body within the world of science, psychiatry's hermeneutical approach is in fact firmly and broadly anchored within hermeneutical tradition.

But how firmly exactly? This question leads us to the scientific nature of the hermeneutical approach, which is not self-evident. It will be argued that the hermeneutical approach – rooted as it is in the 'space of reasons' is scientific in its own unique way, differing from the empiricist approach that searches for physical laws, biological and psychological correlations: 'the realm of law' to be conceived as a more generalised type of natural-scientific explanation (McDowell, 1994). Its form of intelligibility may be different, but is by no means inferior to it. We can and should maintain that either form of intelligibility cannot be reduced to the other as a result of a fundamental difference in their logical structure – while including or excluding responsiveness to meanings and reasons. Yet the hermeneutical scope belonging to the 'space of reasons', is limited: it is the human world and the reality produced by man that are suited to interpretation, not the natural world occurring outside man. A phenomenon of nature may cause puzzlement, which can, however, be resolved by explanation: the rainbow, the stick whose reflected image in the water appears broken, etcetera.

Still, this does not rule out the possibility of the humanities building on knowledge produced by natural science. Indeed, history, archaeology, law and psychopathology all draw upon natural scientific insights. For example, administration of justice benefits from insights gained from the world of physics (ballistography). Similarly, hermeneutical psychiatry may capitalise on general biological and biological-psychiatric knowledge. Yet they do not constitute the core of its scientific effort.

Obviously meaningful action and experience may be explored in a way that does not differ from common lines of research within natural science: cognitive psychology, psychophysiology of emotions, mathematical sociology use a similar approach, and within many branches of the behavioural sciences it is even the dominant approach. And yet, a conceptual divide remains between the nature of what is investigated and the research findings produced. This point was outlined before, in Chapter Four, in the discussion of the issue of operationalisation. By contrast, a conceptually hermeneutical discipline will attempt to stay as close as possible to the realm of meaning that is the theme of its investigation (Geertz, 1973). Rather than eliminate the sphere of meaning, it will actually try to take it into account.

In this respect, hermeneutics offers another point of significance to psychiatry. In sociology or in psychology of mental functioning, subjective elements can be eliminated, as these branches of science deal mostly with (psycho)physiological or group-level phenomena. Psychiatry, however, deals with people who have symptoms and who are actually suffering. Therefore, ignoring subjective factors would be counterproductive. In this sense, the hermeneutical approach complements that which is ignored – justifiably, in its own view – by the empiricist approach. In doing so, it positions itself neither as a competitor nor as a rival. It merely aims to complement, believing that reality involves more than that which can be processed in an empiricist way.[1]

---

[1] In early hermeneutics, this orientation – hermeneutics as a complement or partial alternative to a natural-scientific world view – is dominant. Dilthey interpreted his programme as being both an extension and an alternative to the Kantian approach (De Mul, 2004).

Centred on interpretation or comprehension, psychiatry is also a practice of action. Herein lies a third point of relevance. For example, biological psychiatry is involved in brain research, which may or may not turn out to have practical relevance. Within hermeneutical psychiatry, we recognise a far more intimate relationship with practice, a feature shared with most of the other hermeneutical disciplines. These are predominantly practical disciplines. A hermeneutical discipline par excellence, law proves that legal theory, jurisprudence, and administration of justice are merged seamlessly (Gadamer 1960/1985, pp. 267-278).

Still, a hermeneutical application is essentially different from an application based on natural-scientific knowledge. In the latter case, it is about applying general laws or law-like patterns ('correlations'). Indeed, the field of general psychiatry commonly applies knowledge with regard to laws and law-like patterns or correlations, while drawing up a set of guidelines for diagnostic or (psychopharmaco-)therapeutic ends (derived from group-level knowledge). Again, this raises the question whether individuality is taken into account. By definition, any group-level approach will fail to do justice to the individual aspect. It turns the individual into a nameless non-entity without a history, into a mere carrier of generalised characteristics.[2] Whenever a law-based connection is presupposed, the unique is ignored. As was discussed in the previous chapter, this strategy is based on the assumption of an external relationship among phenomena.

It is essentially different from a hermeneutically oriented practice. Being explorative, interpretative and qualitative in nature, it is not geared towards quantification or standardisation. A science that intends to do justice to the individual – its experience, world-directed thought, and meaningful action – cannot fall back on applying insights originating from a wholly different scientific discipline. By contrast, it finds its origin in actual situations – a specific complaint or a general feeling of discontent. Fundamental, however, is the lack of understanding or the deficit of meaning experienced which manifests itself in a particular situation.

This imperfect situation cannot simply be remedied: first the experience of this deficit needs to be described, namely through diagnostics. This diagnostics may lead to a general rewriting of the situation, in an

---

[2] Granger (1967, p. 185): "A première vue, nous nous trouvons enfermés dans un dilemme: ou il y a connaissance de l'individuel, mais elle n'est pas scientifique, ou bien il y a science du fait humain, mais qui n'atteint pas l'individu".

attempt to shed light on its complexities. Although not opposed to a tendency towards generalisation, hermeneutical diagnostics ultimately aims at understanding the situation itself. Next, any intervention will be based on a set of standards in relation to values and rules that guide and legitimise it.

These three core components effectively constitute a basic definition of the practical hermeneutical approach. After establishing an experienced deficit, diagnostics and subsequent intervention serve to modify the situation based on a set of rules or standards (of a deontological nature). Beginning and ending being defined by an intervention in a situation, we may speak of a cycle, or even a practical cycle. This suggests that a practical discipline, in addition to being individualising and interpretative, it is also normative, deontological, in nature. Yet, the 'interpretative' element remains at the heart of this cycle.

After outlining the relevance of hermeneutics to psychiatry, we shall proceed to discuss the hermeneutical field, and its relationship to psychiatry. This field comprises, subsequently, (1) the object or the domain of interpretation (the 'what'), (2) the way knowledge is collected in the field of psychopathology or psychodiagnostics (the 'how') and (3) a reflection on the philosophical background ('what from'). Three forms of psychodiagnostics, based on three kinds of hermeneutics, will be discussed here. This distinction defines the basic tenets of this chapter.

The Domain: Text and Action

Which field of investigation would be suited to interpretation? An interpretation does not look for causal or external relationships – it attempts to identify internal relationships of meaning that endow a phenomenon with sense vis-à-vis another phenomenon. Phenomena with a mutual internal relationship are not governed by any law, but by the context in which they appear. In this particular case, the context, the unique situation, the individual are incorporated rather than excluded, indispensable as they are to arriving at an explanation in terms of internal relationship. Legal casuistry, literary or historical explanations move within the spheres of specific preconditions for meaning, closed text entities or historical contexts, respectively. What they present is an exhaustive interpretation – depending on the objective – of an individual case: a crime, aberrant behaviour, a story or a historical event. To quote a classic phrase, they are 'idiographic in nature' (Windelband, 1894/1904; Rickert 1902/21). Yet, this does not necessarily imply that any interpretation should be limited to an individual case and would be essentially 'idiographic' in nature, excluding generalities. Cassirer (1924/1971; 1956/1969) countered this limitation by stressing the importance of generalities, of 'forms', which are, however, essentially different from causal generalities. At first glance, this emphasis on 'meaning and form' may seem traditional, but it is still in line with postmodern, deconstructionist modes of interpretation. Deconstructionist or post-structuralist interpretations, while perhaps distorting apparent meanings and forms, will lead to broader meanings and new forms (Derrida, 1972/1982; Lacan 1966/2002).

Two fields would be suited to an interpretative approach: the field of language and the field of action. What does a person say (or write) *and* what does he do? It all boils down to text (the spoken *and* the written word) and action. Will the emphasis on text and action cause the dimension of experience to become obscured? Certainly not – the inner experience is not immediately conveyed, but instead expresses itself through language and action. Only expression can bring out the inner experience. This expression is not a physical event, but an utterance or action that reveals the inner workings of the mind. That is why, in the final reckoning, there is no real conflict between hermeneutics as a theory of interpretation, on the one hand, and phenomenology focused on experience on the other, as was demonstrated by, e.g., Ricœur (1981/2001, pp. 101-130). They mutually presuppose each other's existence. The theme of this chapter being 'interpretation', its emphasis is on hermeneutics, texts and actions. The next chapter, however, will be devoted to the psychic reality, focusing focus on phenomenology and the inner and outer experience.

Texts

Spoken text. Texts constitute the first domain that would be eligible for an interpretative approach. The sounds uttered by a person speaking are not meaningless, but express a meaning or have a meaningful impact. Indeed, a grouping of sounds of letters will effectively convey or express something, referring to a meaning. Even where this does not seem be the case, further exploration may demonstrate that it does. A slip of the tongue may be a mere mispronunciation, but on closer inspection it can also carry a far more complex message: turning the slip of the tongue into a dependent element belonging to a larger body of meaning. So what does happen when a person is speaking?

In any *speech situation*, three components can be distinguished (Ricœur, 1981/2001, pp. 131-145). A subject (speaker) addresses another person (listener), referring to something (a world) – three components: the subject, the other and the world.

In the process, 'something' is being said, which may be referred to as the '*meaning*' of the linguistic expression. By saying 'something' a person will express a particular insight. Next, this person has an intention, and eventually produces an effect. A person saying "It's cold inside" demonstrates insight (it is cold), expresses a wish (for a higher temperature) and produces an effect (another person will turn up the heater). In other words, *meaning* also comes in three components: insight, intention and result.

What exactly defines the relationship between the linguistic expression on the one hand, and its meaning on the other (insight, intention and result)? Is it a cause-effect relationship? The answer must be negative: no external cause-effect relationship exists, only an internal relationship of expression. Rather than *cause* a meaning, the linguistic expression *expresses* it in a particular – linguistic – manner. An internal relationship exists, with the linguistic expression revealing both insight and intention, producing an effect that is not accidental but is intended.

If we wish to investigate the *meaning* of a person's linguistic expression, the key questions would therefore be: what does he *say* content-wise, what does he intend, what does he produce – to which might be added: what form does he use?[3] At the level of content, it may turn out that a slip of the tongue does in fact say something about this person. With respect to form, it may turn out that a remark should be interpreted as ironical. In respect of a person's intention it may turn out that a story is being told in order to convince the other of one's own innocence, the effect of which may consist of a feeling of pity in the listerner.[4] In a diagnostic or psychotherapeutic interview, an attempt will

---

[3] Summarised here is the meaning of a linguistic expression (following Ricœur), which went down in history as the theory of speech acts, going back to Austin (1962/1970) and Searle (1969/1974). Particularly Searle's terminology has found currency. He speaks of propositional, illocutionary and perlocutionary acts, going on to define content, scope and effect of a linguistic expression, respectively. See Searle (1969/1974, pp. 22-25).

[4] Although the boundaries between these aspects need not be sharply defined, a global distinction can be made between semantic analyses of signification, semiotically directed research in respect of the form of linguistic signs and a rhetorical analysis of objectives or intentions (at the language level of sentences, phrases or stories, respectively).

be made to bring out the stratified nature and multiplicity that are inevitably tied to the level of meaning. By contrast, a psychometric approach will in fact rule out multiplicity.

Written text. What has been discussed in the above applies to the spoken word only. Yet, there are major – although not absolute – differences between the spoken and the written word. The spoken word primarily reflects the practical speech setting of the here and now, whereas written language is removed from such a setting. The written word is autonomous and has longevity, as opposed to the spoken word, which is ephemeral by nature – words disappear as they are being uttered, whereas written text is documented by definition: "Scripta manent", "Writings remain".

In the writing setting, we see a threefold separation from the concrete nature of speech. The author will take a step back and the other will yield also, making room for the creation of a world no longer connected to the actual speech setting of the here and now. We may speak of 'three transcendences', or of three generalisations.[5] The author's original intention is no longer decisive to interpretation, as he finds his audience broadened to a general public beyond the individual. He has in fact created room for a new world, with a public potentially encompassing a limitless readership.

In tandem with these three 'transcendences' (in respect of the author, the other, and the world) we observe a change in the field of meaning. Meaning (insight, intention, result and form) undergoes 'objectification'. The text being fixed, with the speaker no longer dominating signification, this privilege is transferred to the 'general other', 'the Other'. This other will decide on the precise meaning of a text (which no longer coincides with the author's subjective intention, but can actually move beyond it).[6] Thus, quite unintentionally, the author may have evoked a

---

[5] The thesis of the three transcendencies (when writing as compared to speech) and its consequences as regards meaning, the central thesis in Ricœur's work during the 1970s and 80s. See Ricœur (1981/2001, pp. 139-140, 145-149). His work on the metaphor (Ricœur, 1975) and on narrativity (Ricœur, 1984) goes back on this distinction.

[6] In this regard, Ricœur qualifies, to some extent, the distinction between speech and writing. See Ricœur (1981/2001), p. 132: "[...] this dialectic (sc. between speaking and writing) is constructed on a dialectic which is more primitive than the opposition of writing to speaking and which is already part of oral discourse qua discourse". Potentially, the three transcendencies may already apply to the field of the spoken word. Admittedly, Ricœur does little to elaborate on this qualification.

poignant image of a period that may go unnoticed as such for generations, without ever being aware of it himself.

Actions

Actions constitute the second domain that would be suited to an interpretative approach. Actions, rituals or facial expressions may be interpreted as manifestations that have meaning and convey a message – they may be interpreted 'as text', while being 'text-analogue' (Taylor, 1985b, pp. 15-58). Although they are not text in the true sense of the word, it may be enlightening to consider them as such. Looking at the nature of the action, a text analogy would be more appropriate than a machine analogy, an action not being reducible to a mechanic movement (Audi, 1993; Kenny, 1963; Ricœur, 1992; Wittgenstein, 1958/1963). We are dealing with a situation involving an actor, another person, and a world in which an action takes place. Action interpreted as text has a meaning (knowing, intending, producing an effect). As a next step, actions may be compared to oral and written texts.

Action compared to spoken text. Insofar as actions are comparable with oral texts, like the spoken word they are 'eventful' in nature. A person will do something, the nature of his action becoming evident from the context, from what he actually intends and knows. We recognise an inner, internal relationship between on the one hand intentions and insights, and actions on the other hand, similar to the internal relationship existing between a linguistic sign or utterance and its meaning. If the intention of an action would have been connected accidentally or causally rather than internally – as has been suggested by Davidson (1980, pp. 3-20) –, its effectuation would have been merely an accidental fact.[7] Yet, if a person has the intention to leave, then his taking leave is not an amazing coincidence, but was simply to be expected. The actual leaving is enclosed in the intention to leave. Wittgenstein writes (1958/1963, § 628): "So one might say: voluntary movement is marked by the absence of surprise". The same applies to the relationship between insight and action. If we do something, we are aware or have some idea of what we are doing. This awareness is embedded in the action itself (Austin, 1961/1970, p. 283). When I'm riding a bicycle, I know that I

[7] Melden, 1961, pp. 43-56; Taylor, 1964, pp. 26-35, Winch, 1958/1976; Von Wright, 1971, pp. 91-107. See for a more detailed discussion Mooij (1991, pp. 13-30, 49-78; 2010, pp. 277-298).

am, an insight that comes with the action of riding the bicycle: an internal relationship does exist between the action and the insight into the action.[8]

In other words, actions embody insights and intentions (reasons, motives), while intentions and insight (reasons, motives) are expressed through actions. Apparently, an internal relationship exists between intentions and insights (reasons, motives) on the one hand, and actions on the other. In view of this relationship of expression, we might say that actions (expressing intentions and insights) convey something, because of which the text or language analogy can be enlightening. This also implies that the space of action, 'the logical space of reasons' is not causally structured, as being opposed to the 'realm of law'. This does not imply, however, that reasons are supposed to be not effective. Reasons are active, effective, albeit it in a non-causal way: by expressing themselves, by guiding action. Beside the nomological and the causal types of explanation of natural events, there is the intentional, non-causal, internal type of explanation of action. Merleau-Ponty writes (1945/1962, p. 259): "The motive is an antecedent which acts only through its significance, and it must be added that it is the decision which affirms the validity of this significance and gives it its force and efficacy". Motives and reasons are meant to be really effective.

Action compared to written text. Actions can be compared to the written word as well as to the spoken word.[9] Like the transition from speaking to writing brings separation from the actual situation and objectification of meaning, compared to spoken texts, a similar separation and objectification will take place in this case. We found that the autonomy of writing deprives the author of his position of privilege that enables him to define the precise meaning of a text. Essentially, his subjective intentions cease to be relevant, and the 'Other' (the reader, the line of generations of readers) will decide what the true meaning is of the text.

A similar process of autonomisation occurs when actions are compared to 'writing'. The action will no longer be interpreted from the context of the actor's actual meanings and insights. Actual intentions recede into the background, the other yields to a 'general other', the actual world gives way to a general world. Finally, the meaning of an action has

---

[8] Anscombe (1957/1963, p. 13, 49) speaks of 'knowledge without observation'.

[9] Ricœur also compares actions to texts, yet in doing so he limits himself to written texts only. See Ricœur (1981/2001, pp. 197-222): "The model of a text: meaningful action considered as a text".

detached itself from the actual situation, becoming more or less fixed. Thus, the environment, regardless of a person's true intentions, may interpret a particular action in its own way. Despite a person's real intention, the environment ('the Other') or a particular branch of science ('Otherness') may choose to interpret a person's behaviour as 'manslaughter', as an 'impulsive act' or as an 'expression of a delusional disorder', although the person involved may see it as an argument gone out of hand, as a mere accident or as an act of self-defence. Rules of experience that prevail in society or in a particular discipline will determine the action's true meaning (nature, scope and result).

This does not apply to a singular action only. An intention is part of a larger objective, while insight is part of a broader or more diffuse insight. Focused, intentional actions are embedded in more complex bodies of action, of customs or rituals a personal character – being the totality of meaningful connections (Jaspers, 1959/1997, pp. 428-430) in which unconscious intentions and unconscious insights also play an essential role.

Individualising and Categorising Investigation

The above comparison between action and text demonstrates that interpretation, contrary to common belief, is in fact objectifiable. Texts and actions are part of a larger objectified body, and interpretation at this level does not necessarily include relating to subjective intentions. Indeed, subjective intentions can be known only if they emerge 'in an objectified way' from texts and actions. In other words, the interpretative strategy towards actions has its own 'objectivity', which goes back to the objectification of the inner world. It is different from the type of objectivity described within the framework of the empiricist approach, which does not take the inner world into account, or rewrites it in terms of independent variables.

Indeed, the interpretative approach that exposes internal relationship does not limit itself to individual cases of a text or text-analogous actions. Other cases can be taken into account as well, in order to develop ideas that proved useful in earlier instances. This represents a categorising rather than a classifying approach. It may help formulate ideas about literary genres, but also about clinical 'genres' like narcissism, histrionics or compulsive behaviour, where a general pattern or structure can be identified or assumed. Like the casuistic activity is referred to as idiographic, this last activity may be labelled as categorising or ideal-typical, because it aims to identify types, categories, or genres (Cassirer, 1956/1969). Since the 'concrete generality' pursued in the categorising approach is fundamentally different from the 'formal generality' presupposed within a causal relationship, the categorising approach may be considered to be an offshoot or derivative from the individualising approach.[10]

Three Paths: Descriptive, Relational and Structural Diagnostics

How would an individualising or categorising acquisition of knowledge be possible in the field of psychopathology of psychodiagnostics? What matters here is not what a person says or does (his texts and actions), but *how* we should interpret what a person says or does. There is more than one way to answer this question. More specifically, any of three mutually complementary 'paths of knowledge acquisition' may be followed.

Descriptive Diagnostics

The first path unfolds from the premise that internal or meaningful relationships can be recognised by identifying with the other. Empathy would enable us to establish the meaning of what a person says or does. This is referred to as the *Einfühlungstheorie* of understanding (Scheler, 1912/1948, p. 105). If we wish to understand what a person feels when he is depressed, we need to be able to empathise with this person. Empathy is needed to understand and describe an experience, but also to understand and describe the reason for an action. If we wish to understand why a person acts the way he does when threatened, we need to be able to identify with the 'other feeling threatened'. In this case, understanding is equivalent to describing meaningful relationships. Empathy is needed to be able to understand and describe.[11]

---

[10] Thus, categorisation is distinguished from classification, causing hermeneutical communality (categorisation) to remain tied to concrete instances (concrete cases), as different from nomological generality (classification).

[11] This point of view has also taken root in the science of history. According to R.G. Collingwood, in order to fully grasp the action of an actor in former days, his underlying thoughts, the interpreter will need to represent these in his own mind. See Collingwood (1939/1978, pp. 107-119), particularly on p. 112: "historical knowledge is the re-enactment in the historian's mind of the thought whose history he is studying".

Initially, this is about the 'possibility to understand', not about actually understanding the experiences and actions of another person. We may fail to understand the inner workings of a psychotic, but we can at least make an attempt. Understanding presupposes the presence of subjectivity and the ability to convey meaning with the person examined, elements that are absent in natural processes or in animal species. What is presupposed, is a 'mind' or an 'I' with an accompanying 'I think, feel, see', etcetera. At this level, phenomenology, in its effort to describe inner and outer experience, will enter the stage. This procedure will be discussed in Chapter Six, but here we are concerned with the possibility of understanding. The fundamental possibility of understanding, of empathy with another person does not necessarily rule out problems in the process of understanding another person's psychic condition. There may be limits to what can be understood through empathy, which is something Jaspers referred to when delimiting understandable from non-understandable delusions (Jaspers, 1997, p. 196, 408, 704).

Besides, a mental condition can also be accepted without actually identifying with the other. Oftentimes, we can simply see if a person is afraid or shocked, without this person telling us. Essential, however, is the fact that the possibility of empathy is presupposed. This approach may be called 'normativisation': based on rules of experience (behavioural standards) the presence of a state of mind is acknowledged, without making further inquiries. Lastly, we may also misinterpret the other's psychic condition. Empathy may be a prerequisite for understanding experience and behaviour, but it is not always needed or may be too limited in its scope. Further verification would then be needed.

The adequacy of the description of what a person experiences and why he acts the way he does should become evident from other messages conveyed as well as from other actions. If the subject reports experiences, e.g., hearing voices, further investigation will have to assess their plausibility: 'He may say that, but is it really true?' If a person claims to have acted out of fear, further testing, further verification will be needed. This requires a complementary and objectifying approach. Intentions and insights (experiences) can be objectified, as they may become evident from the chain of actions. The description of an experience or motive will change into a description of its 'gist'.

This effort can be taken to the extreme, actually causing a description to turn into a rewriting of events. For example, this person need not have actually experienced the very same emotions or convictions if these can be reasonably and generally assumed. We had already established that actions can be compared to written texts and that, based on this finding, the environment (or researchers or the research community) may be able to identify the meaning of the action, even removed or deviating from subjective information provided by the individual. The conclusion can therefore be: "Any person who does that, will do so on purpose, it cannot be otherwise". Or: "You are suffering from a delusion, even though you may disagree". The reason (or 'ratio') of the motive can also be rewritten or reconstructed: "This and this point to the fact that vanity also came into play". This may be referred to as a rational reconstruction. This scheme can be elaborated by including unconscious or implicit objectives next to conscious or explicit objectives, or unconscious insights next to conscious insights. For the very reason that reconstruction or rewriting of reasons – a rational reconstruction – is possible, unconscious motivations can be assumed or reconstructed.

Relational Diagnostics

A second path of investigation starts with a subjective point of view too, but now it is the subjectivity of the investigator. This approach is not based on empathising with the other, but on probing inside one's own mind in an attempt to relate to this other. This represents a relational type of diagnostics, with the investigator trying to gain access to the feelings and thoughts evoked by the other in a particular situation.

The underlying thought is that any person will act and experience based on the situation in which he finds himself. This would apply not only to the subject of investigation, who will act from his present and historically developed background, but also to the investigator, who 'is his own instrument'. From this vantage point, the investigator should have an open mind to the person investigated and, for the duration of the investigation (or treatment), allowing this person to develop a typical relationship with him. He needs to 'immerse himself' in his subject, by truly opening up to this person's world. The investigator interrogates himself, yet by asking questions – "What is it that frightens me in this man?" – he simultaneously interrogates the other and the other's world. By trying to relate to deeper feelings (towards the person involved) the investigator hopes to identify a deeper layer in the other's behaviour and experience. This is actually embedded in the person's actual actions and words, but also transcends them. As was mentioned before, this approach holds an element of 'subjectivity', with investigation focusing on the thoughts and feelings evoked by the other person, which are inevitably stamped by the investigator's own situation or history – by his own 'bias'.

Even here, objectification would be possible. Paradoxical though it may sound, this approach first brings an objectifying correction to the first approach: after all, the other will always be viewed from an individual situation and bias. One needs to be aware of the presence of this bias in order for the reflection on one's own contribution to have a cleansing and objectifying effect (Gadamer, 1960/1985, p. 239). It allows testing and verification in a manner different from the first path, which after all is characterised by reconstruction and rewriting following empathy and description. Here, the correlate of reconstruction would be 'contextual expansion'. The relationships of meaning should become evident from their connections with publicly accessible entities (Winch, 1958/1976). In order to identify the deeper meaning of a story, a historical event, to distinguish a pattern of action, we first need to know its setting, its background, its context and other publicly available elements. Ultimately, this set of situations or a broader context is shaped by the 'world' in which a person lives and which has developed historically. This world will reflect the person's relationship to his natural environment as well as to himself and the other. It also includes that part of the world into which one is cast and where one finds oneself: the family that a person grew up in, the language that one speaks and culture that one lives in. Cultural differences between the subject and the investigator, if any, do not necessarily stand in the way of understanding. Indeed, it is the relational approach that brings out cultural differences and prejudices – both one's own prejudices and that of the other – and may contribute to a possible deepening of understanding.[12]

Structural Diagnostics

The third path builds on these themes, exploring the relationship between the subject – in his present situation, his life history and his family of origin – and the fundamental structures that shape the world and life history. This will expose one's relationship to finiteness, to sexual

[12] To quote Gadamer, a 'tragendes Einverständnis' is required, which may present problems in the case of a hetereogeneous society. The very reason why hermeneutics came into being, in the early 19th century, was the ambition to understand other cultures and cultural expressions, as difference or distance may actually help to deepen understanding: the field of tension between belonging and alienation.

difference, to generational difference and to the notions of difference and lack per se. This type of diagnostics may be referred to as structural, because it explores fundamental structures in the life of a person vis-à-vis his environment in a broad sense. This will lead to a structural analysis or structural diagnostics.

Again, this offers the possibility of testability: this is not about verifying findings obtained through external or internal observation, but about integrating them into an overall structural diagnosis, which is why testing focuses primarily on the structure of the image outlined. The key question should be whether the structure outlines results in an adequate integration of the actual findings, or that it eliminates certain findings. Consequently, rather than produce hard evidence, the onus of testability lies on aspects of feasibility.

Essentially, this characterisation will apply to any of the paths described here.[13] Each of the three empirical-hermeneutical paths allows for, and requires, verification. A high level of objectification may – sometimes – be feasible, but even so objectification will take place on a different level than the objectification pursued by the empiricist approach. The three paths of interpretation were aimed at objectifying subjectivity, while, from the empiricist perspective, objectification is pursued by eliminating (or rewriting) subjectivity as much as possible.

Thus, the three paths outlined share a fundamental feature – they all attempt to identify relationships of meaning: with respect to actual behaviours and experiences, their underlying historical context, as well as structural relationships towards key components of human existence. These three interpretative paths each reflect and anchor a movement within general or philosophical hermeneutics. This anchoring in philosophical hermeneutics will be discussed in some detail.

THREE FORMS OF HERMENEUTICS: OF THE SIGNIFICATION, THE SITUATION AND THE SIGNIFIER

The key concept of hermeneutics is that any mode of experience based solely on natural science will fall short in adequately grasping human reality. From its inception, it has been regarded as complementary. Hermeneutics is associated with meaning and 'subjectivity', with the

---

[13] Ricœur sets great store by the demand of objectifiability within hermeneutics, while also stressing the point that the certainty that can be achieved is found at the level of feasibility or *attestation*.

latter relating to both the object of interpretation and its subject. Acts of speech, actions and cultural products express the state of mind of an actor, and it is up to the interpreter to fully grasp what the actor tries to convey. Herein also lies the close relationship with phenomenology, which emerged more or less simultaneously and has a similar orientation (for a discussion see Chapter Six). They differ fundamentally in the sense that phenomenology takes the primacy of experience or the subject's individual state of mind as a point of departure, acknowledging only at a later stage that this experience is produced through interpretation. Hermeneutics, by contrast, initially centred on the issue of objective interpretation and then went on to include the inescapable subjective elements of interpretation. Thus, since its inception, in the late 19th and early 20th centuries, philosophical hermeneutics has developed in three phases, each reflecting various manifestations of hermeneutics. These phases developed chronologically, but each phase also represents its own unique position, which has retained its validity throughout.

The first path (of empathy and rational reconstruction), it turned out, was predominantly objectifying. It focuses on the way inner feelings and meanings express themselves through speech and action. A dialectics between the interior and the exterior is played out, with the interior expressing itself through the exterior, and the exterior, in turn, shaping the interior. This path constitutes the first phase of hermeneutics. It is defined by attributing or establishing the meaning of actions and texts. 'Hermeneutics of the signification' would adequately describe this type of interpretation. This type of hermeneutics may also include phenomenology, conceived as descriptive psychology (in the sense of Jaspers) or as eidetic exploration (in the sense of Husserl), as Chapter Six will demonstrate. Here our attention is directed to hermeneutics of the signification in its hermeneutical fashion, in a narrowed-down sense.

Hermeneutics of the Signification

This type of hermeneutics was first developed by W. Dilthey (1833-1911). He set out to eliminate any type of bias, addressing the workings of the interior from the dialectics of the interior and exterior, based on the path of empathy by trying to relate to the inner world of the other. By extension, the phrase 'universal sympathy' was even coined. To avoid the pitfall of excess psychologisation and lack of testability, in his later work Dilthey attempted to penetrate a more objectively conceived interior rather than the author's psychic interior – the objective state of mind expressed by the text or the 'spirit' of an age, the disposition of a person. For example, Dilthey writes (1910/1961, p. 236): "The way this mind can be understood cannot be equated with psychological insight. It is actually referring to mental formation of a quintessential structure and order".

Introspection is replaced by interpretation.[14] This shift reflects the tension that has pervaded the field of hermeneutics from the beginning. It is this very tension that drives a psychology-driven and a more objectifying approach, both in need of each other.[15] It does not in any way compromise the fundamental scheme, which allows the interior to become known through expression, without the interior disappearing or being eliminated – a typical feature or behaviourism – by exterior elements, or blending in with them. The interior is important, but so is its 'objectification' through expression. These dynamics are also reflected in interpretation, which focuses on the relationship between partial/whole meaning. A person interpreting will have some expectation of the meaning of a whole, which may or may not be applicable to its constituent parts. Proceeding from a partial phenomenon will lead us to the whole and back to the partial phenomenon, and so this whole/partial structure has a circular nature: the 'circle of understanding'. Premises of a general or more specific nature will always be taken as a starting point. Critics of the circle of understanding argued that anything put in in the way of premises will be reflected in the outcome. However, this criticism is not justified – in part, it is inevitable that premises are taken as a basis, while these premises are also the very object of verification. It makes the 'hermeneutical circle' analogous to the 'empirical circle' of the empirical-analytical, the hypothetical-deductive model. If we wish to interpret a particular behaviour as a typical trait of the Renaissance or as a characteristic of a narcissistic personality structure, this notion will then function as a premise for an overall meaning that needs to be confirmed in some kind of expression or action. That is why the term

---

[14] Dilthey (1910/1961, p. 236): "Das Verstehen dieses Geistes ist nicht psychologische Erkenntnis. Es ist Rückgang auf ein geistiges Gebilde von ein ihm eigenen Stuktur und Gesetzmässigkeit". A summary of this last position is found in the *Aufbau der geschichtlichen Welt,* Dilthey (1910/1961, pp. 230-239), 'Abgrenzung der Geisteswissenschaften'. For a general description of Dilthey's views see De Mul (2004).

[15] With F.D.E. Schleiermacher, arguably the first true representative of hermeneutics, we recognise an opposition between the empathic and the objectifying approaches expressed in the form of a technical (=psychological) *vs* grammatical, opposition or a divinatory *vs* demonstrative mode of understanding.

'circle' is somewhat misleading. A cyclic element is present, but there is no closed circle. Investigation may show that the starting point, prejudice in its concrete and applied form, cannot be implemented fully, and so the premise will have to be refuted or modified. With respect to the example of a narcissistic personality structure, it may turn out that specific actions of the person in question defy interpretation from such a perspective. It is obvious that 'premises' play a key role in the interpretative process, while verification is also possible.

This type of hermeneutics which focuses on establishing meaning is defined by a pursuit for a type of objectivity that is comparable to the objectivity strived for in natural science. The primary goal is to shed one's own prejudices, in order to identify the solution, adopting a *view from nowhere*. This ambition would meet with criticism later on.

Hermeneutics of the Situation

The criticism of the *view from nowhere* was summarised and championed by H.-G. Gadamer (1900-2002). He emphasised that any interpretation will be based on a situation underlying the issue to be addressed. While, in its pursuit for objectivity, the hermeneutics of the signification was guided by the notion that the interpreter should shed his specific prejudices in order to reach an optimally bias-free interpretation, prejudice, in the sense of the interpreter being tied to his individual situation, is now regarded as something positive. This actually stresses the implicit circularity of interpretation even more, because any interpretation will be tied to the viewpoints on which this interpretation is based (Gadamer, 1960/1985, pp. 235-241; Grondin, 2002). Circularity now becomes part of the interpretative process itself. The hermeneutics of the situation found its way into relational diagnostics as well. In this environment, the investigator is supposed to keep an open mind to any experience evoked by the subject. Beyond opening up to the other person's subjectivity, he needs to be aware of his own subjectivity, in order to identify deeper layers in their personality: the situation from which he lives – perhaps without being aware of it himself – his 'prejudices' and his historical background (Gadamer, 1960/1985, pp. 267-273; Grondin, 1994, pp. 71-89). The widening of context strived for brings the need for a type of testing, of verification that is not essentially different from that performed as part of the 'first path'.[16] The relationships assumed should be made feasible based on other grounds than just the emotions evoked by the person studied. Yet, methodological questions regarding the verifiability of interpretations are certainly addressed within this type of hermeneutics, but they are not central to the study. The emphasis is on application, not on testability: what can be learnt from an earlier situation in order to understand the current situation?

This viewpoint is not essentially a new one within hermeneutics. Commonly, a distinction was made among three capacities presupposed in interpretation: the 'subtilitas intelligendi', the 'subtilitas explicandi' and the 'subtilitas applicandi'. What is new is the strong emphasis placed on the importance of its application or concretisation: what is the significance of a particular piece of information to the current situation (Gadamer, 1960/1985, pp. 274-278)? Gadamer based his work on the hermeneutics developed by Heidegger, who – in a certain phase of his philosophical development – pursued an even more fundamental type of hermeneutics: a hermeneutics of existence (Grondin, 1994, pp. 71-103). His tenet was that human *existence itself* is fundamentally determined by 'understanding', which he conceives as a primordial 'being able', covering all types of factual interpretation ('Auslegung'). This fundamental understanding, in the sense of 'being able', is characterised by a for-having, fore-sight and fore-conception (Heidegger, 1927/1962, pp. 188-195, section 32). In this case, the emphasis is on 'fore'. Any type of factual appropriation, any factual insight and any type of grip on a particular subject matter is preceded fundamentally by an even deeper and more establishing gift, anticipation and control. Consequently, any factual interpretation will be based on the possibility of understanding.

However, Gadamer chose a different path: he set out to extend the empirical consequences of the prejudice structure of (any type of understanding) to the field of the humanities (Grondin, 2003, p. 78). This led to a strong emphasis on the inevitability of prejudices in any interpretation, as well on the role of subjectivity on the part of the investigator. He felt that interpretation involved more than a partial/whole structure and a circular nature – a view held by Dilthey – and is in fact also dialogue-oriented (Gadamer, 1960/1985, pp. 333-344). Here, interpretation takes the form of a dialogue – not just in the sense that it

---

[16] Gadamer (1960/1985, p. 237): "The only 'objectivity' here is the confirmation of a fore-meaning in its being worked out. The only thing that characterises the arbitrariness of inappropriate fore-meanings is that they come to nothing in the working-out".

may actually involve a dialogue, as in relational diagnostics. This feature is present at an even more fundamental level, in the sense that the process of interpretation has a question-and-answer structure, making a correct formulation of the question essential. Thus, the text or action becomes a request for interpretation, while interpretation in turn queries text and action for the validity of the prejudice, the premise of the interpretation.

Language becomes of particular significance. Interpretation moves within the medium of language, while language is the medium for any meaningful articulation. With respect to the type of hermeneutics, we may well speak of a universal ambition. This does not mean that hermeneutics can be applied to anything, only that the dimension of meaning depends on language as a universal medium. The theme is 'Language as experience of the world' (Gadamer 1960/1985, p. 397). Yet, this universal nature also has its limitations. Reality is open to interpretation only to the degree that it is 'linguistic' (or language-dependent). These two tenets are summed up nicely by the thesis "*Sein, das verstanden werden kann, ist Sprache*", "Being that can be understood is language" (Gadamer, 1960/1985, p. 432). Anything that exists and can be understood belongs to the order of language (or is language-dependent). However, the following also applies: only something existing that belongs to the order of language (or is language-dependent) can be understood. Brutal reality falls outside its scope.

Also within language itself, the scope of conceptualization and the means of expression are limited. While being the universal medium of understanding, language does impose restrictions. Speaker and interpreter will have to submit to a language, which will always be a specific language. Through its structure and vocabulary, language enables a particular type of speech, while simultaneously excluding other types of speech. No single language offers the possibility of saying anything that is to be said. By definition, language will fall short.[17] The language issue is the main theme of the third type of hermeneutics.

Hermeneutics of the Signifier

This type of hermeneutics deals with the issues presented by language, as elaborated by Lacan (1901-1981). The emphasis is on language and

[17] Grondin (2003, p. 14) stresses that the theme of faulty language – language as being faulty – is also very much alive in hermeneutics, as opposed to what Derrida maintains.

its formal and differential structure, which is determined by terms that are meaningless in themselves ('signifiers'), but produce meaning when combined with other terms (Lacan, 1966/2002, pp. 412-445). Each word is composed of units that have no meaning in themselves (phonemes), but whose combination (into a word) generates meaning next to other units (combined into another word). This will result in a difference of meaning among words: 'moot', 'boot', 'loot', etcetera, according to the principles of structural linguistics developed by Saussure (1916/1986). Meaning turns out not to be a predefined entity, but it emerges during articulation through language and has a derived status. So we are faced with a terminological problem. Hermeneutics found its point of departure in the sphere of content-defined signification, so the introduction of the 'signifier' as an empty and formal term would call the suitability of the term 'hermeneutics of the signifier' into question. Indeed, Lacan would have denied this affiliation most certainly. From a wider perspective, however, this mode of thought appears to be a fresh offshoot from the ancient tree of hermeneutics, even tracing back to its early Romantic roots (Frank, 1997, pp. 79-122). Even in the first type of hermeneutics language is relevant as experience needs to be expressed, and each experience will have pass through the language grid. Next, language manifest itself as a component of the situation into which the person has been thrown (e.g. his mother tongue). Here, with the hermeneutics of the signifier, the emphasis is on the formal structure of language, being a system of differences, with terms ('signifiers') differing among themselves, but also in what they express and define (Pluth, 2007).

Because of the emphasis on the autonomy of language, it goes beyond the interior revealing itself through expression, the view championed by Dilthey. Linguistic expression *shapes* the inner experiences of the mind itself. As we have seen, language constitutes the overall structural entity to which speaker and interpreter need to submit in order to be understood and to understand. To put it in Hegelian terms: the objective mind (of culture) shapes the subjective mind (of the individual). A subject-identity may emerge: That is the gain of the process. However, something is lost in the process as well, and this is where we distance ourselves from the Hegelian view.[18] By definition, language will fall short in expressing the truth: no adequate words exist, "*les mots y manquent*" (Lacan 1973, p.

[18] Lacan has been inspired by Hegel, see Lacan (1966/2002, pp 854-855: 'Hegelian categories'). Hegel has proved to be a source of inspiration for psychoanalysis. See Hyppolite (1957), Mills (2000; 2002), Ver Eecke (2006).

9). Any explanation will call for a new explanation, which calls for a new explanation, and so on. Thus, language brings into being a world that can be expressed through speech, while introducing separation from 'pre-lingual' reality. This results in a twofold lack: language is defined by an interior deficit, which constitutes the first lack. We recognise a deficit of means of expression – interpretation calls for further interpretation. Ultimately – and this describes the second lack – language will fall short in naming what is, in naming reality 'as such' (*an sich*), thus removing us from life in its immediacy, from the primordial unfragmented presence with oneself, the other, and brutal reality (See Chapter Six). This will create a gap between the brutal reality of being, the immediacy of life, the direct presence with the Other on the one hand *and* the language dependent world, with its structural differences and relationships on the other. These structural relationships differ among cultures, with each language and culture expressing these fundamental differences in their own individual way.

This is the type of hermeneutics embraced by structural diagnostics, following from its orientation towards the relationship between an individual human life and the lack: the relationship towards finiteness, insignificance, generational and sexual differences. Structural diagnostics will summarize the insights offered by the hermeneutics of the signification and of the situation, bringing these into context with their relationships towards lack and finiteness. While complementing earlier forms, it also leads to a radicalisation of the hermeneutics of the situation. As opposed to the hermeneutics of the signification, the hermeneutics of the situation emphasises the situational dependency of the interpretation and, consequently, its finiteness. The hermeneutics of the signifier focuses even more strongly on the finiteness of this process, in the sense that self-interpretation of human life is inextricably linked to a lack that can never be remedied.

POSTULATE OF MEANING

The field of hermeneutics, with its defining circular, dialogue- and finiteness-based structure, is underpinned by a fundamental premise: the postulate of meaning. This postulate, an analogue to the postulate of causality that is part of the empiricist approach, underlies the hermeneutical effort in its broadest sense. The postulate of meaning shapes the 'space of reasons', as being opposed to 'the realm of law' (Sellars, 1963). It is a condition of possibility for actual meaning to exist.

However, this postulate does not necessarily presuppose the functioning of a 'totality of meaning', that would enable unimpeded identification of actual meaning – which represents a more or less 'idealistic' view, expressed in Gadamer's suggesting, following a Hegelian line, the possibility of an interpretation without lacunae. The notion of an all-encompassing meaning, one may argue, cannot hold up, in view of the fragmented nature of human knowledge, and so only the notion of a hiatal sense is left as the best feasible option. Sense and meaning can be found or identified, but such an identification will always be faulty, incomplete. The meaning of the spoken and written word, as well as its analogues (actions) can be grasped, but only up to a point. Within this structural (or more sceptical) view, meaning is not a given, but is merely the result of a number of autonomous signifiers.

Viewed either idealistically or sceptically, both varieties presuppose the postulate of meaning that may be defined as the capacity to identify meaning, signs or signifiers. This capacity is, one may argue, dependent on language, whith language itself being a 'symbolic form', a form of symbolisation (Cassirer, 1923/1994a; 1929/1994b). Indeed, language – ordinary or common language – is offering a 'content-wise symbolisation' of the real, constituting the life world. This implies that anything that can be understood belongs to the order of language or is dependent on language (Gadamer, 1960/1975, p. 432). Yet, language is not the only symbolic form in existence. Indeed, it runs parallel with the symbolic form of science, which is precisely refraining from the content-wise linguistic symbolisation offered by common language, constituting the life world.[19] Science presents a formal symbolisation in which reality is analysed into purely formal elements, expressing a particular conception of nature as being predictable and defined by laws: the postulate of causality (see Chapter Four). Thus, the symbolic form of natural science (with its postulate of causality) and the symbolic form of language (with its postulate of meaning) offer two complementary ways of symbolisation.

In a general sense, both are derivatives of the fundamental symbolic function of man, i.e., the ability to produce symbols and interpret them, allowing for both theoretical (natural-scientific) and practical

[19] Cassirer's (1929/1994b, pp. 329-560) concept of science includes natural as well as formal sciences (mathematics). Indeed, one may argue that both the humanities and the formal humanities (linguistics) are dependent on the life world and on the postulate of meaning (Cassirer 1944/1966, pp. 109-136).

(hermeneutical) knowledge to exist, while constituting a scientific reality and the life world, respectively (Cassirer, 1946/1953 and 1929/1994b; Krois, 1987, pp. 33-72; Schwemmer, 1997, pp. 46-61; Orth, 2004, pp. 100-129. Therefore, language and the postulate of meaning associated with, constitutes one of two basic forms of symbolisation (see also Chapter Six).[20]

Historically, the postulate of meaning has been described in various ways. We may think of what Pascal referred to as the '*esprit de finesse*', which differs fundamentally from the '*esprit de géométrie*' (Pascal, 1667/1964, no 1). The '*esprit de finesse*' may even be quite close to Aristotle's *phronèsis* (*prudentia*): practical, individual knowledge as opposed to theoretical knowledge (Gadamer, 1960/1985, pp. 278-279). Although he relates *prudentia* to the ethical and legal domains, where practical decisions should be made in individual cases, this view might be extended to the whole hermeneutical field. Indeed, it is essential that *prudentia* does not imply the application of predefined insights that can simply be put into practice but that these insights emerge from the practical situation in the life world and can be traced back to the life world.

A Case History Taken from Psychopathology

By necessity, the hermeneutical brand of psychiatry bases itself on the postulate of meaning as well as on the capacity of prudence, following all three paths of interpretation mentioned above: the path of empathy and reconstruction, the path of contextual expansion, and the path of structural approach.

Empathy may expose itself to rightful criticism when aspiring to be the one and only form of interpretation, but empathy *is* indispensable. An attempt to relate to the other's position, an identification – faulty or limited though it may be – is required in order to reach optimum understanding of this other. However, because identifying with the other will not result in a shared identity with the other, further testing is needed

[20] With Cassirer, the symbolic function actually manifests itself as a *three-layered* one: *Ausdruck* (in physiognomical perception, in image and myth), *Darstellung* (objectifying intuition, in word and language), and *reine Bedeutung* (the pure meaning and formalism of science). A similar tripartite distinction has been made by Sellars (1963): original image of man (physiognomic perception), manifest image of man (objectifying conceptualization) and the scientific image of man. In Chapter Six the symbolic form related to '*Ausdruck*' will be taken into account.

and is in fact possible through rational reconstruction. Rational reconstruction enables us to reconstruct what a person might reasonably have done – using the broadest possible interpretation of 'reasonably', also including unconscious objectives. As a next step, from the viewpoint of relational diagnostics, its context can be broadened by putting actions and experience into a larger, historical context, to serve as the background or 'prejudice' driving and inspiring a person. The idea would be to put a meaningful connection in a larger, life-historical context, in order to determine whether a minor connection can fit in naturally within a larger entity. Finally, the issue of structural relationships – the relationship towards the lack, finiteness, the difference as such – needs to be addressed.

For example, we were intrigued by a strange development in a person's behaviour (Freud, 1916/1957). He finds himself at a high point in his life, one that he has always pursued. However, rather than enjoy it, he develops a depression, starts making errors and becomes unreliable. Developing an illness, he is no longer able to return to his work and remains a cripple throughout life, both mentally and socially. In order to understand this strange behaviour, we first need to identify with this man as a highly successful person facing a new and daunting challenge. We can imagine feelings of triumph that come with reaching this station in life, as well as the anxiety that may be associated with it: "If only I can keep this up". This allows us to reconstruct the rational of his behaviour, which involves reaching a goal – the coveted position – that brings feelings of both triumph and anxiety. However, the intensity of this person's anxiety cannot be understood, puzzling and perhaps even perplexing the investigator. This feeling of puzzlement – on the side of the investigator – would be enough reason to introduce a new premise in order to close the gap within this process of understanding. The feelings of anxiety may well point to the presence of a deeper emotion: more than just represent an actual competitor, the vanquished opponent might embody an imagined yet threatening opponent. This makes the victory over this person an ambivalent one – it is not only frightening, it is guilt-ridden and perhaps even 'forbidden'. This premise may be tested by including the life history in the analysis in order to widen the context. It turns out the man has a history of avoiding any rivalry with his father, wanting to defeat him but never daring to, choosing the path of passive submission while harbouring feelings of hostility. Thirdly, we might try to identify the nature of the relationship between this man and basic structures – his own insignificance, or finiteness. In this case, any struggle would have the co-meaning of a struggle of life-or-death, which makes each struggle frightening, something to be avoided. Connotations of death, of finiteness are the dominant structural theme here.

It results in the finding that the three types of interpretation are mutually complementary, with each type expressing its own unique brand of hermeneutics. Testing is possible, although methods will differ from empiricist testing methods. The relevant test criteria are twofold, as was shown previously. First and foremost, impressions should be tested against facts pertaining to both action and life history (thus satisfying the correspondence requirement). As a next step, the overall, structural view needs to be tested based on the details and refinement of the investigation as well on the integrative strength of the test design (in order to meet the coherence requirement).[21]

Standards

The possibility of intersubjective testing becomes evident from the key role played by rules in the process of conveying and determination of meaning. The meaning of a word is not defined by statistically identifiable relative frequencies of sounds, but by grammatical and semantic rules. A cultural anthropologist will correlate marriage customs to rules defining group exchange. The process of interpretation or understanding relates to observable actions that are objectifiable and are subject to rules. The introduction of rules effectively introduces a normative entity. Behaviour is defined against a backdrop of rules and can therefore be described as strange, bizarre or inadequate. Indeed, this aspect of strangeness is essential – the interpretative process is driven by experiencing something as strange. This quality of strangeness creates the need for interpretation, while the absence of feelings of strangeness would eliminate the need for explanation. And yet this strangeness will only appear within a framework of familiarity (Gadamer, 1960/1985, p. 262). If we were not more or less familiar with this phenomenon, then interpretation would, in the final reckoning, be impossible. Consequently, standards and frameworks of familiarity will always come into play.

---

[21] This refers to the two current views on truth: the correspondence concept and the coherence concept. The former constitutes a proposition that is true if the content matches the status quo in reality. In the latter case it is true if it is in agreement or not at variance with the whole of propositions that were deemed to be true.

Because of the reference to rules rather than physiological parameters, the normativity involved is a deontological, not teleological in nature (see Chapters One and Two). Dependency on rules implies dependency on culture. Desirable social behaviour is not a natural given, and its interpretation varies widely, the desirability being dependent on culture. This applies also to mental illness, which is to some degree also value-based and culture-dependent (See Chapter Four).

However, psychiatry presents ultimately a different picture, to some extent. The standards we are dealing with have ultimately a different status. Much more than 'desirable social behaviour', the concept of mental disease is linked directly to boundaries within which human existence manifests itself or should manifest itself in order to be defined as human existence. The boundaries are predominantly anthropological in nature. It turns the person with a mental disorder into someone who fails to observe these boundaries, because of his inability to follow the 'fundamental rules of world-understanding' ('*Grundformen des Weltverständnisses*'), which implies a default of symbolisation (Cassirer 1924/1971, p. 70). Tension exists between the way a person behaves and perceives and the way he ought to behave or perceive, between 'actually being' and 'supposed to be'. In this case, normativity is deontological not only in the sense that it relates to cultural values rather than to natural physiological standards – it is deontological in a deeper sense, involving fundamental boundaries, the structural frameworks of human apperception, of world-understanding as such.

This does not necessarily mean that the anthropological standard is fixed or unequivocal – its hermeneutical context will preclude this. The standard that a hermeneutical-anthropological psychiatry focuses on is not a fixed universal standard existing at the level of nature or of cultural values – in fact, it is found at an anthropological level. That is what makes hermeneutical psychiatry – insofar as it is normative – essentially anthropological. This anthropological orientation is not an added feature – it follows logically from its hermeneutical character.

THREE KINDS OF RESEARCH

Conversely, the hermeneutical orientation of psychiatry discussed here paves the way for a particular type of research to come into being: individualising, categorizing and theoretical research that, at a particular level, takes standards into account.

As was indicated above, this primarily concerns casuistic research. The hermeneutical approach in psychiatry brought about in its history a profound interest in casuistry – as was shown in Chapter Two. Within the hermeneutical approach, case studies are valued more highly than could ever be possible within an empiricist environment, where, at best, it could be part of a preliminary stage of 'true' research (Fédida and Villa, 1999). This framework does allow single, so-called N = 1 studies, but even then these studies have a subordinate status. There is a fundamental difference between depicting a patient as a case of some general disorder (a case-record) or describing him as his unique self (a biographical study). From a hermeneutical perspective a mental disorder is rooted in the person's life as a whole and it cannot be isolated from it, because of which a case history grows into a biography (Jaspers, 1959/1997, pp. 671-681). Within the hermeneutical approach, casuistry, while including the patient's life history, represents a fully acknowledged method (see Chapter Eight).

Next to the casuistic type of research, there is yet another type: that of categorising research. It considers a number of cases, focusing on identifying the generic nature or common structure of a type or genre. Essentially, this refers to ideal-typical connections that no single individual case needs to conform to. Such connections should therefore be distinguished from the 'disorders' defined in classifying systems. A categorising approach does not deal with classification, but with the identification of features shared by a variety of cases belonging to one structural category, with the notion of structure referring to a complex system of internal relationships (see Chapter Seven).

A third and final of type of research, theoretical research, deserves mention as an autonomous discipline. The construction of generic structures or types endows categorising research with strong theoretical connotations, but casuistic research too proceeds from fundamental theoretical premises. It is this very orientation of casuistic interpretation and structural construction on a theoretical 'prejudice' that brings the need for an analysis of this 'prejudice', not just as part of the actual interpretative and constructive research, but as a general effort. The major significance of the theoretical aspect qualifies autonomous theoretical research as the third legitimate main type of research within the hermeneutical tradition (see Chapter Six).

In a way, these three types of research, which of course may be extended or refined, together constitute a 'research canon'. Honouring the hermeneutical psychiatric tradition, a connection might also be established with the history of psychiatry, from which this threefold division becomes quite evident. Historically, it was particularly casuistry that reached a high degree of sophistication within psychoanalysis. The psychiatric clinical setting produced numerous categorising studies, e.g., on jealousy, melancoly, delusion, early-stage schizophrenia and symptomless schizophrenia. Moreover, psychiatric theory supplied theoretical studies on, e.g., the psychogenesis and endogenesis of psychoses.[22]

In many ways, the hermeneutical approach is rooted in the psychiatric tradition, but it does raise its own unique and unequivocal issue: the importance and the right of psychic reality. The next chapter will provide an in-depth discussion of its various manifestations.

---

[22] Lacan (1932); Binswanger (1957); Conrad (1958/1987); Tellenbach (1961/1983); Häfner (1961); Blankenburg (1971); Lefort and Lefort (1988); Lambotte (1993/1999).

Six

Psychic Reality and the Symbolic Function in Triplicate

Psychic reality being the central theme of this work, a detailed description of the concept itself cannot be left out. What may be referred to as 'psychic reality' is a cultural asset rather than a naturally given entity. When speaking of psychic reality we distinguish it – implicitly or not – from physical reality. Apparently, we regard the psychic element as an autonomous entity, acknowledging it as a reality. Three levels of psychic reality may be distinguished: intentionality, being in the world, and the language dependent mode of human existence. Mentioned before, in Chapter Three, they will now be discussed in some depth. In addition, we shall devote attention to the issue of what might be presupposed in any of the three levels of psychic reality. In doing so we are considering an agency or a function that enables and supports psychic reality itself. We propose the thesis that psychic reality is ultimately supported by what might be called, following Lacan and the Neo-Kantian philosopher Cassirer, 'the symbolic function of human mind'. By way of introduction, a brief history of the concept of the psyche will be offered first.

A Concise Historical Outline

We might argue that, at the dawn of Western philosophy, it was Plato and Aristotle who first elaborated on the distinction between body and soul – distinctions that to some extent mapped the path philosophy was going to take. Although the former put particular emphasis on an assumed state of separation between body and soul, whereas the latter saw them in their unified aspect, they both left room for the existence of an entity that might be referred to as the 'psyche'.

A Basic Dichotomy: Passion and Reason

Plato defines the psyche as a hierarchical structure, distinguishing three powers conceived as the constituent parts of the soul, which exist at three levels: the principle of reason, below it the power of defence or resistance, and finally, at the lowest level, the power of desire, while both the power of defence and of desire include passions or emotions in their domain (Plato, 2004, *Politeia*, 435 b-c). These passions may come into conflict with each other – ambition may clash with passively directed desires – but eventually the passions, unreasonable as such, can be made to bend to reason. This possibility of conflict may also be played out at a different, more general and ontological level, because Plato experienced overall reality as 'broken' to some degree. Reality does not reveal itself in its entirety, but the present-day world conceals a deeper layer or dimension of reality that holds its true nature and the true extent of life. Consequently, the contrast between reason and emotion lies basically in the fact that man can gain access to this essential dimension of reality by following the path of reason rather than that of emotion.

Essentially, Aristotle adopts a less dualistic view on man and, consequently, a less negative approach towards emotions and desire than does Plato. Like Plato, he distinguishes certain powers of the soul, yet he considers the soul to exist in an state of wholeness. One of these powers is that of *appetite*, or desire, which encompasses the whole of the psyche. More or less in line with Plato, he introduces a threefold subdivision of the power of desire (*orektikon*). First there is the reasonable desire or the reasonable will (*boulèsis*), below it the faculty of aggressive emotions such as resentment, fear, or pride, and lastly the capacity of lust and distress. These three modalities do not belong to the spiritual part of man – the active mind (*nous poiètikos*) as opposed to the soul (*psychè*) – but are more or less subservient to it (Aristotle, 1984, *De anima* , 429a10-11). Where Plato evokes the image of a charioteer reining in passions, emotions and desire, Aristotle stresses the importance of a well-balanced interplay between reason and passion. This harmonious view is in line with the intimate relationship that Aristotle proposes to exist between passions on the one hand and the human body on the other.[1] This harmony-centred view prompted Aristotle to adopt a more positive stance towards feelings and emotions than did Plato. Departing from the ethics of restriction championed by Plato, he advocates an ethics of the proper balance.[2]

---

[1] *De Anima* 403a16: "It seems that all the affections of the soul involve a body-passion, gentleness, fear, pity, courage, joy, loving and hating; in all these there is a concurrent affection of the body".

[2] An explanation of the doctrine of the proper centre can be found in *Ethica Nicomachea* 1105b25-30.

Despite differences in emphasis, the dichotomy between reason or ratio on the one hand, and passion (feelings and desires) on the other, has found currency ever since Plato's and Aristotle's conception of the psyche. Essentially, both Plato's dualism and Aristotle's dual perspective represent different manifestations of the same basic scheme, one that will continue to pervade Western philosophical psychology, despite the constant shifts in emphasis resulting from the advent of new schools of philosophy.

In this regard, the Stoic school of thought, hostile to emotions, was dominated by strong 'Platonic' overtones. In line with dominant Greek views, happiness was considered to be the result of a life of virtue, of perfecting one's personal qualities (prudence, courage, and such), thus relying on a society that nurtures this process of perfection. Yet, Stoicism brought a qualification of this ideal: happiness can and should be found in peace of mind achieved by distancing oneself from the ever emerging concerns brought on by society or fate. Man ought to be guided by reason, and identification of human nature with reason is taken to the extreme, regarding emotions and desires as a disease of the soul that is to be overcome. The reined-in state proposed by Plato or Aristotle's perfect balance is abandoned as an ideal, to be replaced by that of unfeelingness (*apathy*).

The line of philosophy proposed by Epicurus, which is based on the inevitability of pain and suffering, does leave more room for emotion, yet with the ultimate aim of dealing with it in such a way that some degree of peace of mind (*ataraxia*) can be achieved. Despite the essentially anti-Aristotelian nature of Stoicism and Epicureanism, the Aristotelian school of thought was still very much alive. It re-emerged in a most prominent and influential way in the Middle Ages, through Thomas Aquinas, who adopted a somewhat more dualistic view as compared to Aristotle.

These later developments bear testimony once again to the enduring establishment of a Platonic-Aristotelian distinction between a rational and an emotional part of the soul. The separation introduced between reason or understanding on the one hand, and feeling, emotion, passion or desire on the other, proved a lasting influence in the conceptualization of the psychic field within Western culture, which has also taken root in modern psychiatry.

Passions and Reason in Modern Time: Mentalism

The mechanisation of world picture – since Copernicus, Galilei, Descartes – causes the conception of an animated body or embodied soul to give way to the picture of the body as a single and closed mechanism, making the relative unity of body and soul problematic. This process of mechanisation even strengthens the autonomy of the psyche. This mutual autonomisation of the body and the psyche results in an uneasy relationship between the two entities, which is specifically played out in the field of emotions, because of the intimate connection existing between emotion and the body (blushing caused by embarrassment, trembling caused by fear, skin turning white caused by rage) – as was pointed out earlier by Aristotle.

Of course, Descartes did not initiate this movement, but he certainly proved its fervent champion. A part of his effort was devoted to investigating the supposed relationships between emotions (which belong to the domain of the mind) and the body. He considers the passions to be purely passive (Descartes, 1649/1988, art. 2). Emotions are supposed to be the product of events performed by body and perceived by the soul or the mind. Here as elsewhere, Descartes' central problem manifests itself: the inexplicable interaction between the two completely heterogeneous substances of mind and body.

The theme of emotions will find further elaboration with Hume who, however, avoids the inquiry into any possible interaction, limiting the scene to that of the inner, mental world of impressions and ideas. As such, we may speak of 'mentalism'. The basic component of the mind is made up of bodily sensations and sense-perceptions, 'impressions', from which do originate thoughts or 'ideas'. Passions or emotions are considered to be secondary impressions produced in part by the interposition of ideas. It is the thought, the idea of danger, which will produce the emotion of fear. This emotion can result in a new thought which in its turn may produce another emotion: an 'indirect passion' such as pride, vanity, pity, forming the complement to 'direct passions' such as aversion, fear, joy (Hume, 1739-1740/1966, pp. 3-165). This brings a 'soul factory' of associations into being, which might be seen as a duplicate of the external nature, conceived as a mechanism. The connections existing within this soul factory are merely established 'by coincidence' and might have taken other forms as well, which is why they are non-reasonable. Again, passion and reason are opposing forces: reason as the slave of passions.

The coincidental, haphazard character of the associations typifies Hume's basic viewpoint: a mentalistic conception of the psyche. The associations have to be established in a random fashion, because they are part of an inner fabric and are not essentially connected with or focused on the outside world. That is the basic point. Yet experience tells us that emotions and experiences, being part of the individual's interior world, are also essentially connected with the outside world: we are afraid *of* something, are sad *about* something: 'aboutness' being the central theme. Where mentalism fails to bridge – or perhaps even creates – the divide between the outside world and the interior world, the question poses itself whether this divide can be bridged at all. Later schools of thought would develop notions about bridging the divide between the inner and the external world. Following Hume, it was Kant who, in the context of an inquiry into the validity of knowledge, scrutinised the relationship between subjectivity on the one hand, and objectivity on the other. Hegel would carry on this line, putting the onus on the side of subjectivity of the mind, generating objectivity, constituting reality. The British empiricist school, however, continued to follow in Hume's footsteps, well into the 20th century. It was particularly phenomenology that turned this issue into a major field of investigation again, adopting a far more descriptive approach, as opposed to Kant's epistomological effort. Intentionality was to become its central theme.

PHENOMENOLOGY: INTENTIONALITY AND EXPLORATION OF ESSENCE

Phenomenology is a movement within modern 20th-century philosophy that was founded by Edmund Husserl (Zahavi, 2003). Early on, it chose as its motto '*Zurück zu den Sachen selbst*', 'back to things themselves', distancing itself from what we are told by theories, including philosophical theories, in a bid to return to an original experience. Phenomenology sets out to describe, in the most unbiased way possible, what appears to consciousness. This will open up the possibility of a tentative description of the mode of appearance of an object, of a thing. In doing so, we need to consider the fact that a thing can be given only from one side, never in its entirety, from all sides simultaneously: it can be known 'perspectivally' only. For the thing to be perceived in its entirety, we can – or indeed, must – move around it. Also, a thing will present itself within a causal relationship with its environment. Compared to the thing perceived, we identify a difference with the phenomenon of perceiving it, or of remembering or feeling it. We certainly cannot move around this phenomenon. For example, we will not be able to move around the memory of our first car, whereas we could actually walk around the car when we still owned it. In other words, a fundamental difference exists between a thing in its causal relationship to other things, and the psychic aspect as a phenomenon in its intentional involvement with objects (Mooij, 2010, pp. 93-125).

This is the first thesis of phenomenology: the thesis of the intentionality of the psychic. Psychic phenomena engage in an intentional relationship with their objects – they are focused on an object.[3] Herein lies an essential distinction between the physical and the psychic.[4] It also introduces another leading principle of phenomenology: the ambition to describe essential differences, 'essential definitions', much like the essential difference – at least from a phenomenological point of view – that exists between an intentional and a causal relationship.

In addition to an essential difference between causal and intentional relationships, we recognise a difference between external and internal perception. It turns out that external perception is defined by the condition that the object is given perspectivally, but not directly: we cannot see its front and its back simultaneously. What is given directly, turns out not to be the complete object, but a range of appearances outlining (adumbrating) the actual object (Husserl 1983, pp. 86-89, 94-98). By contrast, the inner perception lacks this perspectival attachment, Husserl (1983, pp. 78-81) would argue. The perception of an inner condition (of a feeling) has no front or back, is given immanently, with the feeling itself, and not as an outline. In a sense, we know it 'directly'.[5]

Phenomenological investigation is not concerned with the incidental experiences of an actual consciousness, but with possible modifications of consciousness (perception, memory, fantasy). It performs an eidetic analysis rather than provide an introspective psychology (Kockelmans, 1987). Nonetheless, it is relevant to psychology and psychopathology, in that it renders a contribution to the mapping of the contours of consciousness. It offers a 'regional ontology' (e.g., of the psychic). What

---

[3] The viewpoint of intentionality as a characteristic of the psychic was introduced by Brentano, and further developed by Husserl, yet without implying the 'directedness towards the object' which is in fact intended here (Brentano, 1874/1973, p. 88; Benoist, 2007, p. 87). See also Cassirer (1929/1994b, pp. 227-230).

[4] Conceived by Sellars (1956/1997, § 5) as 'natural' and 'epistemic' facts.

[5] Later Husserl may have become aware of the relativity of this opposition (Welton, 2000, p. 147).

exactly is 'perception', 'thinking', or 'hallucinating'? And what about the basic categories, such as intentionality, intentional involvement? On the foundation created by this regional ontology, this eidetic phenomenology of the psychic, an (empirical) phenomenological psychology, including a phenomenological psychopathology, could be built. It would be 'empirical' in a phenomenological, hermeneutical sense – not in the sense of empiricism. It is an intentional psychology using the instrument of intentional analysis (Owen, 2006, pp. 282-325).

The regional ontology itself, in search of essence, of essential definition, is rooted in experience as well. In that sense, we are not dealing with a reconstruction of the way a phenomenon might come into being (as defined by Kant) or with a justification of the particular use of a term (as defined by Popper). Rather, it is experience itself that, through the exploration of boundaries, will bring out the essential characteristics of a phenomenon (such as perception, memory). Husserl considers this 'intuitive' moment to be defining. In the process, something can be acknowledged as being a definition of essence, without subscribing to Husserl's elaboration – for example, by emphasising its interpretative and provisional character of any eidetic analysis, far more so than Husserl was inclined to do (Mooij, 2010, pp. 129-165).

To illustrate this, Husserl overreached himself when drawing conclusion from the perspectival state of being given to the outside world, based on which an object is nothing more than the correlate of (potentially) mutually complementary perceptions. Based on this finding, in later life he rejected the notion of a '*Ding an sich*', of a reality per se, viewing the world as well as nature as constituted ultimately by (transcendental) consciousness (De Boer, 1978). He developed a kind of philosophical idealism that eventually found only a handful of followers. Yet, the specific nature of this transcendental idealism is still a matter of dispute (Bernet, 2004). Nevertheless, we owe it to phenomenology that some kind of 'exploration of essence' has found support and that the theme of intentionality of the psychic has been acknowledged broadly at last.

Three Levels of Psychic Reality: Intentionality, World, Language and the Lack

Phenomenology allows us to conceptualise intentionality as a first level or layer within psychic reality. 'Intentionality' means that the subject is intentionally involved with its objects and the world, rather than being causally determined by them. This describes the first level. Finding oneself in an world, as well as the world itself, represent the second level of psychic reality. Next, this world is not closed, but has 'gaps' in it – it can assume a state different from its current state. It thus offers a platform for desire and reflection to unfold. The significance of language comes into play here, because language enables a person to distance himself from what is, from that which presents itself. This defines the third level, that of language and of dependence on language of human existence. The three levels are engaged in a 'dialectical' relationship with each other. 'Intentionality' centres on the intentional involvement and thus on the subject-pool, where 'world' is related to the object-pool. Finally, 'language' is the mediator between the subject-pool and the object-pool. Indeed, language – through conceptualisation – adds identity and consistency to the inner experience as well as to the objects of the outside world, because of which they acquire real existence. In the following section, these three levels will be discussed. Chapter Seven makes it more concrete, while adding the description of psychopathological structures.

Intentionality: Two Modalities, Two Domains, Interpretative Nature, Social Embedding

Not every single psychic phenomenon is stamped by intentionality. Experiences of the body proper – proprioception in its true meaning – as well as nociceptive (pain) experiences lack this characteristic. They may be subjectively charged (by the intensity of the pain), but as such they do not refer to anything existing in the world. And yet, they represent merely a small grey area – most of the psychic phenomena are supposed to be both qualitative and intentional (see Chapter Three). Essentially, it is intentionality that defines psychic phenomena, as was discussed before in the discussion of phenomenology: it is its distinguishing mark. This notion was first introduced in respect of the sphere of understanding or, more specifically, of cognition. He who thinks, is thinking of something; he who perceives, perceives something. Yet, intentionality can also be attributed to the affective sphere, with the phenomena of volition being least problematical: a person who wants or pursues, wants or pursues something.[6] We may also speak of an object of desire and of an emotion:

---

[6] In mediaeval scholastics, the object focus was particularly associated with phenomena of volition.

a person who is sad, is sad about something. Even in respect of moods it is quite defendable that a particular mood is intentional, revealing the world from a particular, subjectively biased perspective (as boring, exciting).[7]

It demonstrates that at the level of intentionality – despite its object-relatedness – the emphasis is on the subject-pool. The objects in this case can take a variety of forms: they may be present (in the case of perception), they may be absent or exist no longer (in the case of a fantasy or memory). In each single case the emphasis is on intentional involvement, while its specific nature may vary. An intentional analysis can bring out this difference, and may also show that intentionality is not limited to what is seen actively or is thought consciously. This brings us to the next point, the two modalities of the intentionality.

Two modalities. It turns out that the scope of intentionality is not limited to the sphere of explicit judgment or predication: 'I see a house', 'I feel outrage about this'. A judgment may be preceded by pre-predicative stage – one that affects a person before he actually realises it, causing him to act without actually knowing it. We recognise the distinction between two stages or types of intentionality: a *thematic* and a *non-thematic* stage. This distinction has been phrased differently by various philosophers, but essentially they all refer to the same distinction: predicative *vs* pre-predicative understanding (Heidegger); active intentionality with I-involvement *vs* passive or operative intentionality without I-involvement (Husserl); propositional *vs* expressive representation, viz. (*Darstelllung*) *vs* (*Ausdruck*) (Cassirer).

Like the propositional, thematic type, the non-propositional type of intentionality can be cognitively or affectively oriented. It can be cognitive in the form of 'knowing how' or 'tacit knowledge' without an actual explicit 'knowing that' being involved (Heidegger, 1962, pp. 188-189). Alternatively, it can be affectively oriented, with a perceived object expressing an internal state (Heidegger, 1962, 179-182; Cassirer, 1929/1994b, pp. 68-108). We might speak, with Cassirer, of the 'physiognomy of things': leaves 'dancing', an 'aggressive' car grille, a desolate landscape. Without any active involvement by a reflective and judging 'I', an object is perceived immediately as a totality. It should be noted that also Lacan's concept of 'the imaginary' may be considered to be an

[7] However, see Strasser (1956, p. 110): "Die Stimmung dagegen verweist auf keinen intentionalen Pol". Likewise: Bollnow (1943, p. 20): "Die Stimmungen dagegen haben keinen bestimmten Gegenstand".

equivalent of this (pre-predicative, expressive) domain – while 'the symbolic' leads to reflection and predication (Mooij, 2010, pp. 210-211).

Two domains. Likewise two domains of intentionality can be distinguished: the cognitive and the affective. This distinction derives from a long-standing tradition, unlike the first distinction between the 'two modalities', which is in fact a more recently made one. Indeed, its tradition became evident from the historical review. The distinction may be taken to the extreme, but we can also choose to highlight its inter-relationships: Based on the notion of intentionality, the differences between the two branches will be qualified. From this perspective, there are neither 'thingless emotions' that would originate from an inner experience, nor 'emotionless perceived things' existing in the outside world that might be known entirely objectively. In fact, the notion of intentionality effectively eliminates such a dichotomy. An emotion is always connected with an insight – a person will be sad *about* something. An emotion therefore implies some kind of cognition and the attribution of a value to a situation (Arnold, 1960; Frijda, 1986; Nussbaum, 1986). Then again, the affect is not merely an afterthought of a cognition that is initially presented in a pure form. It is not like a person who first sees an apple and then decides it looks tasty – the apple simply looks tasty or not. An emotion may have a cognitive value. Fear means: 'this is a dangerous situation'. This represents the thesis of the cognitive theory of emotions, even leading to the notion of the 'rationality of emotions' (De Sousa, 1980).

This does not imply that the cognition would be a true one, certainly not. An emotion can delude us – the situation may turn out not to be dangerous at all. Thus, the emotion can be a source of knowledge but at the same time a source of misguidance or self-deceit. Lacan (1966/2002, pp. 140-141) strongly emphasised the deceitful power of emotions (Soler, 2011, pp. 3-11). This does not mean that feelings are always deceitful, but mistrust is justified.[8] Hegel (1807/1979, pp. 221-228) was also aware of this possibility of deceit and self-deceit, which prompted him to introduce the concept of 'the law of the heart and the frenzy of self-conceit' ('*Gesetz des Herzen*'), in which he criticises a 'culture of emotion' that would define emotion as a source of truth and authenticity. And yet this qualification – the possibility of deceit – does not essentially detract from the formal connection between emotion and cognition. We

---

[8] Contrary to what is commonly thought of (Green, 1973), Lacan provides a very rich theory of affects (Soler, 2011).

should accept as a fact that emotions carry insights with them, acknowledging that these insights may be true or not true and even misguiding.

In addition to being closely related, feelings and knowledge have one more element in common. Both are internally related to action, being also a type of intentional relationship. There is a subject with an intentional involvement, while doing something (eating, running). This 'something' (eating, running) is the intentional object that matches an intentional description: I am throwing a ball, I am having a meal, etcetera. When throwing a ball, I am aware of this and I want to throw it (it does not happen by accident). Thus, having a belief and intentions (volition) is essential to any type of intentional action. It is supported by a knowing and a wanting, with a belief and a volition prompting the action, while, conversely, the action performed retrospectively defines the belief and the volition. This point was discussed in Chapter Five and was elaborated in the discussion of the hermeneutical and Anglo-Saxon philosophy of action.

Perception is interpretative. The definition of human intentionality can take on yet another level of meaning. The thesis of intentionality is that 'to see' means 'to see something'. We can actually take this a step further: 'to see something' means 'to see something as something'. Unlike having a *sense datum*-experience – 'here now red' – seeing holds an element of interpretation, a notion that finds general support within phenomenology (Maldiney, 1961, p. 50). From the perspective of classical analytical philosophy Sellars (1956/1997) countered the 'Myth of the Given'. The same point was raised by Wittgenstein as well: When we see a cube-like image in a textbook, with the accompanying legend describing it as a cube, a die or a wire-frame, we will actually see the object matching the interpretation before us (Wittgenstein, 1958/63, II, section XI). Perception thus become dependent on our interpretation and, consequently, on the language in which we interpret. Obviously this does not apply to perception and cognition only, but also to emotions and action. An insight, an emotion or action can be put into words – they pass through the language grid.

Social embedding. This state of dependence on language has yet another consequence, namely that intentional phenomena essentially are not private events to which the subject would have exclusive access, contrary to what Hume proposed in his theory of mentalism. Being part of a social practice, intentional phenomena obey intersubjective rules of validity. Perception is about a publicly accessible entity within the public domain of language, where normative criteria apply and discussion is possible: "You're right about this, you're wrong about that". This also applies to psychic phenomena that seem to unfold inside a closed inner world, e.g., fantasies or fears that no-one else will actually notice, or pain that is kept hidden. Yet if they can be known in principle only by me, then even I cannot know them. Indeed, knowledge presupposes articulation and third-party testing, and it is impossible for such procedures to take place with regard to private events that can only be discussed within a private language (Wittgenstein, 1958/1963, §§ 244-266). Thus, all psychic phenomena, including those belonging to the less manifest side of psychic reality, can be articulated or narrated. Unlike the mentalist view held by Hume, the psychic is not a self-absorbed interior world, but is in fact involved with the world, turning it into a commonly shared world as well. This leads us to the second level of psychic reality: the world.

World

The concept of 'world' may relate to objects in their broadest sense, and, consequently, to the 'sum of all objects' as well as to the 'horizon' within which a person perceives these objects or deals with them: the situation in which a person finds himself, his reference point or horizon of understanding. It causes man to live in a world, in a situation defined by himself, which he shapes from within his intentional relationships. In turn, he finds himself in a situation which he has not created but that will nonetheless determine him and his thoughts, feelings or actions: man shapes his world and is shaped by it as well. This point of view was put forward by hermeneutical phenomenology, and developed as a concept in Heidegger's early work (1927/1962).

Man designs his own world while also being 'thrown' into the world. This world holds 'objects', in the broadest sense of the word: objects of nature, plants and animals, as well as fellow-subjects or fellow human beings. All these objects are contained in the overall medium of space and time. Moreover, people engage in an intersubjective relationship with each other. Therefore, the fundamental structuring moments are shaped at least by the relationship with space and time that a person can enter into, and by the relationship established by associating with others as well as with oneself. This world is not just my world – insofar as it is my world, it belongs to others as well. This issue was raised before, within the context of intentionality, but is now presented with a slightly different emphasis, namely on the significance of the situative bias of each single intentional phenomenon.

Indeed, this bias can be taken a step further: intentional relationships (thinking, feeling, acting) are determined not only subjectively and situatively, but also by the external structure of a culture. This leads us the third level: anything that is described as an experience and is interpreted from within the situation, can be made to fit into a structure. An action will not qualify as an action until it has been deemed valid as such, based on specified terms. The degree of suitability for being included or being equipped with a structure concerns the third level within the range of intentional relationship, world, and structure. At a structural level, we may assume that language occupies a position of privilege, as it constitutes its actual core. In Hegelian terms, it is the domain of the 'objective mind' – marked by language – that shapes and adds structure to the 'subjective mind'.

Language and the Lack: Dividedness, Desire and Reflection

Certainly, this significance of the 'objective mind', of language and culture, is not a new finding. We already found that perception and emotion, as well as action, first need to pass through the language grid to be known or identified. However, the emphasis will now be put on its *consequences* at the level of the subject, the subjective mind as such. This point will be elaborated within the framework of structural analysis, particularly that of the structural psychoanalysis developed by Lacan.

Subjective dividedness was to be its first consequence. Language bestows identity upon the subject: I am John, I am a teacher, an uncle, etcetera. According to this line of thought, language provides the qualifications for a subject without the individual subject becoming completely identified by it. It is the generic nature of terms that precludes the individuality, the particularity, of the subject from being phrased. The introduction of language causes the subject to be split into a subject that is what it claims to be and a subject that fails to become part of it: a subject of the statement and a subject of the enunciation (Lacan 1966/2002, p. 581, 676). The result is subjective dividedness: it is this subjective dividedness that can be equalized with the distinction between the conscious and the unconsciousness as formulated by Lacan (*vide infra*).

Desire is the second consequence. Indeed, a loss will also result – any experience passes through the language grid and will therefore be marked by it: A linguistic symbol will present something that is actually absent. Reality is put 'at a distance' and its immediate experience becomes lost. The resulting void allows meaningful intentional relationships, including those of desire, to take root, allowing a world to be formed. Indeed, something is lost in the process: the immediate reality and the enjoyment associated with it – *la Chose, das Ding* (Lacan, 1986/1992, p. 102-103, 117). Thus, the medium of language leads to the institution of a dimension of absence, of loss and lack, allowing meaning to be established. Therefore Žižek could write (1992/2008, p. 154): "You cannot have both meaning and enjoyment." This loss will invite the subject to redirect its quest to the lost object, which will, however, never be found because it was lost at the actual moment of symbolisation. The experience of a lack as a lack will result in a desire to remedy it, which demonstrates the intimate relationship between 'language' and 'desire'. This desire manifests itself in the form of a demand, with a specific demand ("I want chocolate") expressing the desire ("I want attention"), while also leaving a remainder, which will prompt the next demand ("I want white chocolate"). Any answer to the demand will fall short in respect of satisfying the desire (Chiesa, 2007, pp. 151-156). This dialectics of a (conscious) demand and an (unconscious) desire constitutes a rewriting of the dividedness, described before as the distinction between the conscious and the unconscious.

The origin of the desire will preclude the desire itself from being satisfied fully. This desire is nothing more than a generic term used to indicate this relationship. Indeed, the desire is the product of a lack, a hole in one's existence, centred on a lost 'object'. This process of symbolisation and separation – according to Lacan – will cause the subject to loose that particular part of itself that, if reclaimed, would return it to the fullness of life – like the loss of a mother's breast which would initially belong to its suckling child rather than to the mother itself. It is lost in the process of separation, leaving a gap ('*objet-trou*') that defines the outlines of what give partial pleasure, to be exemplified by the partial objects: the breast and scybala, the gaze and the voice (Lacan, 1973/1986, pp. 187-200). This 'object' – the object *a* – might be described as the 'cause' of the desire, being its anchor point. It cannot be perceived empirically and actually eludes perception – it cannot even be imagined – but it does add colour and desirability to what is perceived.[9]

[9] The object has ceased to exist, taking on a 'transcendental function' instead. Lacan emphasised this transcendental function when making reference to Kant. He speaks of an '*objectalité*' in order to delineate this 'object' from actual objects. Lacan (2004), pp.

Basically, this 'object' is part of a construct that establishes a relationship between the subject and the objects of desire. This construct may be called a *phantasm* – a product of imagination. This phantasm represents a window on the world, rather than an escape from it. This phantasm structures both the affective world of perception and the relational world, because the framework of the phantasm will define what is meaningful within this world, and which particular ties with the relational world are considered valid. It adds a unique shape to the desire of any individual man or woman, making it consistent as well as recognisable: this is his or her desire. The phantasm supports desire. In return, the phantasm and phantasmatic imagination are nourished by desire. Thus, the phantasm and the phantasmatic imagination represent the deepest, most meaningful essence of a subject's psychic reality, 'the kernel of the subject's being' (Žižek, 1992/2008, p, 162). The desire, with phantasmatic imagination as its anchor point, is the outcome of the introduction of language as a 'fracturing' medium. In addition to adding dividedness and the dimension of the lack and desire, the language dependent and 'broken' nature of human existence has yet another consequence: the possibility of reflection.

Reflection, made possible by language, is the final, (although not the most basic) component of psychic reality. "Is what I desire a true desire, or am I only fooling myself?" "Is what I see really what I think I see, or am I just imagining it?" The reason is that language not only refers to the world, shaping it, but also presupposes the presence of other language users. If a language were to apply to me only, it cannot apply to me either; if a world were to exist unto me only, it could not exist. This point – the impossibility of a private language – was discussed before, within the context of intentionality, but is now approached from a slightly different angle. The emphasis now is on the difference of perspective rather than the sharing of a perspective with others. Identifying with another person's viewpoints, with a different perspective, offers the possibility of developing a new take on the matter. Another person's subjective perspective – reflecting this person's unique frame of mind, views and desires – will thus become manifest. In fact, it will result in a whole new insight.

248-249: "Pour vous en donner le relief dans son point vif, je dirai que l'objectalité est le correlat d'une coupure. Mais, paradoxalement, c'est là que ce même formalisme, au sens ancien du terme, rejoint son effet. Cet effet, méconnu dans la Critique de la raison pure, rend compte pourtant de ce formalisme". See also Baas (1992, pp. 22-82).

It produces something else as well – next to offering categories that allow the world to be structured into, e.g., houses, people or animals – language supplies its formal modalities: it is possible, it is certain, necessary, it is not so. The modalities of possibility, certainty, denial, etcetera are introduced (Sellars, 1956/1997, §29, §31). Thanks to the modalities offered by language, what is presented by experience can be 'thought away', 'crossed out': what is, 'may' exist, but then again it 'may' *not* exist. We see a given, factual world give way to a possible, virtual world. Therefore, thanks to language (1) we can adopt the other's perspective, and (2) we can vary and modalise the very thing that experience presents us with. Combined, these two aspects of language would make reflection possible, in a sense: varying, qualifying experience – what can exist, may as well not exist, what exists can be thought away, 'crossed out' – *and* by choosing to adopt the other's perspective.

Two tours. In other words: firstly, through the symbolic function, language allows us to enter the world of intentional relationships, while secondly the subsequent process of reflection provides us with the option to distance ourselves, to free ourselves from the confines of this world. Lacan (1966/2002, pp. 712-717) will speak of a dialectics of alienation and separation, of an introduction into language (alienation) and of being able to relate to language (separation). This theme of the 'two tours', the 'two moments of the process of symbolisation' will be elaborated more extensively later on, in Chapter Seven.

It is precisely this inner distance, this possibility of reflection, which allows us to engage in a relationship with ourselves, to observe both ourselves and the world from an external vantage point: Our position in the world is both 'ego-centric' and 'ec-centric'. We may argue that this inner distance is comparable to what has traditionally been referred to as 'freedom of will', in its broadest sense: the capacity to reflect, to deliberate.

Psychic Reality and the Symbolic Function: Cassirer and Lacan

Until yet the investigation was about a subject position characterised subjective dividedness, by desire and object loss, and by the possibility of reflection, all of these representing consequences of the language-dependent mode of human existence. Summing up, the 'exteriority' of the 'objective mind' involves the 'broken' aspect of the 'subjective mind'. There remains yet another issue, which concerns the *origin* rather than the 'consequences' of language. As a matter of fact, three questions may arise. What is presupposed in language, making language actually possible? Next to it, what is presupposed in intentionality, and finally what may be presupposed in the world constitution? It will turn out what is presupposed relates to the symbolic function of man, manifesting itself on these three levels of psychic reality.

At the level of *language* one may presuppose a subject being able to speak, or at least being able to use linguistic signs and signifiers, and to recognise the representative function of linguistic signs and signifiers. Essentially, a linguistic sign represents something that is absent in itself. We can use the word or signifier 'cow' to refer to a real cow, an entity which differs from the word 'cow', the word 'cow' not being the cow itself. As opposed to the mentalism according to Hume or to representationalism (the Augustian picture of language), however, this is not done directly: here we have the word 'cow', and there we have the object of cow, 'here the word, there the meaning, the money and the cow you can buy with it' (Wittgenstein 1958/1963, §120). This takes place in an indirect rather than a direct manner. Initially, the terms or linguistic signs do not refer to an object, but to each other. Indeed, language is a structure that defines its elements through their difference with other elements from the linguistic system, which besides receive their actual meaning from within the social context in which they are used (Saussure, 1916/1986). Meanings are not given beforehand, but are established through differential inference and contextual relationships. Terms – signifiers – generate meaning *within a linguistic system* in relationship to other terms, as well as *within a social infrastructure*: this *we* call a cow, a calf, a bull, a heifer, etcetera.

This process does not apply to perception and cognition alone, but also to emotions and action. Even physical arousals, excitements are determined through the connection established with the objective form of language. Cassirer (1946/1953) writes p. 88: "they (viz. myth and language) are both resolutions of an inner tension, the representation of subjective impulses and excitations in definite objective forms and figures".[10] The connection with the organism is also crucial to Lacan: The signifier transforms the immediacy of life, '*immanence vitale*',

[10] Cassirer (1946/1953) writes p. 36: "the inner excitement which was a mere subjective state has vanished, and has been resolved into the objective form of myth or of speech." See also Cassirer (1956/1969, pp. 87, 105, 107, 123, 148, 149).

'*tension vitale*' into articulated demands (Lacan, 1960-1961).[11] The cry of the baby expressing his vital tension, will be answered by a response of the (m)Other 'let me feed you' ('*laisse-toi nourir*'). The mother will interpret and symbolize the child's vital tension, while putting it into words and stamping by that his inner experience ('Oh yes, I am hungry, that must be true'), yet leaving a remainder of another aspect of the experience not being phrased.[12]

Taking the detour of a language system – supported by the social infrastructure of a language community – allows an external object or an inner experience to be referenced: thirst, hunger, cow, bull, heifer, etcetera. Crucial is the 'inferential structure' of language (Cassirer, 1923/1994a) or its differential structure (Lacan, 1966/2002, pp. 412-441) enabling reference to be made. Therefore, this reference is not a direct but an indirect one, being established inferentially and differentially within the frame of language. In language, a function thus becomes manifest that transcends the frontiers of language itself: an external event or an internal experience will be put into words, will be symbolized. We may speak of a symbolic function, one that is expressed at the level of language – i.e., the third level. Yet, the symbolic function will also manifest itself at both other levels: that of intentionality and the world.[13]

At the level of *intentionality,* once again we recognise an indirect, mediated course which, however, now follows the path of the signification rather than of the signifier. It turned out that while seeing something, we also see 'something' 'as something'. Perception is interpretative. To put it differently: before receiving linguistic underpinning, perception or consciousness is already symbolic in nature (Cassirer, 1929/1994b, pp. 371, 377). Cassirer (1923/1994a, p. 42) refers to the 'natural symbolic of consciousness' ("natürliche" Symbolik des

---

[11] The primal repressed ('*l'urverdrängt* ') relates to '*ce qui est vivant de cet être*' (sc. *du sujet*) – 'being that is alive' (Lacan 1966/2002, p. 581), 'the living part of that being' (Lacan, 1966/1977, p. 288). Lacan declared in 1972: "Ce qui est refoulé, c'est la vie". See Mooij (2008, 201).

[12] Lacan (1966/2002, p. 549): "In my view, the subject has to arise from the given state of the signifiers that cover him [*le recouvrent*] in an Other which is their transcendental locus".

[13] The term 'symbolic function' was derived from the 'philosophy of symbolic forms' developed by the Neo-Kantian philosopher Ernst Cassirer. Its elaboration here, distinguishing sharply between world and the real, owes a great deal to Lacan's theory of the symbolic order. See for Cassirer: Krois (1987), Lofts (1997), Schwemmer (1997), Kreis (2010). See for a comparison between Cassirer and Lacan: Lofts (1994) and Mooij (2010, pp. 7-10, 147-156, 206-213).

Bewusstseins'). A content of consciousness will receive identity only in relationship to other contents of consciousness, while also including the whole formal frame of consciousness. A thing can be given or be present only through referring to other things, and by representing a concept which refers to other concepts. The phenomenon of day, while referring to the phenomenon of night, represents the concept of 'day' which is referring to the concept of 'night'.[14] A thing is actually present or given and can be present only through representing something else (viz., a concept, a meaning) in a mediated way. Not only language, intentionality also is made possible by the symbolic function: the function of representation (representation token in a broad sense). Or, to put it differently: Apperception informs perception. Thus, perception takes on an objective form, it is stamped by objectivity. We may refer to this as a semantic theory of objectivity: semantic, because – at the level of consciousness, where language (ideal-typically) is not yet involved – we should speak of 'meanings' rather than of 'signifiers'.

Following Lacan, however, we might add that even these phenomena and meanings associated with, are already 'differential' in nature, effectively functioning as signifiers. For example: within the natural continuum of light intensity, with all its gradations, the term 'day' does *posit* the phenomenon of day, and consequently the difference between day and non-day, thus allowing the phenomenon of night to present itself (Lacan, 1981/1993). The phenomenon of the day refers to the concept of 'day', as well as to the differential pair of day (+) and *non*-day (-), while being transformed into a signifier itself. The phenomena of experience and external objects are not only conceptually charged, but are already and more fundamentally differential in nature. They are both inferentially organised, with perceptions derived from concepts (according to Cassirer), and differentially structured (+/-) (according to Lacan). For instance, man and woman are not so much conceptual or content-wise opposed, but are primarily differentially opposed (+/-), with men having a phallus (+) and women not having one (-). Next to that, the conceptual content of 'being an man' or 'being a woman', may vary with time and culture. The 'empty' formal difference provides the foundation, based on

---

[14] Here lies another difference between Lacan en Cassirer. Cassirer (1929/1994b, pp. 222-238) emphasises the equiprimordiality of 'form' and 'content' via the concept of 'symbolic pregnance'. See Krois (1987, pp. 52-56). Lacan (1966/2002, pp. 20-21, 228-229), however, is according priority or supremacy to the form ('the signifier') over the content ('the signified'). That constitutes, *in nuce,* the basic difference between the two.

which conceptual 'fulfilment' may be played out later on (phrased in Husserlian terminology).

Thirdly, at the level of the *world including intersubjectivity*, the symbolic function manifests itself as well, protecting man from being exposed to the space and time of the real, by interpreting these as occurring in an objective, subjective, and mediating way, also allowing man to engage in a relationship both with himself and with others based on a specific structure of desire (see Chapter Seven). Indeed, the world does not coincide with reality per se. Thus, on the levels of the world, intentionality and language, a function manifests itself that transcends their own frontiers: the symbolic function.

THREE MODALITIES OF SYMBOLISATION: CASSIRER

In addition to these three levels of psychic reality – intentionality, world, language – there exists yet another threesome. Rather than being related to the content of the three levels, they refer to the three stages of symbolisation. Indeed, we found that intentionality can function either pre-predicatively (in an expressive or imaginary way) or predicatively (propositionally, symbolically): the entity of perception presents itself physiognomically or in an objectified manner, respectively. A third type of symbolisation may be added, as the entity of perception can also be formalised (this water coming from the tap is H_20).

These three forms, three stages of symbolisation apply not only to the level of intentionality, but indeed to any level. The world also can be interpreted in a pre-predicative (physiognomical, imaginary) or predicative fashion (articulated, symbolically), or can be formalised. Ultimately, the threefold distinction can be made to apply to the level of language. In doing so, we might pay heed to fixed (imaginary) meaningful entities, to the contextual quality of meaning made dependent on differential articulation, and to formal linguistic structure (Cassirer, 1923/1994a, pp.124-300). As a result, each of the 'three levels' can function according to these 'three modalities', these three forms of symbolisation.

These forms of symbolisation correspond with the threefold distinction introduced by Cassirer: expressive representation, propositional representation (objectifying intuition), pure meaning (*Ausdruck, Darstellung, reine Bedeutung*), which he subsequently connects with the cultural manifestations of myth (expression), language (representation in a narrowed down sense) and science (pure meanings), respectively. Globally, this threefold distinction matches Lacan's distinction between an imaginary order and a symbolic order, extended with the order of formalisation (‘*logique*’, ‘*petites lettres*’, ‘*mathèmes*’).[15] Like the ‘three levels’, the ‘three modalities’ have an intersubjective infrastructure similar to the one proposed by Cassirer (Kreis, 2010). What applied to the three levels obviously also applies to the modes of symbolisation contained within it (Cassirer, 1944/1966, p. 130, 223).

Excurs. A threefold distinction in the field of modalities is not that uncommon, as it makes a case for the validity of introducing a threefold distinction as such. With Kant (1783/2002), whose philosophical views prompted him to interpret thought as ‘judging’, we recognise a threefold distinction among subjective judgments of perception, objective judgment of experience and a formal judgment of understanding: ‘Wahrnehmungsurteil, Erfahrungsurteil, Verstandesurteil’ (Ueling, 1996). Actually, Cassirer reintroduces this distinction. We might also consider the ‘other phenomenology’, namely that developed by Hegel (1807/1979). Again, in his theory he distinguishes three forms: sense, perception and understanding. More specifically, the primal directedness towards an object, its objectification, and their formal underlying principles: ‘sinnliches Bewusstsein (Meinen), Wahrnehmen, Verstand’. What Hegel adds is intersubjective depth structure (Brandon, 2001, pp. 32-35), by being the first to connect the intersubjective dimension, the practical domain, with the theoretical domain: the pragmatic turn, initiated by Hegel, later on to be strengthened by pragmatism itself and especially by the ‘linguistic turn’ in philosophy. Indeed, symbolisation or world disclosure is established in an intersubjective manner.

Following Cassirer, we can distinguish an evolution in these three types of symbolisation (or representation). In fact, they may well be conceived as stages or grades of the process of symbolisation. Expressive representation (*Ausdruck*, the imaginary, myth) would then constitute the

---

[15] Formalism (logic, or science) is not an autonomous order in Lacan’s view, but he does acknowledge its unique form. The third category he introduces – in addition to the imaginary and the symbolic – refers to the real. Cassirer does not feel this need, with the real being resorbed by symbolic forms. In his logicist period (from the late 1960s onwards) Lacan also moves towards this direction, when equating ‘structure’ (logic, topology, Borromean knots) with the real, turning into more than just a model. It also disqualifies the supremacy, the priority of the symbolic, as the three orders are supposed to be equiprimordial (in line with Cassirer). Lacan (2005) writes (p. 231): “[...] le réel apporte l’élément qui peut les (sc. l’imaginaire et le symbolique) tenir ensemble.” On closer inspection, it seems that the later Lacan, the so-called ‘Lacan of the real’ is more of an idealist than the term would suggest.

first stage, as a type of proto-symbolisation, leading to the generation of images and meaningful entities. Propositional representation (*Darstellung*, the symbolic, language) would then be the second stage, generating distinction and limitation. Pure meanings (*reine Bedeutung, petites lettres*) are the third stage, facilitating the formalistic approach of modern science.

This highlights an essential difference between the first two forms of symbolisation on the one hand and the third form on the other. The first two forms lead to the creation of a life world (including cultural activities such as morality, law, art, etcetera) as well as a bodily determined subjectivity.[16] It presupposes the traditional image of man, e.g. 'manifest image of man' (Sellars, 1963), the 'life world' (Husserl, 1953/1970b), including its conceptual infrastructure (Strawson, 1974) – albeit in a modified and in a modern form that includes subjective dividedness (see Chapter Five and this Chapter). Yet, there is an essential difference with the 'scientific image of man'. Despite a formal, differential underpinning (Lacan), the symbolisations generated in the life world are content-oriented (*see supra*). The focus of the third form, however, leads to a process of symbolisation in which phenomena are analysed in formal elements, precisely by refraining from a description of everyday reality (see Chapters One and Four). It shapes today's formal science, with its unique symbolic form. Rather than a situated body-subject it presupposes the presence of an anonymous general '*Bewusstsein überhaupt*', a consciousness per se – a view from nowhere, from infinity. In summary: The third form of symbolisation reflects a modern asset, spawned by modernity, and actually constitutes its very core, in every aspect (Koyré, 1957). Eventually, the emergence of modern science will transform retroactively the life world – 'that water from the tap is H_20' – by giving it a modern figure.

In order to identify the nature of the personal subjectivity within the life world, however, only *the first two forms* (the first two stages) are relevant, which follows from the foregoing. Moreover, significant as much is the difference between both forms – between the 'order of the image' and the 'order of the word', between 'totality of meaning' and 'formal difference'. This applies also to the genesis of personal

---

[16] There is some debate as to the exact number of (legitimate) symbolic forms with Cassirer (Krois, 1987; Lofts, 1997). Failing to interpret them content-wise, as Cassirer was inclined to do, the problem will eliminate itself. All we have left with then are three forms, going back to *Ausdruck, Darstellung, reine Bedeutung*.

subjectivity: the perspective of development. The relevance of two stages – two tours, two moments – and their mutual differences have already briefly been mentioned and will re-emerge more extensively in the next chapter, in a variety of contexts: the issue of space and time, of inter-subjectivity, of psychosis.[17] However, we should not forget that, in order to grasp the overall concept of the fullness of human subjectivity, which also includes scientific consciousness ('Bewusstsein überhaupt') the *third form* (grade, stage), and consequently, the threefold overall symbolisation, inevitably presents itself.

THREE DIMENSIONS OF THE SYMBOLIC FUNCTION: LACAN

When describing the three modalities (of symbolisation) and the three levels (of the psychic reality), the question poses itself whether they can actually be realised – that essentially is a transcendental question. This is the dominant issue of these paragraphs. Rather than inquire into the factuality of a course of events, we look for their conditions of possibility. This type of question goes back to Kant (1781/1965). In which cases can we speak of valid scientific knowledge and what is presupposed with generalised types of world disclosure? Kant sought for a static answer to this question, in a non-empirical but transcendental consciousness. Hegel (1807/1979), by contrast, dynamically positioned it in the dialectic evolution of the mind. Cassirer, returning to a static approach, located it in the symbolic, representative quality of the human spirit, giving it a dynamic form: its three modes (*Ausdruck, Darstellung, Bedeutung*). To these we might add: the three levels of the psychic reality (intentionality, world, subject position). What is presupposed by the three modalities of symbolisation and the three levels of psychic reality, is, we might summarise, the symbolic function: the function representation in the broadest possible sense.

Indeed, the symbolic function enables the transformation of the real per se into a scientific world, but primarily into a life world, which implies a three-tiered psychic reality and (first of all) the two primary forms of symbolisation (associated with the imaginary and the symbolic). However, this symbolic function should not be interpreted ontologically, as if dealing with an actual sphere of reality, but only in a functional way

---

[17] This is the issue addressed by Lacan usually under the heading alienation/separation (see Chapter Seven).

(Cassirer, 1910/2000; Kreis, 2010).[18] For a psychic reality to exist – on three levels, with initially two (and next three) forms of symbolization – the path of symbolisation will be followed. It protects man from being exposed to brutal reality of being, to the immediacy of life and to the immediate presence with the other. It precludes the impossible enjoyment that such an immediate presence would offer.

We see a threefold transformation taking place: in respect of (1) the *immediacy of life*, (2) the *immediate presence toward reality,* (3) *and the immediate presence with the other.* The immediacy of life (i.e., the arousals of the body) – Lacan's '*immanence vitale*', Cassirer's '*Unmittelbarkeit des Lebens*' – are transformed into the intentionality of experience. Next, the 'real' of the external nature is transformed into a temporal-spatial world. Lastly, the immediate presence with the primordial Other is replaced by intersubjectivity. Thus, we see a subjective, objective and intersubjective world taking shape. *The three levels of psychic reality and the three modalities of symbolisation associated with it are interwoven with and dependent on the three dimensions of the symbolic function.*[19]

There is always the intermediate form of interpretation or representation (Cassirer, 1929/1994b, p. 359). Lacan (1966/2002, p. 346) speaks of 'the omnipresence for human beings of the symbolic function stamped on the flesh'. This transformation of brutal reality, the real into a meaningful world presupposes, in a sense, a 'fundamental symbolisation' supporting any actual symbolisation, thus enabling objective validity of the world as world (Kreis, 2010, p. 231). Symbolization puts brutal reality, the real at a certain remove, thus creating a meaningful world of objects and subjects, with which we enter into a relationship because they exist unto-us. And yet there is no reason to believe, as did Hegel or the Neo-Kantians and Cassirer, that progress of formal scientific knowledge (Cohen) or the sum of all cultural symbolisations (Cassirer) would reveal reality in its true form – not even approxi-

---

[18] Heidegger's (1929/1973, pp. 246-268) criticism, in the Davos talks, that Cassirer properly specified the *terminus ad quem* (culture) while failing to define the *terminus a quo* (the mind), eventually turns out to be unjustified, for want of autonomous terms: only objectified relations exist. See with regard to the Davos talks Gordon (2010).

[19] Cassirer (1923/1994a, p.51) writes: "Für sie (sc. die Philosophie) [...] ist das Paradies der reinen Unmittelbarkeit verschlossen". Lacan's equivalent statement is as follows (Lacan, 1966/2002, p. 696): "We must keep in mind that jouissance is prohibited [*interdite*] to whoever speaks, as such". Cassirer's '*Paradies der reinen Unmittelbarkeit*' is the equivalent of Lacan's '*Jouissance*'.

matively or asymptotically (Cassirer, Cohen, and Natorp, 1998). According to Lacan, such an asymptotic 'point of reconciliation' cannot exist, such a possibility would simply fall outside our scope. Most certainly, it can never hope to represent a sum total. The fundamental difference between Cassirer and Lacan is that Cassirer's symbolic forms, in line with Neo-Kantianism, fully absorb reality, turning reality into a mere correlate of symbolizing consciousness, whereas Lacan defines the remaining aspects as essential. Brutal reality will reveal itself in what does *not* work properly (*ne marche pas*), what does function as an impasse, an impossibility, as a non-integratable remainder, as a traumatic nucleus. Consequently, the real can be defined as pre-existing to symbolisation (real $_1$), as well as partly excluded (real $_2$), whilst allowing symbolisation into a world, as a result of the process (Balmès, 1999, p. 62-64; Fink, 1995, p. 27).

Besides, symbolisation of the real runs parallel with the renunciation of a non-mediated presence and the enjoyment associated with it, viz. in a threefold manner: (1) a primordial *Jouissance du corps*, the *Jouissance* of the living (Miller, 2007, p. 141), related to the immediacy of life, (2) *Jouissance de l'être* (Lacan, 1966/2002, p. 694), related to the external real, and (3) *Jouissance de l'Autre,* related to the immediate presence with the primordial Other. Still it does allow for a limited and restrained form of ('phallic') pleasure, as a result of the process. In this form the real does not manifest itself as an impossibility or an impasse but as a threat of an invasion, of a return of the excluded, the impossible, *Jouissance* itself.

Both forms of the real are tied together in the process of symbolisation, one being the reverse side of the other. Indeed, any symbolisation, appropriation of the signifier ('*Einbeziehung ins Ich*', primordial '*Bejahung*') runs parallel with an expulsion of primordial enjoyment, expelling it from the subject ('*Austossung aus dem Ich*') – see Lacan (1966/2002, pp. 323-324). It makes that in both cases the real is conceived as being 'internally excluded', i.e. excluded, internally, by the symbolic. In summary: The real, as understood by Lacan, can be defined in a primarily static form, as pre-existing to symbolisation (real$_1$), partly excluded (real $_2$) which stills allows for symbolisation – taken together 'cold real', – *and* a primarily dynamic form of the real, access to which is denied by the symbolic in an active way ('hot real'), being constituted itself in the process of symbolisation, yet allowing for a limited, restrained form of enjoyment (Balmès, 1999, pp. 68-73; Rabinovitch, 1998, pp. 25-53).

Contrary to Lacan's view, which is steeped in conflict and loss, Cassirer's mode of thinking appears to be dominated by harmony. The argument in favour of Lacan is not so much that the symbolic function according to Cassirer would be supposedly dependent on and drawing upon an 'energy of the spirit' – see Heidegger's criticism – but is dependent on and only effective within a external and limited linguistic and symbolic order, which needs to be accepted ('*la bourse ou la vie*'). It functions in a arbitrary and differential way (Lacan), stamping the organism, the flesh of the subject, from the outside, while inherently bringing limitation and 'castration' – a more pertinent, indeed Lacanian, criticism of Cassirer. Having said this, it by no means compromises the transcendental effects of the symbolic function. Indeed, any actual attempt at framing or enclosing is bound to leave a remainder, because brutal reality can be expressed in a variety of ways. This results in a divide between brutal reality (the real) and its interpretation (the world), which also functions as a safeguard for the multiplicity of modes of interpretation to exist.[20] Apparently, the symbolic function has a transcendental task, which lies at the heart of intentional phenomena, of being in a meaningful world and in a language-dependent mode of existence, and of threefold quality of symbolisation. Once again, it fulfils a 'transcendental function'.

THE AFFECTIVE

Would this emphasising of intentionality (and of the constituted nature of the perceptive world, the significance of language and the symbolic function in general) not result in an overstating of the significance of 'activity' within psychic reality? Would this not lead to an understatement of 'passiveness'? Passiveness was mentioned before, while discussing a primal form of intentionality which precedes a thematic, judging type of intentionality: a passive, pre-predicative form.

In addition, the affective type of intentionality could bring out the importance of passivity even more. Yet this is not self-evident. For

[20] The 'gap' ('*béance*') theme refers to a fundamental notion of Lacan that has been phrased in a number of ways. Here it is referring to the separation between brutal existence (*le réel*) and its phrasing (through symbolic systems), without any guarantee of harmony occurring between phrasing and being. In doing this Lacan is stressing the very theme of modernity (more than Cassirer was capable of): denying harmony. Indeed, Lacan is more of a Kantian than of Neo-Kantian.

instance, it turned out that emotions are closely connected to cognitions – cognition and affect being intertwined: a point of view represented by the cognitivistic theory of emotions. Emotions are supposed to evaluate a situation. In that sense they are also related to cognitions. i.e., to activity. Emotions trigger an action, i.e., they change the tendency to act, making the connection with activity even stronger. Fear causes flight behaviour, rage produces an attack, fright leads to a freeze response. Moreover, we are able to 'manipulate' our emotions: avoid them, cover them up with opposite behaviour, or ward them off by displaying similar emotions, e.g., in a more intense form, so as to prevent us from experiencing the more subtle but also more painful variety. Emotions offer insight but may also present a form of self-deceit, as was emphasized by Lacan. To some extent, what psychoanalysis refers to as self-defence even goes back to this possibility of self-deceit. Up to a point, we can even control affective experiences: producing an emotion that leads to a 'magical' transformation of the world (Sartre, 1939; Schafer, 1976, pp. 271-294). All this describes the active side of emotions.

Nonetheless, the passive aspect which has traditionally been attributed to emotions is still relevant. Up to a point, emotions are also associated with something that befalls us and which we cannot control. This passiveness makes them absolute somehow, turning them into something we find difficult to escape from. Moreover, emotions are often complex, blending into each other or changing radically, which makes them obscure in a way. Sometimes, perhaps even often, love is associated with admiration and can eventually turn into hate. This prompted Lacan to coin the phrase 'hainamoration', which is composed of 'haine, amour, admiration'.

And then there is the element of time. Emotions can fluctuate, but strong emotions may linger for a long time, making it difficult for us to adapt to a new situation, as we find ourselves unable to get a hold on them. Indeed, profound emotions seem to elude time, manifesting themselves in an expected and violent way, apparently taking us by surprise. Or else they cannot be coped with, haunting us for a long time. In each of these cases we are engaged in a passive relationship – we don't affect emotions, emotions affect us. Apparently this is a key feature of emotions, and traditionally it has been regarded as such. This leads to a qualification of the more rationalist, 'cognitive' view of emotions. As such, the passive component is also given due credit.

What contributed to this qualification are recent developments in the field of emotion research that highlight their biological background. The biological component of emotions was never entirely ignored – neither by Aristotle nor by Descartes – but was not always given proper attention either. The cerebral organisation of emotionality turned out to be much more complex than had previously been thought.[21] For example, an anxiety-mediating system was identified that is hardly situation-specific but which exercises a powerful effect nonetheless. Next to it operates a less overt but much more specific and slowly operating system, with the two systems functioning in a mutually balancing fashion (LeDoux, 1996/1998). This more or less reflects the distinction between primary and secondary emotions. Primary emotions (such as anxiety) represent more or less innate, non-specific dispositions, while secondary emotions (such as anger) are types of emotional experience and action tied to the individual life experience. In addition to these two kinds of emotions, feelings can be distinguished that are potentially nuanced and are of a reflexive nature, such as feelings of guilt and shame (Damasio, 1994).

The neurobiology of emotions and emotional life offers an area of research that spawns new insights and clarifies facts that are already known. The concept of dual anxiety mediation systems illustrates why certain behavioural patterns are not easily influenced or are likely to return in stress situations. Then again, the difference in levels between the biological substrate and the subjective experience itself should not be ignored either. The two levels cannot be equalised nor are they causally related, but are supposed to be engaged in a type of 'founding/being-founded relationship' (Merleau-Ponty, 1945/1962, p. 394) with the biological substrate creating the conditions for subjectivity, including emotional subjectivity, to exist, as was outlined before (Merleau-Ponty, 1945/1962, p. 394) (see Chapter Three).

Biological research of emotions will strengthen the notion that the brain, through lower organizational levels, is in constant interaction with its environment, mediating a type of proto-subjectivity that precedes a more personalized form.[22] The notion of plasticity of the brain and of environmental control highlights the value of 'life events' and, more generally, of life history, which more or less bears out the relevant points made by psychoanalysis. Moreover, copious references to 'unconscious'

---

[21] From the 1950s onwards a three-tiered structure of reptile, mammal and specific human brain organization has been assumed – the so-called triune brain. See MacLean (1980).

[22] This may be an elaboration of the theory of the 'embodied mind' developed by Damasio, Varela and others. See also Chapter Three.

representations and emotions within biological views on emotions make the step to a psychoanalytical approach a small one indeed.

In fact, this step was already taken in the description of the third level, the language-dependent mode of existence of man, and the associated subjective position of dividedness and desire: the untold and the unfulfillable, as two dimensions of the unconscious in the psychoanalytical sense. In a more complementary fashion, the conscious/unconscious distinction introduced in the above can then be explained further.

Conscious and Unconscious

The path taken by psychoanalysis was certainly not the path chosen by neurobiology or experimental psychology. In fact, it adopted a more classical distinction, viz., between reasonable and unreasonable, assuming nevertheless that certain 'unreasonable' feelings and thoughts had a 'reasonable' nucleus, be it in a wider and unconscious sense.

The classic distinction between formal and material object is useful in this respect. The formal object of perception of, e.g., a triangle, is what makes a triangle a triangle. The material object is the triangle actually perceived. Similarly, in respect of emotions we can distinguish between a material and a formal object. The material object of anxiety is that which actually triggers this emotion. The formal object represents the daunting aspect of the material object: the imminence of an anticipated overwhelming danger.[23] This distinction will allow us to identify a discrepancy between the formal object and the material object. Indeed, in some cases there appears to be an apparent mismatch between the material object and the formal object. Thus, fear seems ill-matched to the material object 'mouse', considering the formal object of fear (anticipation of an imminent and overwhelming danger). Apparently, emotions – as well as desires and other phenomena from the affective sphere – can be viewed as imaginary (or imagined) and can therefore be criticised as being less rational (De Sousa, 1980).

Based on this distinction, the notion of the unconscious can be clarified further. It may be assumed that the formal object of an image can be linked to incongruous objects. A person may be afraid of a mouse, or show no fear when threatened by a gun. A person may see any elderly male person as an authority figure, and come into conflict with this

---

[23] See, in line with mediaeval scholastics, Kenny (1963, pp. 187-203).

person, or turn a blind eye to other qualities of the same person. In this respect, it may be useful to speak of unconscious representations and unconscious emotions. In this particular case, the link between the formal and the material object has partially been lost. Formally, unconscious hate is still hate, but it is inappropriately focused on particular individuals. An unconscious representation of an authority figure would be a case in point, but again it is inappropriately linked to a particular individual.

To put it differently: as far as the aspect of representation is concerned, the unconscious consists of a chain of representations cycling like a news ticker bar, stamping (material) objects. Where conscious intentionality has become 'dysfunctional', an unconscious signifying chain may be set in motion. We may also speak of an 'unconscious ideology' as the set of beliefs that focus individual orientation, resisting new or differing insights – a shadow cabinet if you like. A constant in this respect are hidden beliefs such as: "If I'm successful, things will take a turn for the worse", or "No matter what I do, it's all pointless anyway", and "If I commit myself to a person, I'll be abandoned, so I won't commit myself or I'll break off the relationship once things become uncomfortable", or the idea "An intimate relationship will be too overwhelming, so I'd better engage in multiple relationships", and so on. In fact, these represent more or less unconscious beliefs or fantasies that dominate both perceptions and actions. Ultimately, this is where the phantasm notion comes into its own. For example: When the (unconscious) basic phantasm is framed as "The Other is overwhelming", this may lead to sexual fantasies of deriving pleasure from being overwhelmed, but also to a conscious attitude of keeping oneself at a distance of other people. The phantasm is (in part) an unconscious formation, while offering a reverse side towards consciousness. Thus once again, the phantasm is not a fantasy that causes us to stray from reality, but the framework itself that defines what may be experienced as desirable or threatening, in any case as meaningful within relational reality.

Since insights and the emotions associated with them may be 'unreasonable', as in the present case, the same may apply to desires, only more poignantly so. Desires also have an object: e.g., the formal object of a desire is an absent 'good'. Conscious desires, demands, are focused on a possible and accessible object. Unconscious desires can drive conscious desires, e.g. demands, but they can also thwart them, when striving for full retrieval of something that was left and cannot possibly be retrieved: it is the 'real', 'impossible' core of the unconscious. It is this very impossibility that makes the desires in the sense described ultimately deserving of this epithet. The search for something lost in the past – an unmediated presence and rest produced by precluding it – which is also unattainable and therefore 'unreasonable' as a pursuit. It makes any satisfaction disappointing: what happens in reality fails to fulfil the unconscious desire, the unconscious imagination. As was observed before, unconscious desires thwart conscious demands, while also controlling them, as a result of their being partially stamped by the lack produced by precluding an immediate presence. This prompted Freud to write that finding an object (of love) also represents, to some extent at least, the recovering of an original object. Any object that gives satisfaction will thus become a substitute-object of an original and lost object, which is turned into an ultimate and impossible goal – the desire for the impossible object that, being lost, constitutes the 'cause' of the desire itself – Lacan's object *a*.[24]

Like psychic reality is defined by intentionality, the unconscious, as an alternative realm of psychic reality, is shaped by intentionality with an impasse structure (Mooij, 1991, pp. 54-55). Not being eliminated, intentionality will continue to exercise its effects. Indeed, this is more than just a privately accessible entity, because unconscious representations and desires reflect something that can be expressed and put into words, be it in a circumspect manner (even though this cannot actually be realised): this constitutes the narrative aspect of the unconscious, being structured as a language, as a discourse ('*discours de l'Autre*'). Demands reflect a desire, with the desire expressing itself while leaving an unsaid remainder.

CONCLUSION

It turns out that the unconscious brings an extension of the psychic reality, which follows logically from the definition of the psychic in terms of linguistic intentionality. It is not simply a twofold intentionality that shapes psychic reality: propositional and non-propositional, cognitive and affective, conscious and unconscious – in other words, the subject-pool. Indeed, it is also shaped by what it focuses on: its objects, the world as a whole – the object-pool. Both pools are spanned by the

---

[24] Freud writes (1905/1953b, p. 222-223): "Finding an object is actually retrieving it".

exterior order of language and culture, which serves to bestow identity. This process is associated with dividedness on the subject side and loss on the object side, leading to a subject position, which is characterised by dividedness, by desire and by the possibility of reflection. This represents a retrograde effect (*après coup*) of the 'objective mind' of language and culture, of the symbolic order, on the organism, the proto-subject, which becomes a subjective mind and a subjective body. It precludes an immediate presence to brutal reality, to the other and to the own body. It may be referred to as an (impossible) '*Jouissance de l'être*', '*Jouissance de l'Autre*', '*Jouissance du corps*'. This transformation of a primordial reality into a meaningful, shared world unto-me presupposes a structuring principle – an alternative sphere which is transcendental rather than empirical. Instead of forming a deeper layer of reality, it should be conceived as serving a functional purpose only: It does not 'exist' substantially, but can be reconstructed as a supporting function. This principle can be defined as the 'symbolic function' allowing the complete range of actual symbolisations of intentionality ('seeing' in the sense of 'seeing as'), being in the world, and the intersubjective structure of desire.

In the next chapter, these three levels will be elaborated, whilst indicating how disruptions may occur that lead us to the field of psychopathology: normality and neurosis, the personality disorder and the psychotic structure. This may demonstrate that the 'transcendental' sphere, the symbolic function itself, can be profoundly affected, as may be the case with psychotic disorders. In a way, psychosis is characterised by a non-operational symbolic function, to the degree that it results in the impossibility of reflection – the psychotic finding himself incapable of engaging in free, reflective use of language (obviously within the boundaries imposed by the rules of language). This becomes manifest in the field of intentionality and world shaping, in the form of hallucinations or delusions, where any claims to intersubjective validity and objectivity are effectively dropped.

Between normality, with its effective symbolic function, and psychosis, defined by a defective symbolic function, lies the field of the personality disorder, in which the symbolic function in the sense of the possibility to reflect is present, only in a deficient form. This leads us to the threefold distinction of psychopathological structural forms which will be discussed in the next chapter, between normality (including the neurotic structure), the personality disorder and the psychotic structure.

Seven

Three Psychopathological Structures and Nine Subject Positions

The first step in psychiatric diagnostics is to assess the '*status praesens psychicus*', or current mental status. Assessment focuses on establishing the presence or absence of symptoms such as consciousness disorders, mood disorders, hallucinations or delusional disorders (Wing, Cooper, and Sartorius, 1974). These symptoms can then be consolidated into mental conditions or syndromes which are defined based on current classification systems. Abnormal behavioural patterns occurring within the context of a personality disorder can also be categorised. This procedure may be driven by underlying nosological motives, defining a symptom as the expression of a hypothetical pathology. Alternatively, it may support a more pragmatic objective. The two approaches, outlined in Chapter Four, have one feature in common: They externalise the various phenomena whenever possible, isolating them and abstracting them from any inner connection with other phenomena, being empiricist or tending towards empiricism. Moreover, nosologically oriented systems tend to expand, as a result of the ongoing subdivision of groups of phenomena into even smaller units. Within a pragmatic context, we also witnessed the development of a range of behavioural evaluation scales supporting psychometric research – e.g., 'anxiety scales', 'depression scales', scales measuring aggressive behaviour, and so forth.

A type of diagnostics that does not abstract inner relationships or relationships of meaning is the hermeneutical approach, in its broad sense. It introduces a distinction from the empiricist approach, as was discussed in previous chapters, notably in Chapter Five. The empiricist approach is certainly valid – particularly for the sake of standardisation – but the hermeneutical approach also has its place for purposes of individualisation, categorization and exploration.

Three Levels of Psychic Reality

A hermeneutical diagnostics may be individualizing in itself, but some general guidelines are needed nonetheless. Three levels may be distinguished, as was discussed before (in Chapters Three and Six) within the context of the psychic reality: the level of intentionality (focused on the world), of the intended world, and of language and lack. First and foremost, the psychic is dominated by intentionality. Feelings and thoughts are about 'something'. A person feels sad about something, is thinking of something, is seeing something. Intentionality may reveal itself either through propositional, thematic functioning, with an active involvement of the 'I', or can be non-propositional in nature, without any 'I-involvement': A road may be perceived in an objectifying manner as being two metres wide, or be experienced subjectively as 'too narrow' or 'wide enough'. A higher organisational level is attained when, in the field of perception, a world of perception is constructed – one that holds 'objects' in the broadest sense of the word (artefacts, plants, animals, people). Space and time, as well as intersubjectivity, are key categories. The third level includes the introduction of language and lack, taking account of desire (produced by a primary lack) and of the capacity to reflect.

This discussion will draw implicitly on the three types of hermeneutics which, in their empirical and philosophical manifestation, were specified before (in Chapter Five): the hermeneutics of the signification, of the situation and of the signifier. The hermeneutics of the signification the descriptive phenomenology in the sense of the early Husserl and the hermeneutics developed by Dilthey addresses the meaning of phenomena in a more or less objectified sense. The hermeneutics of the situation – hermeneutics in a narrowed down sense – stresses the connection between the process of meaning-giving and situation in which this process occurs, thus pointing to the state of embedding which characterises meaning within the broad context of a world. The third type of hermeneutics – the hermeneutics of the signifier – emphasises the inextricable bond between subjective and situational determined meaning giving process on the one hand and the pre-existence of language on the other hand, bringing separation and distinction, lack and desire into being.

There is a specific, homological relationship between the three levels and the three forms of hermeneutics. The three levels concern empirical-hermeneutical relationships, which can subsequently be approached from one of the three types of hermeneutics (of the signification, of the situation and of the signifier) in their empirical manifestation (descriptive, relational and structural diagnostics). The analysis of intentional phenomena (the first level) is eminently suited to an approach from the hermeneutics of the signification; the analysis of the world (the second level) can be approached most effectively from the hermeneutics of the situation while, finally, the analysis of the intersubjective structure of desire (i.e., the third level) is best discussed from the hermeneutics of the signifier. Thus, the three levels of the psychic reality each reflect the three types of hermeneutics.

THREE PATHOLOGICAL STRUCTURES: NEUROSIS, PERSONALITY DISORDER AND PSYCHOSIS

There is another side to this as well, as each level involves specific standards, norms. These standards or norms allow a particular way of experiencing, of situational involvement, and of linguistic phrasing to be described as 'abnormal' or even as 'pathological'. Moreover, such a normative, 'deontological' description may be derived from the categorization employed within traditional psychopathology. This does not necessarily mean that the abnormal types described have to coincide fully with traditional pathological categories, although reference to them will be made. Still, it will turn out that traditional psychopathology continues to offer a highly useful guide for discussion. After all, traditional psychopathology distinguishes fundamentally among, respectively, neurosis, personality disorders and psychosis. These types of disorder may be conceived as many structures that differ fundamentally from one another. Unlike the neurotic disorder, the psychotic disorder is characterised by loss of reality. At a halfway, intermediate position we find a third structure that shares features with both the neurotic structure and the psychotic structure, without actually being reducible to either.

Traditional psychopathology even refines this position into a threefold subdivision for each single structure (neurosis, personality disorder, psychosis). The *neurotic structure* is subdivided into hysteria (histrionics), obsessive neurosis (compulsive neurosis) and phobia (avoidance behaviour). The *structure of the personality disorder* has been commonly subdivided into perversion, psychopathy (which corresponds partly to what is now called the narcissistic personality disorder) and the dependent condition ('Süchtigkeit'), which bears strong similarities to the current qualification of borderline personality disorder).[1] Traditionally, the *psychotic structure* is also characterised by a

---

[1] In early psychiatry, the term 'abnormal personality' was more common than the present-day term 'personality disorder'. See Schneider (1950/1955, p. 23): "Abnorme Persönlichkeiten sind von den mit guten Gründen als krankhaft postulierten zycklothymen und schizophrenen Psychosen gründsätzlich scharf zu trennen".

threefold subdivision: schizophrenia, melancholy/mania and paranoia. Each of these conditions will be discussed later on in more detail. It should be borne in mind however, that this chapter does not intend to offer an exhaustive description of what, either today or at any one time in the past, is or was defined as a mental disorder. Rather, the focus is only on the kind of mental disorder that is suited to an interpretation based on these three pathological structures – neurosis, personality disorder, psychosis – each of them including three pathological positions.

Explanation

A few commenting notes. The condition that today is defined as mood disorder can be categorised into a variety of structures, depending on the context in which they occur: neurotic depression (dysthymia), *psychopathische Verstimmung*, melancholy, etcetera. Within the structural framework, the mood disorder therefore does not represent an autonomous position or structure. The same applies to dissociative disorders, which may occur within each structure (of a neurosis, a personality disorder or a psychosis) without actually qualifying as a structural unit. Most likely, somatoform disorders do not qualify as a structural unit either. However, if an underlying alexithymia (viz., being incapable of naming meaning, implying a symbolisation disorder) is present, such a disorder could rightfully be included into a structure (once its presence has been confirmed). The same probably applies to the gamut of autistic disorders, a minor part of which may be categorised as psychotic. ADHD disorder do not represent a position in itself but may contribute to the development of a position (e.g., of a personality disorder).

The Symbolic Function

The three structures (neurosis, personality disorder and psychosis) combined with the three levels (intentionality, world, and desire) and the three types of hermeneutics) (signification, situation, signifier) offer a guide for the present discussion. This represents an empirical investigation, concerning an empirical sphere, i.e., in its broad, hermeneutical sense.

Figuratively, at the level below the empirical sphere, we can also distinguish a transcendental sphere – such as discussed in Chapter Six. The 'transcendental' sphere is affording the conditions of possibility for engaging in intentional relationships, of designing a world, of a language-dependent mode of existence. Fundamental here is the act of symbolisation, which enables the constitution of a world – a shared world – and removes man from the brutal reality of being, transforming it into a world characterised by a distance to immediate reality. Symbolization also implies a separation, in a threefold sense. Symbolization puts reality-per-se at a distance, subjectifying it. Reality-per-se becomes a world-unto-myself. By extension, the intersubjective domain is concerned, as symbolization will result in the preclusion of an immediate presence to a primordial other: Through the introduction of separation and distinction, it enables individuals to engage in intersubjective relationships. Thirdly, it affects the level of the body, as the (real) physiological body of meaningless 'arousals' (the organism) is transformed into a body-subject transected by language and culture, into a body-unto-me (Cassirer, Lacan).

The distinction between the two spheres – empirical and 'transcendental' – may be legitimate, but should not be absolutised. The two spheres may be distinct, but are not separate. The distinction is functional rather than ontological. Describing a certain cognitive phenomenon, e.g., a hallucination, will have a predictive value for the way intentional phenomena are (transcendentally) established. Describing a person's world also brings anticipation of a state of affairs that will be addressed from the transcendental perspective in a more explicit way: by introducing the structuring principle of the symbolic function.

A formal difference between the two spheres does exist, however. The first sphere refers to phenomena and their embedding within a structural whole, whereas the symbolic function relates to its conditions of possibility. Or, to phrase it differently: If we focus on the structuring moments of the former, we ponder on what is offered by the experience of the empiry – in its broadest hermeneutical sense – whereas the latter will cause us to meditate on its condition of possibility. Thus, the distinction into two spheres, in addition to supporting our line of reasoning, is also essential in that it reflects two different hierarchical structures: the phenomena and their embedding within a structural whole, and a structuring principle.

Initially, this distinction between the empirical and the transcendental spheres will only be touched upon briefly. As was argued before, the two spheres are distinct, but not separate. The transcendental sphere (of the structuring principle of the symbolic function) will be dealt with explicitly as part of the general discussion of the psychosis, but only as a minor point in the section dealing with neurosis and personality disorder. The underlying motive is that the deactivation of the symbolic function in the psychotic condition 'negatively' demonstrates what it achieves and brings about positively in ordinary life. Inevitably, only a basic, 'essayist' version of such a design can be offered at best (see also the table in the Appendix outlining the psychopathological structures).

THE FIRST LEVEL: TWO DOMAINS AND TWO TYPES OF INTENTIONALITY

The history of ideas regarding the psychic reality discussed in Chapter Six shows that two fundamental domains of intentionality have traditionally been distinguished: a cognitively focused and an affective one (including the sphere of desire).

A key role in the *affective sphere* is played by mood or basic mindset. It can be either positive or negative, stable or unstable. Representing a basic mindset, more than putting its stamp only on a part of the world, it actually pervades and reveals the world in its entirety. A mood gives access to the world: it has a function of disclosure – not to be contaminated with offering truth, while eventually offering deceit. This also applies to emotion which – as opposed to unveiling a global world, as in the case of a mood – is focused on specific intentional objects and events contained in this world. Next to it, a mood and emotions will develop in a comparatively autonomous, wayward fashion: their intensity increases and, after peaking, may diminish spontaneously again (Hell, 1994/2002, pp. 259-261). This relative autonomy, waywardness causes the affective domain of mood and emotions to escape, to some extent, from the experiencing subject's hold.

Both aspects – a world-disclosing nature and autonomy, waywardness – apply to desire as well. Yet, as opposed to emotions and mood, desire does not relate to something that exist, but to something that does *not* exist. It relates to the lacks and holes characterising the world as it presents itself to a person. Although the desire is focused on a negativity, on something that does not exist, it subsequently acquires meaning through the creation of fantasies or phantasms, which together represent the framework that gives desire its concrete shape. Whether or not structured by a fantasy or phantasm, the desire itself is characterised consistently by a lack or absence, and therefore by a form of non-being. The alarming nature of the lack, the 'hole in existence' gives desire its urgency: the lack must be remedied, the hole must be filled. Essential in this respect is the degree to which a person can tolerate, renounce or negate boundaries, can live with a life characterised by a lack.

The affective branch of intentionality can be matched with a particular type of the body, of the body proper: a passive or needful, enjoying body. In addition to this 'supporting', 'anonymous' body, a more active and instrumental type of body proper can be distinguished. Within this modality, the body functions as an entity that walks, looks and grasps, that takes a stance. As such, the body will act in an active and instrumental way – it appears and creates situations (Zutt, 1938/1963a).

This second, active form of the body can be matched with the second, active domain type of intentionality – the *cognitive* type. The cognitive should also be understood in its broadest sense, ranging from the cognitive awareness of one's own body to abstract mental faculties. Within this sphere, however, perception plays a key role, if only because the 'faculty of understanding' has to rely on what is offered by perception. Significantly, perception shows things that are not offered 'purely', as a conglomerate of colours and tones, but as anthropomorphic and physiognomical entities of meaning (Zutt, 1955/1963c; Cassirer, 1929/1994). Apples are not red first and then tasty, cars look fast or slow at a single glance. Although the body performs an active function within this modality – it looks, observes – the world of perception does have some degree of autonomy as well. The meaningful entities – the kind or threatening aspect of the world – will reveal themselves: the world has an specific 'face'.

We speak of the physiognomic character of the world of perception, as a type of non-propositional intentionality: Before the world is objectified, the path of pre-reflexive, non-propositional intentionality will cause us to experience it as a self-evident presence. This type of intentionality has been defined in different ways by a number of authors.[2] Invariably, they refer to the sphere preceding reflexive, propositional intentionality (see also Chapter Six).

Not only has the subject a non-propositional, pre-reflexive experience of the world, it has a similar experience of itself: a pre-reflexive self-awareness. As a next step, this type of self-awareness will be associated

---

[2] The range of definitions offered is as follows: passive, operative, without I-involvement *vs* thematic (Husserl, 1970/1949, section 38, p. 80); pre-predicative *vs* predicative (Heidegger, 1962, section 32, p. 189); preobjective *vs* objective (Merleau-Ponty); mythical, physiognomic, expressive *Ausdruck vs*, representation, *Darstellung* (Cassirer, 1944/1966, pp. 76, 116, 132); imaginary *vs* symbolic (Lacan, 1966/2002).

with a pre-reflexive other-awareness. I experience like others experience, mirroring takes place through social attunement. Pre-reflexive (specular) self-awareness, other-awareness and world-awareness go hand in hand (Stanghellini, 2007, pp. 135-143). Combined, these three elements constitute the core of what is sometimes referred to as '*ipseity*': a non-propositional, non-thematic type of intentionality. This point is well worth remembering. We might tentatively equate this non-propositional sphere with what Lacan calls the imaginary order, and '*ipseity*' with the figure of an imaginary ego, '*moi*', as Lacan would define it (Mooij, 2010, pp. 210-212).

However, this '*ipseity*', (or '*moi*', in Lacanian terms) may be defective. This deficit in respect of pre-reflexive self-awareness, world-awareness, other-awareness leads to excess reflection or hyper-reflection, bringing objectification of experiences that are commonly lived pre-reflexively. To some extent, it serves to offset the lack of lived experience, be it in an alienating fashion (Sass and Parnas, 2007, pp. 69-71; Stanghellini, 2007, pp. 139-141). It has been argued that schizophrenia is characterised, among other things, by an inadequate pre-reflexive intentionality, which can subsequently be compensated by hyper-reflection (which combines to form the specific '*ipseity*' disturbance in schizophrenia). It is inward-looking in nature, 'scanning' inner life that exists, but contact with which has been lost. In addition to the agonising complaint of melancholy – "I feel that I don't feel" – a lack of contact is being felt – "I don't feel that I feel" (Stanghellini, 2007, p. 143).

Within the context of this hyper-reflexia, the schizophrenic person becomes aware, in a thematic fashion, of things that will normally occur 'automatically', without thought. It demonstrates that schizophrenia has philosophical significance, as it will engage, without prompting, in the act of artifice of the phenomenological *epochè* (Depraz, 2001).

Explanation of the Gaze and the Mood

Following this discussion of disturbance of pre-reflexive type of intentionality, we may devote some attention to disturbances of the two domains of intentionality, viz., cognition and affect. Firstly: the field of cognition. Within this field, perception, visual perception, is significant to psychopathology, particularly in relation to the theme of the 'look', the 'gaze'. Some examples may help illustrate this. Within the hysterical position, visual perception and the other's look play a key role (Nasio,

1990/1995, pp. 179-189). It all comes down to being seen, to appear before the other, showing a perfectness that does not actually exist. In the case of a compulsive neurosis, we see a different type of preoccupation with perception, taking the form of control, dissection, precision. The other's gaze may also be an object of fear, representing a phobic object, avoiding the other's desire as it manifests itself in the gaze. Within the sphere of perversion, we recognise the two opposing forces of voyeurism and exhibitionism, reducing either oneself or the other to the gaze (Bonnet, 1981). Finally, a psychosis may be associated with delusional feelings of being pursued by the other's gaze, or of being watched in a hallucinatory fashion.

If the gaze can manifest itself in a variety of ways, we may wonder how the gaze, should be defined in the first place. Any attempt at describing it will result in a loss of objectification. Objectification will put the eye centre stage – but the eye is not the same as the gaze, it is only the carrier.[3] The gaze passes from the inside to the outside, essentially leaving the body through a hole. Similarly, the physiognomy of the world perception also endows objects with a gaze, according to Merleau-Ponty Sartre and Lacan (Leguil, 2012, pp. 267-306). As such, the gaze is part of the objects leaving the body (e.g., the voice).[4] Thus, the gaze uniquely and intangibly refers to the other. The other appears by virtue of the act of being looked at.

In addition, the other manifests itself also through the process of looking. Following Lacan, we might say that, also in our way of looking, we submit to the Other's gaze. The subject's being looked at by the other, is even its primary mode of existence. Like the discourse of the Other defines our speech, it is the Other's gaze that determines our view. Apparently, this state of affairs reflects a fundamental passiveness of the subject in relation to the Other, a submission to the Other, which may also be disturbed pathologically. Remember the delusional perception of

---

[3] Zutt (1957, p. 352): "Das Auge ist ja nicht der Blick, es ist nur der Träger des Blicks. Auch andere Gegenstände – Sartre hat darauf hingewiesen – können Träger des Blickes werden (andere Lücken!); z.B. kann der offene Laden an einem Gebäude, der Lichtschein einer Lampe, mich in die Verfassung des Erblickten, des von einem Blick Betroffenen versetzen". Also Blankenburg (1971, p. 108).

[4] Lacan introduces the gaze within the framework of his theory of partial objects, object *a*. They constitute the fabric of an affective bond. A person may find himself attracted by the other's gaze (or voice): the desire focuses on (the other's) gaze. With respect to this issue, Lacan is oriented on Merleau-Ponty rather than on Sartre. See Lacan (1973/1986, pp. 67-122).

a person who mistakenly feels watched by another person (Kulenkampff, 1956). Or the type of hallucination that causes a person to see something (or hear something, in the case of an acoustic hallucination) which, according to the classical definition of a hallucination, 'does not exist'. Rather than hearing active voices or seeing images, it involves being looked at passively or being addressed by an inescapable other (Henry, 2001).

It makes the omnipotent gaze of the other (produced by a hallucination or delusional perception) particularly overwhelming. This omnipotent other is not actually another person. The very fact that the subject finds itself unable to escape the gaze is evidence of a loss of an autonomous position, resulting in a fundamental elimination of boundaries (Kulenkampff, 1956). This loss of position suggests that this type of intentionality – cognition in its overall meaning – is fundamentally disrupted.

A possible disturbance of the second domain of intentionality, viz., affectivity, can be illustrated by focusing on mood, a field in which Binswanger first developed his *Daseinsanalyse*. We are referring to mania, the manic episode, which can clinically be described as a condition characterised by the patient being delusional, in combination with inflated self-esteem (which also may reach delusional proportions) and motor or verbal disinhibition. With regard to this last point – disinhibition – in the field of thought we might speak of a 'flight of ideas', with the maniac's thoughts moving from one to another in a desultory fashion, at a rate faster than can be articulated. Still, we are not dealing with a specific type of thought disorder or cognitive disorder. Often, the manic patient will talk much ('Rededrang'), without actually pondering his words. Both perception and action are desultory, unfocused, not particularly serious, 'playful' in nature, in turn causing existence itself to become desultory, fleeting, something not to be taken seriously. Thus, the focus seems to be on a mood, rather than on a formal thought disorder or race of thought. All things are taken lightly, nothing is taken seriously. Binswanger (1931-1932/2000; Ey, 1954, pp. 70-86) spoke of mood optimism and joy of existence, although the latter term is not particularly apt, with real joy being absent.

And yet Binswanger's concern was not with describing an affective intentionality disorder, but with typifying a specific form of being-in-the-world, viz., the manic form, as deviating from 'the norm', exposing an uninhibited fashion, lacking a point of gravitation or focus. Apparently, we are able to distinguish intentionalities – as various types of directedness – as well as worlds – as objects of directedness – but in fact they do refer to one another. Which brings us to the second level: the world.

Second Level: The World (Relationship with Space and Time)

If the world can be conceived as the sum of all that we focus on, or as its horizon, it follows that a number of basic shaping or structural moments can be distinguished: the structural moments 'time and space' and 'oneself and the other'. Man is always engaged in a relationship with space and time, with others as well as with himself. In anything I feel or conceive with regard to the world, I'm engaging in some form of relationship with objects in space and time, as well as with fellow subjects. This brings us to our first point of discussion: the relationship towards space and time.

Being able to occupy *space* has traditionally been regarded as an essential quality of matter. For example, Descartes conceived the mental substance as thought, and the material substance as extensiveness. In line with the emerging natural sciences (Galileï), he conceives matter as 'res extensa'. Anything that occupies space and has extensiveness, by definition can be measured and calculated. Heidegger speaks about things being 'present-at-hand': to the degree that they are present-at-hand, they are both measurable and objectifiable. In addition to being present-at-hand, they can be ready-to-hand, e.g., when functioning as utensils that reflect the world in which they are used (Heidegger, 1927/1962, p. 135). Anything that is present-at-hand, will occupy a particular objective position. By contrast, what is ready-to-hand, is characterised by its proximity, which should not interpreted as referring to a small geographical present-at-hand distance, but to a proximity in the form of 'being close'. Things with which I feel a connection, are close to me. However, this dichotomy is not sufficient and, on further inspection, the concept of 'space' could actually fall into three subtypes.

External, Internal and Dimensional Space

First, there is the objective (physical, geometrical, external) space. This space is homogenous, and the shortest distance between any two points is always a line. Next, there is the subjective (inner or internal) space. Binswanger spoke of 'orientierter Raum'. The central point of orientation is the 'here', from which follow 'there', 'higher', 'lower', etcetera. This is the space that presents itself within consciousness: It is not homogenous, but is oriented from a vantage point ('here'). Its being oriented separates the subjective space from the objective space, but it is still focused on the outside, the objective space. That is why a person in principle can be mistaken about his orientation, or why his orientation may be distorted somehow. This may be the case with neurological disorders (e.g., apraxia, where a person reaches incorrectly for objects, or agnosia, where a person fails to recognise certain objects)[5] It is also witnessed in psychiatric disorders. In the case of severe psychotic disorders, it may even lead to a reversal of the left-right orientation, the left-right orientation being a fundamental aspect of the subjective space (Kusters, 2004).

The nature of the relationship between the objective space and the subjective space presents a fundamental problem, which has traditionally been addressed from the philosophy of space. One may argue that a third or mediating type of space could well be imagined and is even necessary. This third type of space may arise from the spatial quality of the subject itself, according to Heidegger.[6] And following Merleau-Ponty (1945/1962, pp. 98-147) we could say that this concept of space is seated in the body itself. Manifesting itself as a body proper, a bodily subject, the subject both occupies space and is subjectively (pre-predicative, pre-consciously) aware of this fact. This dual position serves to create the link between objective space and subjective space, one may argue. This allows an 'intentional arc' (Merleau-Ponty) to be strung between the spatial subject and spatial objects. Moreover, this 'third form of space' brings a limitation, as the infinite physical space is transformed into a limited, closed and human spatial world holding a spatially situated *finite* bodily subject.

This third space would enable man to live from each of the three dimensions, which run parallel to those of physical space (height, width, depth) as well as to their correlates in subjective space. And yet they differ in a fundamental way. What we find here, are not objective relations in the external world or their correlatives in subjective experience, but the dimensionality of life itself, the dimensions from which man lives his individual and limited life: the width of the plane,

---

[5] See the discussion of the Schn(eider) case in M. Cassirer (1929/1994b, pp. 181-184) and (Merleau-Ponty (1945/1962, pp. 98-147).

[6] Heidegger (1987), p. 105: "Das Dasein des Menschen ist in sich räumlich in dem Sinne des Einräumens von Raum und der Verräumlichung des Daseins in seiner Leiblichkeit".

the elevation, and the central point from which the central perspective is shaped. Binswanger (1932/1955, pp. 176-220; 1988, pp. 49-123) spoke of a 'gestimmter Raum' and an associated 'Bewegungsrichtung'. This 'third space' can truly be defined as 'dimensional space' or as the 'spatiality' of the subject.

Next, what is the significance of this distinction between objective (external) and subjective (internal) and dimensional space to the theory of symbolisation – a central theme in our enquiry? Introducing subjective and objective space constitutes a first step in the process of symbolisation that transforms the brutal reality of being into a spatial world. The introduction of dimensional space is a second step, connecting objective space and subjective space, while curbing ('castrating') both of them in the process, as the dimensional time originates from the spatial quality of a *finite* bodily subject. Because the second stage brings limitation, dimensional space could justifiably be defined also as 'symbolic space': 'symbolic' in the sense of introducing limitation and restriction. Dimensional space, symbolic (form of) space, and the spatiality of the subject are thus equivalent terms.

What is its relevance to psychopathology? Spatial awareness can be disturbed, and so can dimensional space likewise. It may be that a subject primarily shapes his life with an emphasis on only one dimension: a height perspective, a central perspective or a marginal perspective – which is the case with neurotic disturbances, as will be demonstrated later on. Alternatively, a subject may shape his life, while one of the three dimension being weakened – which is the case with personality disorders. Thirdly, one of the dimensions of the dimensional space may implode, as in the case of psychotic disorders. As a result, the connecting function of the dimensional, symbolic space that engages the objective space with the subjective space, has been rendered inactive entirely. It brings a decay of both the objective space and the subjective space, as their mutual bonds have been severed. Ultimately, the subject finds itself thrown into the 'space of the real', beyond any symbolisation, which shows itself as a pseudo-external space. Alternatively, the subject may become overwhelmed by boundless space consciousness, that fails to take account of objectivity – as is evidenced, for instance, by a reversed left-right orientation

External, Internal and Dimensional Time

Time can be analysed in a similar manner. First of all there is objective (physical, cosmological, external) time, which proceeds in a linear fashion, with a t_1 and a t_2, a before and after, on its time axis. It more or less reflects the concept of time proposed by Aristotle.[7] This concept of physical time corresponds with physical space.

Secondly, there is a subjective (inner, internal) time, characterised by an awareness of present, future and past. This represents the internal time consciousness following Saint Augustine and particularly Husserl (1928/1964). It distinguishes three 'ecstasies': present, past en future. The present is not the t_1 on the time axis, but a 'now' which also has duration (through retentions and protentions): there is a 'later', a future that is expected and an 'earlier' past remembered. Subjective time, inner time, internal time consciousness, is oriented from a 'now-point' (as subjective space is oriented from a 'here'). Yet, external time and internal time are separate, but are also related. Objective, physical time, as expressed on the linear time axis, presupposes the presence of a subject, while the ecstasies of subjective, inner time presuppose the presence of a line, and consequently an axis, holding t_1 and t_2, both a 'before' and an 'after' (Ricœur, 1984, p. 21).

There is yet another, third time variety, one that mediates between objective and subjective time: the dimensional time, the temporality of the subject – analogous to the 'third form of space' (the dimensional space, spatiality of the subject). The subject perceives time (in a subjective manner), then it becomes objective 'within-time', '*inner-zeitig*', but ultimately finds itself to be both temporal and finite.[8] It lives within a limited time span (between birth and death) on the objective time axis, while being subjectively aware of its own mortality. This dual position serves to establish the link between objective time and subjective time, limiting both in the process. Objective time is transformed into calendar time, which refers to the dates of birth and death. Subjective time (inner time consciousness), on the other hand,

---

[7] Aristotle (1984, *Fysica IV* 219 b 1-2).

[8] The temporality of *Dasein* represents Heidegger's fundamental line of thought in *Sein und Zeit*. In this regard, his views will not change, see Heidegger (1987, p. 61). In this respect he puts emphasis on the significance of time to psychopathology; Heidegger (1987, p. 229): "Auch bei allen pathologischen Phänomenen sind immer die drei zeitlichen Ekstasen zu berücksichtigen und deren jeweiligen Modifikationen".

stretching into the infinite, is transformed into a finite life-historical time. Man thus is able to live from each of the dimensions or ecstasies of this life-historical time: from a finite future, a present with a duration, the facticity of the past. That is why this 'third type of time' can justifiably be referred to as 'dimensional time' or as 'temporality of the subject'.

What is the significance of this distinction between objective (external) and subjective (internal) and dimensional time to the theory of symbolisation? The answer is comparable to the one offered within the context of space. Introducing subjective and objective time constitutes a first step in the process of symbolisation that transforms the brutal reality of being into a temporal world. The introduction of dimensional time represents a second step, connecting objective time and subjective time, while curbing ('castrating') both of them in the process. Because the second stage also brings limitation, dimensional time may well be referred to as 'symbolic (form of) time': 'symbolic' in the sense of implying limitation or restriction. Dimensional time, symbolic (form of) time, temporality of the subject are thus equivalent terms.

What is the relevance to psychopathology? Dimensional time, like time consciousness, can be disturbed. A person may over-express a dimension (past, present or future), as in the case of the neurotic disorder or he may under-express a dimension, as in the case of the personality disorder, which will be discussed later. Alternatively, one of the dimensions of the dimensional time may implode altogether, as in the case of a psychosis, as a result of which objective time and subjective time become disconnected. This will lead to a loss of objectification (no or an impaired object constitution within calendar time) as well as a loss of subjectification (no or an impaired subject constitution as a finite subject in life-historical time). The subject has become prisoner of the 'time of the real', which escapes symbolisation, of pseudo-external time (fragmented, disconnected, or continuously excessive). Or, one may fall prey to unhinged, pseudo-subjective time, a pseudo-inner time consciousness removed from objectivity (a perpetual now, *nunc stans*).[9]

Underlying these disruptions, which will be discussed in the next section, is a successful, a partially successful, and an unsuccessful symbolic transformation of brutal reality into a meaningful world

[9] The distinction introduced in the above between objective, external space and time *and* a pseudo-external space and time – a 'space and time of the real' – had not yet been made by Mooij (2010, pp. 61, 62), where these both concepts were still supposed to coincide.

characterised by structural moments of space and time, of subjects and objects: the symbolic function. The structural moments of the world itself reflect the empirical world itself as a product of either successful, partially successful, and unsuccessful symbolisation. Its description will take us to the domain of psychopathology.

When investigating the various types of relationships we find that a subject can engage in with the structural moments of time and space (dimensional, symbolic space and dimensional, symbolic time). Traditional psychopathology may offer some degree of guidance, particularly when it comes to distinguishing between hysteria, obsessive neurosis (compulsive behaviour) and phobia (avoidance behaviour). The table in the Appendix outlining the psychopathological structures may be helpful in gaining a quick insight into the various types of relationship.

Neurosis: Hysteric, Obsessive, Phobic Position

Essentially, the neurotic structure is characterised by an enlargement of character traits that would still be recognisable to the average person, or by the presence of symptoms (e.g., of lack of power, of compulsion and anxiety) that the average person can relate to. It represents a modification of normality without exceeding its boundaries, presenting three forms: the hysteric, the obsessive and the phobic position. In respect of space and time coordinates we may therefore expect dimensional space and time to be intact, be it accompanied by an undue emphasis on one of the three dimensions of both forms – while leaving objective, external and subjective, internal time and space intact. For instance, there are no disturbances in the field of consciousness of time en space.

The *hysterical* or histrionic position is characterised by a lack of satisfaction, an overall feeling of being wronged, harbouring a grudge that has its roots in the past: hysterical 'vindication' or spite (Israël, 1976/2001, Verhaeghe, 1998). The emphasis put on feelings of spite, of being wronged in the life, points to an undue emphasis on the past. Feelings of spite go back to a wrong or injustice suffered in the past. Seen from a spatial perspective, the dominant dimension represents the 'centre'. The hysterical person is supposed to display self-centred behaviour, causing him to draw attention to himself, putting himself at the forefront. Rather than keep to the edges of the field of presence, he is always looking for the centre, living in an egotistic, self-centred or 'centric' manner.

The *obsessional* or compulsive neurotic position is characterised by an elevated orientation, offering an overall, commanding view of events. There is a predisposition towards living from a '*point from nowhere*' aimed at attaining both maximum overview and objectivity. In addition, there is a strong preoccupation with measurable and knowable aspects, with precision. As Heidegger formulated it, things are found in the sphere of being present-at-hand, of the objectifiable, rather than in the sphere of being ready-to-hand, of proximity. It defines the future as the predominant dimension. As the obsessive personality focuses on control, he needs to anticipate future events, in order to prepare for contingencies, postponing or moderating his actions, if necessary.

Within the *phobic* or avoiding position, rather than looking for an elevated or central position, the subject prefers a marginal vantage point (Charbonneau, 2004, p. 125) in order to fade into the background. The central position or being in a central position is particularly intimidating (notably in the case of agoraphobia), causing the person to avoid such situations. An elevated position is also experienced as daunting as in the case of acrophobia (Zutt, 1938/1963, pp. 389-390).The phobic person is wary of danger, yet without actually dealing with it in a compulsive manner. Rather than occupy the vantage point of a commander overlooking the battlefield, developing future-oriented strategies, he focuses on impending danger, driven by 'anxious expectation'. First and foremost, he lives from the dimension of the present.

Personality Disorder: Perverse, Narcissistic, Borderline Position

The structure of a personality disorder occupies a position halfway between a neurotic structure and a psychotic structure (Kernberg, 1984). The world of the personality disorder is less alien that than of the psychosis, but more unfamiliar than that of the neurosis. The phenomena as such may be similar to those seen in the neurotic structure, but their anchor points are different, which in itself is cause enough for provoking feelings of alienation. It will appear that its relationships differ in a structurally fundamental way from both other structures.

Like the neurotic structure is characterised by an overemphasis on one of the dimensions of dimensional (symbolic) space and time, the structure of the personality disorder is defective in that one of the dimensions of both forms is demonstrably weakened or suppressed – while leaving objective (external) and subjective (internal) space and time intact. For example, in principle there are no disturbances of internal consciousness of space and time, unless in very severe (almost psychotic) cases. Once again, three positions can be distinguished, corresponding to the distinctions made in classical psychopathology. Each represents a negative 'mirror image' – an inversion – of the corresponding position within the neurotic structure: perversion, narcissism and the borderline position.

A remark beforehand: If reference is made to Lacan, it is worth realising that he recognises only one position within this field, to which he besides attributes the quality of a structure: the perverse structure. He rejects the construct of the borderline position, while mostly ignoring the narcissistic personality structure. This is no reason why we should not discuss these figures within the present structure – particularly because of their intimate relationship with the perverse position. A second remark beforehand: The perverse position reflects perverse issues occurring within the framework of a (serious) personality disorder – corresponding to the DSM-type of paraphilia. That is why a clear distinction is needed from perverse traits or perverse configuration phenomena (perversities) associated with a neurotic structure (Freud, 1991; Kernberg, 2006; Socarides, 2004) or manifesting themselves within a psychotic structure. In a perverse position in its strict sense the perverse configuration is not limited to certain areas of the personality, but pervades the whole structure of the subject. Yet, this does not mean that the line between both is a clear cut one or is easily to draw.

The *perverse* position may be conceived as related to that of to the hysterical one, being more or less its 'negative'. As opposed to hysteria, the past is being considered irrelevant and is effectively ignored. This irrelevance of past events ('let bygones be bygones') makes it understandable why psychotherapy, focusing as it does on the past, turns out to be problematic and is often avoided by the perverse subject. Issues such as abnormal behaviour traits are above all taken as a matter of fact, and there is no desire to look for its origins in the family situation (Bonnet, 1993). Also, a non-ability to engage in lasting intimate relationships may point to a defective bond with the past, being to threatening. Indeed, intimacy presupposes an open attitude towards the past, which is a shared past. Spatiality is characterised by a partial rejection of centricity, as well as a preference for a centric/eccentric position. The pervert has an inclination to appear out of nowhere, drawing attention to himself, only to vanish into thin air afterwards. Again, we see a preference for anonymity and elusiveness. Think of the exhibitionist appearing, exposing himself and disappearing, without leaving a trace.

The *narcissistic* position is equivalent to the narcissistic personality disorder, and it may be conceived as the 'negative' of the obsessive personality, as its very opposite, even though similar in theme. A recurring and remarkable feature is the lack of foresight, the failure to anticipate future possibilities. Based on this defect, crimes – if it ever comes to that – tend to be ill prepared, ultimately resulting in failure, which cannot be put down to low intellectual ability: It reflects the feelings of grandiosity and impulsiveness. Also, the anticipatory abilities with regard to what the future may bring, expressing itself in having future-oriented ideals, is mostly underdeveloped. As can be expected, the neglect of the future is associated on the level of spatiality with a deficient dimension of height, leading to a lack in having 'overview'. Indeed, overview may be weak, sometimes even to the point of distorting the view of reality, leading to illusions such as 'no one can catch me', what is obviously not the case. In severe cases reality-testing may be effectively compromised.

The *borderline* position appears to be a modern variety of what traditionally has been called the 'dependent attitude' or 'Süchtigkeit' (Von Gebsattel, 1954, pp. 220-237). It offers a 'negative', in a sense, of the phobic or avoiding position. While the phobic person lives a marginal life, avoiding contact, the borderline personality moves just outside the boundaries (that still contain the neurotic, phobic person, as a result of his condition). He is looking for a limitless contact, characterised – both in terms of relationships and substance abuse – by excessiveness.

From the perspective of dimensional (symbolic) time there is weakening of the dimension of the present, which will even affect – also in less severe cases – inner time consciousness. An inner void is felt, which is rooted in chronic depersonalisation. Normally, the present retains what has just happened (retention), while anticipating what is going to happen (protention), turning the present into something considerably more than a flimsy separator between a past that is no more and a future that is yet to come (Husserl, 1928/1964). Indeed, the present holds an element of duration and, as a result, also some element of being, with its retentions and protentions providing a 'foundation in reality'. A weakening of the function of the present manifests itself clinically in phenomena of derealisation and depersonalisation (associated with feelings of alienation towards external reality or towards oneself). This depersonalization, chronic or not, is a almost quintessential characteristic of the dependent condition (and of the borderline personality position). It contributes to the development of addictions, as psychoactive agents provide a temporary relief from the inner void to counteract the dearth of experience. Search for excitement or the pain of automutilation – pain for having the feeling of 'being there' – is in fact an effective means of combating it. Depersonalisation, by virtue of the 'rush' used to combat it, brings out the significance of 'the moment', demonstrating that the temporal dimension of the present constitutes the weakest link here (Mooij, 2010, pp. 75-91).

Psychosis: Schizophrenic, Melancholic, Paranoid Position

The psychotic condition is characterised by a loss of reality testing, paving the way for delusions and hallucinations to occur. Indeed, a delusion has traditionally been described as an 'incorrigible error', implying the loss of reality testing. A hallucination is described as an 'objectless perception', which also implies the absence of any degree of reality testing. And yet the concept of psychosis within the present context is more limited than the one offered above. A psychotic condition per se is a non-specific concept, considering that psychotic symptoms can occur with anyone (e.g., in the case of a serious infection or sensory deprivation), or that a person may develop a full-blown psychotic state or episode, e.g., in the case of a hysterical position (Libbrecht, 2001; Maleval, 1981/1991) and a borderline position. The proposed concept relates only to psychotic conditions that are presumed to reflect an underlying psychotic structure (Van Heule, 2011). Decompensation of this structure may be associated with psychotic phenomena, possibly leading to manifest psychosis. However, the psychotic symptoms may not become manifest if the psychotic structure is adequately supported by care offered by the environment, by specific symptoms having a stabilizing function, by a specific way of living – later on called '*sinthome*' (Lacan, 2005). In these cases, following Lacan, we may speak of 'supplementation' (Lacan, 1966/2002, p. 484; 1981/1993; 2005).

As indicated in the above, psychosis in its narrow sense has traditionally been subdivided into three subcategories: schizophrenia, melancholy, and paranoia. It should be noted, by the way, that Lacan does not embrace this tripartite division, instead considering the paranoia to be the psychosis par excellence. He does address melancholy and mania, but hardly mentions the schizophrenic position. This, of course, does not preclude integration of these categories. Each of these positions is supposed to be associated with a specific dysfunction with regard to space and time relationships (spatiality, temporality). However, there is a fundamental difference with the neurotic structures, also with those that fall within the range of personality disorders. These disorders are characterised, respectively, by an undue emphasis on one dimension (in the case of a neurotic disorder) or by a weakening of a dimension (in the case of a personality disorder), but in either case dimensional time and dimensional space are not compromised. In the case of a psychosis, however a particular dimension of dimensional time or space has become quite inoperative (or at least highly dysfunctional). As a result, the possibility to operate from the affected dimension is lost, the patient no longer being to live from the present, the future, the past, etcetera. This, incapability consequently affects the function of dimensional space and time as such – its function being to establish a relationship between objective space and subjective space. This loss of function results in a rupture of the connection between subjective and objective time and space. It will lead to a form of (spatial and temporal) consciousness that no longer takes account of spatial and temporal objectivity, as it is no longer connected with an experiencing subject.

The *schizophrenic* position is derived from a somewhat controversial yet well-established conception of mental disorder: schizophrenia (Blom, 2003). Within schizophrenia, conditions occur that are characterised by so-called 'positive symptoms' (such as hallucinations and delusions), and conditions characterized by a prevalence of 'negative symptoms' (such as loss of affection and loss of social competence): the symptomless types of schizophrenia. It may well be that the positive symptoms are in fact a reaction to more fundamental negative symptoms, with the positive symptoms obscuring the negative symptoms. In the early 20th century, it was Bleuler who captured the essence of the symptomless type of schizophrenia by introducing the term 'autism' (which should be distinguished from a type of autism that refers to disorders from the autistic spectrum, characterised by impaired social interaction and communication skills). The schizophrenic form of autism is in line with what Minkowski (1927/1997, p. 132), following Bleuler and particularly influenced by Henri Bergson's philosophy of life, described as '*perte de contact vital avec la réalité*', where the poignant character of the relationship with reality is lost altogether.

Dimensional space will be defective. We see a loss of the ability to occupy an active central position and to synthesize, from a central perspective, a spatial world, the patient having the idea that everything that happens is referring to him. The ability for having a central position being lost, the centrality of dimensional space is obviously defective. Conrad (1958/1987) spoke of a so-called 'Ptolemeic shift', which results in the schizophrenic ceasing to function as an active centre, being relegated to the role of passive centre: '*die passive Mitte der Welt*'. Quite appositely, a patient says: "It feels as though everything revolves around me".[10]

Internal space consciousness may be, in less severe cases, still intact, depending on the schizophrenic's knowledge of his whereabouts. Yet this may lead in extreme psychotic bouts to a disturbed spatial awareness the point where even the left-right orientation may be reversed. Admittedly, these are extreme cases, but the perspectival structure of the world becomes almost necessarily flawed. This type of disturbance has been touched on briefly before – in the discussion of a disturbance of pre-reflexive, operative intentionality, as a result of which the subject's pre-reflexive involvement both with himself and with the world is disrupted (ultimately leading to the phenomenon of hyper-reflection): an '*ipseity*' disturbance that could be put on equal footing with a defective '*moi-ici*' in Minkowski's sense. Here the implications on the level of space consciousness are displayed. In Minkowski's terminology one might say that his 'me-here', his '*moi-ici*' – 'I am here, this is what I am doing' –, is absent or defective (Minkowski, 1927/1997, p. 94). If the '*moi-ici*' as a structuring principle is absent or is seriously compromised, the perspectival structure of the world becomes flawed, resulting in an unstable relationship between foreground/background or figure/background (Wiggins and Schwartz, 2007). Besides, the figure-background relationship organizes the sphere of perception, leading to a categorization of what is offered by perception. Disruption of this relationship leads to a deluge of stimuli that are not subject to signification or categorization, exposing the subject to raw reality: a *pseudo external space*. This onslaught of unfiltered reality stimuli facilitates the occurrence of hallucinations (as positive symptoms). Removing oneself implies a withdrawal, with possible subsequent functional decay and loss of interest (as negative symptoms), regardless of the question which has 'primacy' here: the undue distance or the undue proximity to the real

---

[10] Conrad (1958/1987, p. 76): "Ich habe das Gefühl, alles drehe sich um mich."

(Hell, 1993). Hallucinations may then result from 'weakness zones' in a perceptive field (Rosolato, 1985, pp. 274-289).

Temporality is also disturbed, viz., with respect to the past (Kraus, 2007). What is impaired here is not primarily the capacity to have memories of the past – inner time consciousness –, but the past's supporting power – *dimensional time* –, insofar as the past supports the present, providing for the continuity of action and experience – although, in a derived sense, it may manifest itself also in the field of internal time consciousness; see below. That which should be a self-evident given, now needs to be recreated time and again. There is no 'retrograde continuity'. In Heideggerian terminology: the aspect of 'being already' ('*Je-schon*'), has been deactivated in part. This lack of a supporting self-evidence (the 'being-already') may lead to hyper-reflectivity likewise, because all that should happen 'by itself' and presented as a natural self-evident given, now needs to be 'invented'. This phenomenon of hyper-reflection was raised before, in the discussion of a disruption of the pre-predicative intentionality and an 'ipseity' disturbance associated with, also having consequences on the level of space; see above. The point is now discussed related to the issue of time.

In the 1970s, Blankenburg came up with a very apt description, '*Der Verlust der natürlichen Selbstverständlichkeit*', the loss of self-evidence, suggesting that all that we consider 'self-evident', underlying our thoughts, actions and social interactions, will lose its power and becomes problematic. He quotes one of his female patients saying:

> What's wrong with me? So insignificant a thing, so funny, so important, but we cannot live without it. I had never grown up. I was simply there, belonging, but not really present. I simply lack the natural capacity to take things for granted.[11]

This exemplifies that the bonds with a supporting and continuity-giving past ('having been', '*Gewesenheit*') have become frayed. When there is no durable past, there is no future either: If there is no 'where from', there is no 'where to' either. Yet the lack of a future outlook – 'being

---

[11] Blankenburg (1971, p. 42): "Was fehlt mir eigentlich? So etwas Kleines, so komisch, so etwas Wichtiges, ohne das man aber nicht Leben kann. Ich war nicht gewachsen. Ich war einfach da, nur hingehört, aber nicht dabei. Das ist wohl die natürliche Selbstverständlichkeit die mir fehlt". And she continues: "Ich war nicht gewachsen. Jeder Mensch muss wissen wie er sich verhält. Mir haben die Grundlagen gefehlt". See also Blankenburg (1971, pp. 21, 60, 77, 100-104).

able' in Heidegger's sense – as such is rooted in and derived from the loss of the relationship with the past, in the form of 'having been', the past of dimensional time.[12]

As a result – particularly with the occurrence of positive symptoms – *the internal time consciousness* of schizophrenics may become disturbed also, similarly the way in which subjective space, the space consciousness, could be affected – such as has been discussed before. This disturbance of the internal time might even result in time reversal: The future has happened already before in inner experience. Alternatively, a disturbance of the external, objective time may occur, the patient being overwhelmed by a *real, quasi-linear time*, taking the shape of fragmented or frozen time: The clock is not ticking but has stopped (Kusters, 2004). Both types of disturbances – concerning internal and external time – reflect the rupture between internal and external time, the connection of both having to be provided by the dimensional, symbolic time, with the decay of this form of time causing these disruptions.

The *melancholic* position has traditionally been associated with a deficient relationship, not with the past but – paradoxical though it may seem at first glance – with the future. Particular melancholy has commonly been approached from the time perspective (Straus, 1928/1963; Von Gebsattel, 1954, pp. 1-18). From a modern perspective, it is important to distinguish between traditional melancholy and what is today referred to as depressive disorder or mood disorder. Traditional melancholy lives on in the 'depressive disorder with psychotic characteristics', but this traditional form involves a broader spectrum, including the milder types of depression, viz., in cases where the themes of loss and guilt are particularly relevant. Tellenbach, for example, described the '*Typus melancholicus*' as a personality structure that to some degree would predispose towards psychotic melancholy, which is strongly dominated by conscience and conscientiousness, as a result of which a person fails to capitalise on his possibilities. Tellenbach (1961/1983) speaks of 'Inkludenz' and 'Remanenz', while also pointing to the relationship with compulsive neurosis (Tatossian, 1992). Depressive disorders seen today will usually have a different background and are connected more strongly with a feeling of being underrated by others and a loss of self-esteem rather than with feelings of guilt and

---

[12] Heidegger writes (1927/1962, p. 326): "Only in so far as Dasein *is* as an 'I-*am*-as-having-been', can Dasein come towards itself futurally in such a way that it comes *back*."

failing in respect of a norm (Ehrenberg, 2009; Juranville, 2005, p. 42). Commonly, these present-day, 'postmodern' depressive conditions lack structural unity but are likely to occur within the context of, e.g., a neurotic structure, or even in the absence of any psychopathological structure (Lantéri-Laura, 2003).

If we refer to melancholy here, we use the definition of traditional melancholy (a serious depressive disorder with or without psychotic symptoms), to the degree where matters of guilt and loss are involved. As mentioned before, the key issue has always been about time. Hardly surprising, because a melancholy person will first and foremost complain about having committed a major – as well as an irreparable and fatal – mistake. He is a prisoner of the past, which has an absolute hold over him. This fixation on the past has been interpreted as the result of being barred from the future. This state of being locked up can be interpreted in two ways. A life's philosophy-oriented psychopathology would conceive this being barred from the future as the absence of a life power which normally functions as a forward-driving force, a 'vis a tergo' in life.[13] A melancholic person cannot accomplish anything, because there is no life power that enables him to do so.

Alternatively, this being barred from the future can be explained on the basis of the phenomenological-anthropological time perspective, which puts *dimensionality of time* centre stage. According to this line of thought, the reason why a melancholic person will not accomplish anything is that 'being able' implies some anticipation or future-oriented action – the very thing he is incapable of. To the degree where he is barred from the future, the past will take over. Since, from a dimensional viewpoint, the past can never be dealt with definitely, as it can always be revised from a finite future, the hold exercised by the past will never be truly absolute. However, once revision of the past from the future and from future possibilities is no longer possible, revision will not be possible either and so the past will reign supreme, overwhelmingly. A melancholy subject thus falls prey to his past, where all is loss and any loss will be irreparable. The incorrigible nature of any delusion occurring originates, it could be surmised, from this state of preclusion of the future.[14]

---

[13] A critique of the life-philosophical approach of the time issue (as being too limited) is presented by the philosopher M. Theunissen (1991, pp. 222-224, 236-238).

[14] Maldiney (1991) writes (p. 65): "Le présent du mélancolique va au passé et vient du passé. Mais sans devenir. "

The decay of the dimensionality of time may cause also subjective time (internal time consciousness) and objective time (or linear time) to become unhinged, shedding their mutual connections. The flow of *internal time consciousness* declines, even seems to grind to a halt, which is experienced as tormenting to a high degree. And what remains, is a *pseudo-linear time,* without involvement of a subject that can hold on to something. This is reflected in the now classic complaint voiced by one of Von Gebsattel's patients: "All the time I'm thinking about time passing by, I can't help it".[15] Time proceeds in a straight line from past to future, with both past and present disappearing without a trace, leaving only the sheer negativity of a constant loss: Only decay is left, nothing is retained, while access to the future is denied.

The *spatial correlate* of an absent future dimension (from the perspective of dimensional, symbolic time) will be the absence of a height dimension (from the perspective of dimensional, symbolic space), reflecting the incapacity to rise above a given situation in order to put an absolutised situation into perspective. The traditional complaint phrased metaphorically by the melancholic person would support that notion. The hopelessness is experienced as being inside a bottomless pit, without any hope of escape. This is also reflected in the field of subjective space (spatial awareness): the subject feels locked in, with the walls closing in on him, perhaps even crushing him. Thus, not only the theme of the 'future', but also that of the 'height' will lead to a homology among obsessive neurosis, narcissism and melancholy.

Finally, also the *paranoid* position is associated with a time-space problem, not in the domain of future or height, but with regard to 'present' and 'boundary'. We are referring to the traditional paranoia concept, which in classical psychopathological literature was distinguished from schizophrenia, and is today described as 'delusional disorder' (Radden, 2007). Therefore, this does not represent a paranoid type of schizophrenia. During a paranoid delusion the subject will feel pursued and wronged. He clings on to some past event which he expects to re-experience time and again. Life becomes an endless cycle in which the past continues into the future, unchanged. A 'short circuit' has occurred between past and future, with an elimination or implosion of the

[15] Von Gebsattel (1954, p. 2): "Ich muss unaufhörlich denken, dass die Zeit vergeht". The quotation continues as follows: "Während ich jetzt mit Ihnen spreche, denke ich bei jedem Wort: 'vorbei', 'vorbei', 'vorbei'". This sentence rather perfectly conveys the negativity 'contributed' by time.

present. The future becomes an identical copy of a frozen past. The distance created by the present, a result of the durative aspect that any present carries, has been reduced to zero. Like the decay of the future leaving the melancholic person trapped in the past, the paranoid person is at the mercy of the future which, with the present in decay, becomes a copy of the past. Ultimately this will lead to a decay of objective, external time as such and the subject falling prey to a quasi-linear time, without any personal involvement. The paranoid person has become prisoner of a linear time shaped like a closed circle. Rather than the constant loss of the melancholic, we see the constant recurrence of the immutable: what happens is always the same.

Just as the present, according to the traditional philosophy of time, has been represented as a 'boundary' ('*peras*'), i.e., between present and future, so the decay of the present is reflected spatially in the decay of the dimension of the delimited plane. Likewise, traditional psychopathology has often associated paranoia with 'delimitation': "This process of fading of boundaries, their degree of permeability and blurring may be referred to as *Entgrenzung*" (Kulenkampff, 1963, p. 204). Thus, not only the theme of the 'present' but also that of the 'boundary' will lead to a homology among phobia, the borderline position and paranoia.

SECOND LEVEL REVISITED: THE WORLD (RELATIONSHIP UNTO THE OTHER AND UNTO ONESELF)

The relationship unto the other and unto oneself creates another potential rapport. The world is structured not only by time and space, but also intersubjectively. We meet others and position ourselves relative to them, while in turn we become 'the other' to others. The relationship with the other and, consequently, with ourselves, can be regarded as another structuring moment for the world.

Intersubjectivity: Two Traditions

At a factual level, intersubjectivity takes the form of an interaction as well as dialogue (with the other and with oneself). This is the level addressed by Gadamer (1960/1985, p. 358), interpreting a conversation as a fusion of horizons between two participants (see Chapter Five). He thus presupposes the presence of subjects already individualised. The next question concerns the conditions of possibility of intersubjectivity rather than its factuality, leading us from Gadamer to Heidegger. With

Heidegger (1927/1962, section 26, pp.153-168) the subject, the '*Dasein*', is essentially solitary in nature. The other will only appear as a 'Being-with' ('*Mitsein*') of the 'Being-in-the world' ('*in-der-Welt-sein*'), as 'They'. The other merely occupies a subordinate position. This was the major objection raised by Binswanger against Heidegger's philosophy. In that respect, there is no essential difference with Husserl, because the latter also adopts a solipsistic viewpoint: The subject constitutes the world. To some degree, the other will appear as an empirical other, constituted by the subject, while partly functioning as a co-constituent. Husserl's complex theory of intersubjectivity – the analogical apperception – turns precisely on this aspect (Husserl, 1950/1970a, pp. 108-112, section 50).

Counterpoint to his solipsistic approach is the dialogical tradition in line with, e.g., Buber and Binswanger, which constitutes the other major tradition in the field of the philosophy intersubjectivity (Theunissen, 1984). Buber states: "*Ich werde am Du*", which thesis is problematic in itself, is self-contradictory. If we are not entitled to say that an 'I' exists before meeting a 'you', the 'I' will not become an 'I' unless in a relationship with 'you'. And yet, the concept of 'meeting' presupposes the autonomy of two subjects

Wittgenstein may help us break this deadlock, namely through his criticism of the impossibility of a private language (Wittgenstein, 1958/1963, §§ 244-266). The point made here is that anything that applies to me alone would lose its validity even to me, because any validity would then be forfeited. Indeed, anyone who would aspire to think about himself from a point given to himself only, would fail to end up with himself. Thought, perception and action presuppose a publicly accessible entity, viz., language and culture, which is sustained by the Other manifesting itself as a collection of others. This point has been raised before, in Chapter Six.

Imaginary and Symbolic Relationships

Lacan can provide a useful addition in this respect: This primacy of language, of Otherness and the Other, is also expressed in the life-historical perspective (Homer, 2005; Bailly, 2009; Levine, 2008). Initially, a child cannot identify with 'itself', the 'self' still being a void; instead it identifies with an image of itself offered by the outside world – the first image being its mirror image (Lacan, 1966/2002, pp. 93-81). This identification process is mediated by the image and is therefore referred to as imaginary. It is also imaginary because it is fictitious, producing an image of wholeness and unity that is beyond the child's grasp. This connection with unity and grandeur gives the imaginary identification a narcissistic twist. The child imagines itself to be greater and more powerful that it actually is and, seeing itself as a unified entity, denies its own dependence on others. The relationship with others is also narcissistic, mirroring in nature. Feelings of grandeur and rivalry are typical of this type of relationship, with the other being mimicked, representing a mirror-image other: an imaginary, little other, an 'other-similar' (Nobus, 1998; Thieberge, 1999; Widmer, 2006; Nasio, 2007).

Rather than being confined to early childhood, this pattern of mirrored relationships will be at the heart of any relationship following a pattern of imitation or 'mimesis' (Girard, 1986). Thus the imaginary dimension seems to be a constant in human relationships. In any situation where people mirror's each other behaviour, we recognise an imaginary or dual relationship pattern. The other becomes an other-similar ('*autre-semblable*') or a second powerful Other, in regard of which the subject becomes dependent and submissive, in order not to lose attention, love or admiration.

The transition from a dual, dyadic to a triangular, triadic relational pattern constitutes a new step. Its developing proceeds in a synchronous (simultaneous) rather than a diachronous (sequential) fashion. In fact, we are dealing with two steps, similar to the time and space issue: a pre-symbolic and a symbolic phase. A first step is entering the exteriority of language, – which step is partly imaginary, mimetic in nature or is, at least, supported by the imaginary. The process of learning to speak, of internalizing the exteriority of language by mimicking the Other's speech, brings the child into a position of submission to the Other, to language of the Other (Otherness). Lacan (1973/1986, pp. 203-212) refers to this as 'alienation'. At the same time, by speaking and symbolizing, a distance is created towards an immediate presence (of physical reality, of the primordial other and oneself) and all associated enjoyment (*Jouissance*). It transforms the real into a world that is also shaped by language, holding subjects that abide by rules of language and action. The acknowledgment of this state of affairs and the acknowledgment of the rules as being rules (and not commands), constitute the second step. Lacan (1973/1986, pp. 203-212) speaks of 'separation': In fact there is no commanding Other, the Other itself is lacking, is deficient; there is no ultimate, guarantee nor guarantor for the validity of rules; there is no 'Other of the Other' (Richardson, 1983). These acknowledgments signify the transition from the first step, 'the entry in language' – initially supported by the imaginary – to the second step – supported by a true insight in the very nature of the symbolic.

Where a dual relation pattern typifies the order of the imaginary, the symbolic order is defined by a triangular relational pattern. Here the relationship between both parties is determined by a third term (a rule or law) governing the interaction between parties, similar to rules of a game structuring relationships between participants without imposing them (Mooij, 1991). More specifically: There is a difference between parents and children, between men and women – a sexual and generational difference, which will turn out to be decisive. There is a Law, the Law-of-the-Father, the Name-of-the Father, dictating that a mother should *not* engage in a type of exclusive relationship with her child (Mooij, 1975/2001, pp. 134-147; Mooij, 1993; Nasio, 2005, pp. 30-96; Verhaeghe, 2009).[16] The same applies to the child. This step constitutes the second moment of the paternal metaphor: It should *not* have an exclusive relationship with his or her mother, with the primary Other, it is not entitled to have or to be 'everything' to the (m)Other – metaphorically spoken: to be her 'imaginary phallus', the child trying to fill the lack in the (m)Other perceived in her absence. This position constitutes the first moment of the paternal metaphor, to be relinquished by the second moment, the second step: the decisive acceptance of the lack, while giving it a symbolic-phallic signature. This new position arrived at enables desires (supported by a phantasm) and future-oriented ideals to come into being. The inaugural renunciation of the immediate presence has now been sealed by establishing these supportive psychic configurations. Without eliminating the imaginary dimension, it is put into perspective, turning the Other into more than just the 'other-similar', an 'other-peer' (or an imaginary other): an Other that is potentially different and essential.

The above use of the word 'phases' may be somewhat misleading. as the symbolic dimension is not only introduced at a later point in time, but also underlies the imaginary dimension. Indeed, its very first manifestation is the Other acknowledging the child "That is you" (Lacan, 1966/2002, p. 568; Le Gaufey, 1997, pp. 81-105). That is what defines the 'primacy of the other' within the sphere of intersubjectivity.

---

[16] Lacan (1966/2002, p. 485): "[...] the Name-of-the Father [...] being the signifier which, in the Other, qua locus of the signifier, is the signifier of the Other qua locus of the law".

It makes that the 'relationship towards the other and towards oneself', this second dimension of the world, is best discussed combined with the issue of the desire from the third level: that of language and the lack, and the possibility to reflect. The distinction between imaginary and symbolic relationships, between dual and triangular relationships, will emerge as a matter of course.

THIRD LEVEL: LANGUAGE, THE LACK AND THE LAW

As was demonstrated, the introduction of language, renouncing the primordial condition, brings renunciation of an immediate presence and an associated 'complete' and impossible enjoyment (Braunstein, 2003). Human desire is shaped as part of this trajectory in which man distances himself from some immediacy or immediate pleasure, going down a road of postponement and longing, taking account of the pleasures of others, of the prevailing rules and the Law. This road is defined by 'how' he distances himself from this original enjoyment as well as 'the degree to which' he distances himself from it.

'How' he distances himself is expressed in the 'morsels of pleasure' which he has preserved from this great all-embracing enjoyment, storing them in his inner being and constructing a mould that will only fit those elements that produce pleasure. Lacan coined the phrase 'phantasm' to describe this construct, defining it as the subjective structure of desire that determines what can be desired and what produces a feeling of pleasure or, more generally, a sense of purpose. Thus a phantasm will structure both the affective world of perception and the relational world, as the framework of the phantasm will define what is meaningful within this world, and what particular ties with the relational world are considered valid.[17]

There is also a 'degree to which' one can distance oneself. It leaves its mark on the subject position, not primarily with respect to the phantasm's content, but in a formal way. This distance may be ideal, in which case we find ourselves in the field or 'bandwidth' of normality, shaped by the neurotic position. We recognise a structure of desire, supported by a phantasm that effectively keeps immediate enjoyment at bay. This distance can be medial, undermining the structure of desire as a result of immediate enjoyment manifesting itself, taking the shape of

---

[17] Lacan (1966/2002, p. 487, n. 14): "[...] the field of the reality [...] is sustained only by the extraction of object *a*, which nevertheless gives it its frame".

enjoyment of the Other that needs to be served. This is the field of the personality disorder. Then again, the distance may become too small, resulting in the subject being possibly overwhelmed by a reality from which he cannot distance himself. This constitutes the psychotic structure, lacking the unity that would produce the phantasm, which creates the need for a remedy, a social or a psychic supplement or support ('*sinthome*') (Lacan, 2005) to prevent actual psychotic decompensation.[18]

However, the content of an individual phantasmatic figure ('the how'), if present, is defining and specific for this highly particular subject. In other words, it does not lend itself to specifying a psychopathological structure, as opposed to the 'degree' to which the subject distances itself from immediate enjoyment in the case of a neurosis or normality, personality disorder and psychosis. These disorders will be discussed within the framework of desire, without making reference to individually different phantasmatic figurations. It should be noticed, once again, that the description of psychopathological structures and positions is merely of an ideal-typical nature. A particular psychopathological structure or position may not be found in a pure form, but a structural outline does offer a framework that allows a coherent organisation and interpretation of psychopathological phenomena. Also in this case, the table in the Appendix outlining the psychopathological structures may be elucidating.

NEUROSIS: ACKNOWLEDGEMENT OF THE LACK

The neurosis falls within the contours of normality, in that no fundamental disruption of the relationship between the subject and the world occurs (as opposed to the Psychotic structure), but that it is characterised by an undue emphasis on one or more structural components. The status of the desire with an inherent lack is still intact, but the this lack can be maintained, but in a variety of ways (see also Dor, 1997; Fink, 1997; Julien, 2000; Schokker and Schokker, 2000; Soler, 1998; Van Haute, 2001; Vergote, 1980; Verhaeghe, 2008).

---

[18] One may argue that Lacan later on, in the 1970s, even seems to have abandoned the concept of 'phantasm' in favour of that of '*sinthome*' (Morel, 2008, pp. 39-54). Yet these psychic formations appear rather to be complementary, providing a degree of separation (neurosis) or offering a remedy in case of a basic failure in establishing separation (psychosis).

Traditionally, the *hysterical* or histrionic position has been characterised by spurious and egotistical behaviour, associated with symptoms expressing impotence or faintness, e.g., psychogenic paralysis and dissociation (including various type of consciousness loss). The hysterical person is focused on other people, aiming at getting attention using theatrical means, in an egocentric way. Consequently, the world of the hysterical person is 'populated': the subject observes and wishes to be observed, thus expressing a voyeuristic and exhibitionist trait. There is an urge to kindle desire within the other, in order for him to desire the subject in turn. The objective is to stress the lack in the other prompting this desire, to 'seduce' the other. The subject's desire is the other's desire, causing the other to desire him or her: Am I desirable to him, am I desirable to her? It highlights the theme of sexual differentiation, a prominent one in the hysteric's mind. What defines being a 'man', or a 'woman', what does it mean to be a 'woman to a man', 'a man to a woman'? What exactly is an ideal man, an ideal woman?

There is a desire for perfection (a perfect man or woman that must exist somewhere), which is of course bound to lead to disappointment and lasting dissatisfaction with what one is or may hope to get (Miller, 2011, pp. 141-147, 150-159). It defines the hysterical person's desire as a desire for a desire that can never be satisfied (Lacan, 1966/2002, pp. 521-524; 1998, pp. 355-370). Rather than deny the lack that is inherent in desire, the person nourishes it, be it in a specific manner. This comes at a price, because the subject, being focused on the desire for him or her, pays little heed to its own deeper desires. This may result in a lasting 'identity weakness', manifesting itself in what the other perceives as 'spuriousness'.

The *obsessive* or compulsive neurotic position is dominated by a different strategy aimed at maintaining desire. The other is not seduced, but is controlled. Typical character traits are order, perfectionism and control, sometimes extended with compulsive actions or thoughts, and excessive doubt. The conscientious attitude points to the presence of strict ethics, possibly dominated by feelings of guilt. The subject imposes strict ethics on both itself and the other, allowing very little leeway. As a result, the world of the obsessive person is sparsely populated. What is asked of the other, is also asked of oneself. The strategy focuses on transforming the unpredictable nature of (the other's and the subject's own) desire into the predictability of a formulated demand (i.e., the demands made on oneself or on the other). Full anticipation and control counteracts desire, while obscuring one's own lack as well the other's.

Preferably, an impossibility is pointed out – this or that cannot or should not be done. It defines the obsessive person's desire as a desire for a desire that is impossible (Lacan, 1966/2002, pp. 526-527; 1998, pp. 405-421). Highlighting impossibilities means maintaining both the desire and the lack, be it in a highly specific manner, not by going down the road of dissatisfaction, as in the case of hysterics, but by pursuing an impossible desire. This strategy also comes at a price. By merely intending to receive desire in the form of a demand, both the other's desire and one's own desire is suppressed. The associated aggressive tendency that includes sadistic feelings must not become patent, because this would make the desire overly explicit. It may lead to (auto-)sadistic processing, with inward directed aggression and, and to auto-sadistic fantasies. This discord in regard of one's own aggression leads to an inner contradiction that has a paralysing effect on the subject, which can be typified as doubting, overbearing and forceful – compulsive, in other words.

The *phobic* or avoiding position is cognate with obsessive behaviour, while also having distinguishing characteristics. From the present perspective, the difference is that in the case of obsessional neurosis, the conflict-ridden relationship with desire is played out predominantly at an internal level (only to be externalised as a next step), where the phobic person experiences danger as coming primarily from the outside world. The character is defined by the urge to avoid contact with others, whilst simultaneously submitting oneself to their judgment. This may include symptoms such as panic attacks and specific phobias, such as agoraphobia or claustrophobia. The urge to avoid people is often prompted by feelings of inferiority towards others. A 'moral masochistic' element, as phrased by Freud, can also be discerned: "Don't pay any attention to me, just ignore me, I'm not important".

The strategy focuses on submission to the other, to ensure that the other will have no demands to make and thus will not pose a danger. In the process, it is not denied that the other lacks something and wishes contact, but the contact with the other is fragile and critical. Anxiety is caused by being at the centre of attention (as in agoraphobia), being unable to leave (in the case of claustrophobia), or revealing one's own desires (erythrophobia, fear of blushing).

In the process, the other's desire and the subject itself are respected and maintained, be it in a specific manner, namely by avoiding the other. Making himself subservient to the other will kindle a desire, yet the subject will negate both himself and his desire. And if he wishes something for himself, he will express his wish preferably as something inevitable, in order to obscure his own desire as much as possible. In this case, the desire is for an inevitable desire.[19] This strategy also has a downside. The act of submission to the other, as a defence against the unpredictable nature of the other's desire, will effectively erase his own desire. It will make the subject feel small, dependent, inferior and frightened, leaving him with a 'hollow' feeling, which may lead to the development of phobic symptoms or transient paranoid reactions.

Explanation

Lacan's theory may actually lend theoretical support to this tripartite distinction between hysteria, obsessive neurosis and phobia. The symbolic order exposes basic positions which, at their most general level, reflect sexual and generation differences: male/female, parent/child. This difference is defined by the common denominator of 'phallus'. From this perspective, the symbolic order becomes 'phallic'. Apparently, an unifying principle exists for men, but not for women. From it follows, we could say: "*La femme n'existe pas*", "The Woman does not exist". Moreover, the symbolic does not reflect any natural fixed order, and so there is no such thing as a natural orientation of men towards women, or women towards men. From this follows: "*Il n'y pas de rapport sexuel*", "There is no sexual relationship". In the final analysis, the symbolic order becomes arbitrary, there are no guarantees. Consequently, we could say that there is no Other of the Other: "*Il n'y a pas l'Autre de l'Autre*" or "*L'Autre n'existe pas*". "The Other does not exist". They represent three basic propositions of the symbolic order, and we might assume that each of the three neurotic subjective positions refutes one basic proposition, their pathological content depending on a specific refusal. The hysterical position refutes "*La femme n'existe pas*": an ideal woman *does* exist. The obsessive position refutes the "*Il n'y a pas de rapport sexuel*": there *is* order, not chaos. Finally, the phobic position rejects the requirement of autonomy as an implication of "*L'Autrė n'existe pas*":

---

[19] Commonly, Lacan limits himself to introducing a dichotomy (hysteria and compulsive neurosis); the position of the phobia may vary. In his earlier work he referred to phobia as a distinct and equal figure (Lacan, 1966/2002, p. 88, 432), but later he will abandon that (Lacan, 2006, p. 307). See also Fink (1997, pp. 116, 163-164). This definition of the desire of the phobic position is not found with Lacan, but is instead derived from an analogy with the hysteric and obsessive positions.

the Other *does* exist, and he is supposed to tell me what is good for me. By the same token, this theme is also reflected in associated disorders. Take for example the problematic relationship with 'the' woman in the case of perversion, or the '*pousse à la femme*' in schizophrenia (see below); the issue or order within psychopathy and melancholy; or the dependency problems seen in borderline position and paranoia.

To the extent that this manifestation of the symbolic represents the symbolic order of modernity based on the third proposition ('*L'Autre n'existe pas*'), we might say that defining 'dependence' as a pathology is a typically 'modern' manoeuvre which is not likely to work with premodern cultures. This points to the cultural relativity of at least this type of psychiatric disorder (the avoiding personality disorder, the borderline personality).

PERSONALITY DISORDER: DISAVOWAL OF THE LACK

The field of the personality disorder will get a more detailed discussion here – compared to that of neurosis – and a widening scope will be provided. Indeed, the traditional Lacanian perspective is limiting this field to perversion only (as was mentioned before). Yet perversion will retain a basic position, the other positions (narcissistic and borderline) being interpreted as its modification. Generally spoken, in the case of the personality disorder, the lack is neither masked nor emphasised – in which case it is presupposed – but is both acknowledged and not acknowledged – it is 'disavowed'. First of all, this leads to a specific relationship towards the Law. The person knows about the Law, but does not draw conclusions from it, is not willing to pay the price. He both acknowledges and disavows the Law: it can be mocked (perversion), broken (narcissistic position) or obscured (borderline position). The Law, the fundamental Law, refers to the gender difference, which in this case brings a splitting in the attitude towards sexual difference, which is acknowledged but also not acknowledged. This is reflected in the relationship towards pleasure which, in this case is not phallically related to a gender difference. Instead it takes a more primordial form of enjoyment (connected with anxiety and death), more closely related to a forbidden, impossible *Jouissance*. The experience of this primordial type of enjoyment as 'forbidden' (and by that as inviting to be transgressed) and not as simply 'being impossible', constitutes already a 'pathological' interpretation, this type of enjoyment being characterized by its impossibility in essence. The subjective position also differs from that of the neurosis, characterised as it is by a penchant for an object-position leading to desubjectification (depersonalisation, feelings of emptiness). This concerns the third and last consequence of the disavowal of the lack. This bias towards the object-position, turning away from a subject-position, will disrupt any intersubjective relationship. It is reflected in the social domain which, contrary to the neurotic case, is problematic in the case of the personality disorder, as it often includes an antisocial component (impulsiveness, lack of control, not taking responsibility, externalizing).

The *perverse* position is associated with abnormal sexual behaviour (paraphilia), but such behaviour does not necessarily point to the presence of a perverse position, as was discussed in the above. It would be appropriate to distinguish between a perverse position on the one hand, and 'perverse traits' (André, 1993; Clavreul, 1980; Freud, 1991) or 'perversities', as these manifestations may well be called, considering that they may occur with all other positions associated with each of the two other structures (neurotic *and* psychotic). Commonly, perverse traits are part of the neurotic position, as was demonstrated before. However, a perverse position means that the perverse theme pervades the person's life, at every level of the subjective position. Its character is essentially perverse, is dominated by a perverse theme, not merely limiting itself to a sexual scenario. A sexual component may even be absent: For example, certain types of swindle or fraud are instigated by a perverse position of the perpetrator.

We already saw that perversion is found on the side of hysteria, but in this case the disturbed relationship with the other is taken one step further – more than just seduce the other, the subject will attempt to 'break' him or her. The pervert is going 'too far' in seducing the other, causing the relationship to be defined by 'betrayal'. Firstly, because of the choice for an object-position, the burden of subjectivity (dividedness, desire) will be on the side of the other. The other will feel abused subjectively, but the strategy focuses on getting the other to collaborate, turning him into an accomplice who chose his own fate: "She said 'yes'", "She asked for it", "She actually enjoyed it". This may be happening only in the person's imagination and in a distorted perception or even in reality, as in the case of swindle. A desire is foisted on the person being tricked, a desire that may be far removed from his own true desire, but which he nonetheless appropriates with time and which he supports. This may turn him into a accomplice of something he also rejects. The desire in this configuration is not absent, but finds itself predominantly on the side of the other. The perverse subject rather positions itself as a non-desiring subject, as a mere instrument geared towards fulfilling the Other's enjoyment (Lacan, 2006, p. 185).

As a consequence – the second characteristic of perversion – the emphasis is no longer on desire but on immediate enjoyment, in relation to the primordial Other (which desire is supposed to keep at arm's length). As opposed to the psychotic case, however, the subject is not overwhelmed by this enjoyment but actually seeks it out (Lacan, 1966/2002, pp. 645-670; 1994, pp. 95-150; 2006, pp. 247-264). It is the enjoyment of the Other that has to be served: 'sexual service of the mother' (Lacan, 1966/2002, p. 723). This has two consequences. Serving the Other's enjoyment implicitly cuts the subject off from its own (phallic) pleasure: this brings anger. Next to it, serving the Other's enjoyment – and the intrusion of the Other – will make any degree of dependency threatening, whilst offering the opportunity of abuse. This causes anxiety (brought on by uncomfortably close proximity). Thus, the enjoyment of the Other and the servitude need to be directed, to be staged. Feelings of sexual enjoyment, not being connected to sexual difference anymore, are closely tied to anger and anxiety. This explains its great intensity of sexual enjoyment, making it existentially far more significant than in the neurotic case, regardless of its varieties. The Other may be embodied by the actual other, the partner, but may also be unconnected to him, being the 'cause of the Other' whose needs are served by the subject: Its greatness needs to be both honoured and supported (Lacan 2006, p. 253). The pervert may act as a true believer, as a fundamentalist providing succour and attributing infallibility to the Other whom he serves (God, Allah, Freedom of speech).

The relationship to the Law is also characterised by a split: it is acknowledged and not-acknowledged. This is a third characteristic. There may be a third person lurking in the shadow, an impotent spectator, sometimes a game has be played with the authorities, who are being fooled. The Law also is directed and has to be staged. The overall picture is dominated by *splitting* (in respect of the lack, the Law, the gender difference, the subject position) in perversion, which supports the intermediate position of perversion between neurosis and psychosis.[20]

---

[20] This 'object character' of the pervert in relationship building is strongly emphasised by Lacan, which seems to be a fortunate choice. Cf. Lacan (1966/2002, pp. 653-654) and Lacan (2004, p. 222, 255). The distinction between the 'subject character' of the neurotic position and the 'object character' of the perverse position corresponds to the

The *narcissistic* position or, rather, the position of the narcissistic personality disorder, offers a modification of the disruption of subjective relationships which, in this case, is in line with the theme of obsession, only as its opposite or counterpart. Rather than a temptation developing into a – sometimes enacted – rape, it represents control developing into enforcement, with excess of control resulting in a disruption of preservation of order, which the obsessive person is looking for. While narcissism is in line with obsession, it also represents its inversion (its perversion).

In this case, the lack is both acknowledged and not acknowledged – a general characteristic of a personality disorder. The narcissistic personality disorder expresses itself as a disavowal of one's own insignificance which is transferred to the other, thus turning him into the main carrier of suffering, of subjectivity. Again, the perpetrator is not functioning as a 'subject', but rather as an object, a walking instrument that, e.g., during a robbery, derives its power from carrying a gun, which is supposed to put fear into the other in order to turn him into the carrier of subjectivity. The subject is attacked by a perpetrator, by an 'object' that forces something upon the subject, in this case against the will of the subject itself. This type of 'frightening and intimidating' experience can be seen in less dramatic situations as well, as in the case of a narcissistic manager bullying his staff. In both cases the narcissist forces the other (the victim, his subordinate) to perform actions it would never have done voluntarily, but which the other does nonetheless, who is afterwards left with feelings of embarrassment and shame for having committed or undergone them. The breaking of the social bond does not involve the mode of betrayal – as in the case of perversion – but the mode of violence.

Next to it, the centre of gravity, not being tied to enjoyment, is about grandiosity. In Freudian terms: the main theme is not libido, but narcissism. The ideals are highly ambitious, mirroring self-overrating, and are not accompanied by the realization that they need to be fulfilled at some point in the future. They take the form of 'having already been fulfilled' – which may mask an excessively low self-esteem. They do not represent (symbolic) ego-ideals, but are a manifestation of an

---

traditional distinction between what is sometimes referred to as the 'autoplastistic' type of neurosis, and the 'heteroplastic' type of the personality disorder: the neurotic person is suffering himself (being on the side of subjectivity), the person with the personality disorder will cause the other to suffer (on whose side subjectivity is found).

(imaginary) ideal-ego. Indeed, the aim is to deny one's own lack or insignificance, which realization is yet not entirely absent but is obscured by feelings of grandiosity (Kohut, 1971).

Once again, the Law is broken in the process – the Law is acknowledged, but only in part, in a specific way. This is the third characteristic, with the value of the Law being minimized, played down. It brings a disruption of intersubjective relationships, charging the victim with dividedness, subjectivity and anxiety to the point where it will succumb. A variety of the perverse position can be recognised here, taking the form of desexualised perversion or 'desexualised sadism' (like sadism plays a parallel role as 'perverse trait' in obsessional neurosis). Enjoyment is acquired, but it lacks a sexual content: the enjoyment looked for involves violence.

Excurs on psychopathy. How should we define the relationship between the narcissistic personality disorder and psychopathy (Cleckley, 1941/1976; Hare, 1991)? Rather than represent a position, psychopathy refers to a variation on the position of the narcissistic personality disorder (a strongly inflated self-esteem) with a strong tendency towards manipulation and intimidation. The type of psychopathy proposed by Hare – PCL-R score > 30 points – would then reflect a low-level personality functioning (strongly dominated by a lack of control, impulsive behaviour, externalisation, etc.). This comparatively rare variety can be conceived as psychopathy version 1. In addition, another high-level variety might be distinguished (not being highlighted by Hare): the psychopathic manager, the property developer, etc. – who causes great damage but still succeeds in escaping prosecution for tangible crimes: psychopathy version 2. Finally, there are so-called 'psychopathic traits' – reflecting a PCL-R score of 20-30 – that, in light of these relevant facts, might better be described as anti-social traits. This concept of 'psychopathic traits' – psychopathy version 3 – is comparable to that of 'perverse traits', 'neuroticism', 'alexithymia', etc.

The *borderline* position is characterised by an intricate relationship between the subject and the other, occurring in line with the phobic theme, be it as its opposite. The phobic position will cause the subject to see the other as a threat or danger, while also attributing him or her responsibility for the subject's well-being. However, individual responsibility, which is still present in the position of a phobia, is denied in the borderline position. The type of bond that takes the form of 'I depend on you/ you are responsible for me' of the phobic position is replaced by the bond type defined as 'I am yours/you are mine'. The distance maintained in the phobic position tends to disappear in the borderline position, thus offering an inversion (perversion) of the phobic theme.

The lack is disavowed in the sense that it is both acknowledged and not acknowledged. It is acknowledged in that the subject is willing to fill the lack with the other – recognizing the existence of a lack. Then again, the lack is not acknowledged as the subject thinks he is capable of filling the lack entirely, so that a world without a lack may exist. The objective is for the person to make himself small, transforming himself into an object while turning the other into a subject that can be made whole: The choice for an object-position is recognizable in this case of personality disorder as well. Once again, the issue of desire (and its inherent unfulfillable quality) yields to that of enjoyment – the Other's enjoyment. It makes itself subservient to the Other's enjoyment.

Consequently – representing a second characteristic – the centre of gravity in this case is neither sexual enjoyment nor narcissism but the relationship towards the Other, in a search for (non-)separation, whilst being in itself another manifestation of the enjoyment of the Other. The strategy is different from that of perversion ('staging and betrayal') or of narcissism ('intimidation and violence') and takes the form of 'entanglement and power'. Indeed, power is a major factor here also. To the extent that the other can be made whole and his need is satisfied, he becomes omnipotent. And yet this position of omnipotence is bestowed by the complementing subject in order to give the subject, in its turn, power over the other. This power is tied to the restriction that the subject is capable of exercising power only in the role of complementing object. Thus, both can imprison each other in a dual or symbiotic stranglehold, playing out a struggle for power, constantly switching between roles: powerful or powerless person, tormentor or victim.

The Law requiring separation is alternately acknowledged and denied, being concealed, covered up, in a relationship of enmeshment. This is the third characteristic. It reflects a masochistic theme, which does not merely take the form of an enacted fantasy or demonstrable character trait – as a 'perverse trait' presenting itself in the phobic position – but of a full-blown manifestation, the borderline position and the phobic position being connected by the theme of masochism. As in the case of narcissism, we may speak of a variety of the perverse position: In the borderline position, the variety is not defined by 'desexualized sadism' but by 'desexualised masochism'. The subject is making itself dependent on the other, handing itself over to the other completely. Indeed, the aim is to deny one's own limitations, thus enabling boundlessness and excessiveness to take over (Mooij, 2010, pp. 75-93).

PSYCHOSIS: FORECLOSURE OF THE LACK

The psychosis differs fundamentally from the psychopathological structures discussed before, in the sense that the structure-giving subjectivity referred to in the foregoing (limitedness, desire, dividedness) in those cases is acknowledged, at least in part. In the case of the psychotic structure, this quality of the subject itself is compromised, as was already demonstrated in the discussion of the topic of space and time: the elimination of a human, finite form space and time – as a result of the decay of the dimensional, symbolic space and time (spatiality, temporality). Parallel to this, the relationship with the other is upset in a more fundamental way compared to the structures previously discussed. Whether or not there actually is another, is irrelevant – there always is. The real question is whether there is a 'space' in which the other can appear. To fulfil that condition, figuratively speaking there needs to be at least one 'vacant chair' or 'empty spot' to be occupied by an actual other.

The modality of being-in-the-world as being with others is absent, its self-evident nature is lost, or needs to be rebuilt or reclaimed, as it were, with every encounter. If the other makes his presence known, however – despite the fact that there is no 'empty spot' in which he can appear in his limited guise – the subject will find himself at the mercy of a superiorly omnipotent other. As opposed to the case of the neurotic person or the person with a personality disorder, the other will appear without any lack whatsoever, as a result of which the subject cannot possibly escape him during his paranoid delusion or hallucination. The corresponding subjective position would be the loss of one's own position in respect of the other's position. To some extent the subject will lose his hold on itself, its 'inner anchor', finding itself thrown at the mercy of the omnipotent other. Blankenburg (1971) speaks of a loss of '*Selbststand*'. Summarising this in Lacanian terms, the psychotic structure is characterised by a fragmented and incoherent body image (a deficient imaginary), by an impaired differentiation towards the mother as primary symbolic Other and a weakening of the Law (symbolic deficiency), and, at a bodily and real level, by maintenance of the *object a*, not being lost (Lacan, 1966/2002, pp. 445-488; 1993; 2005, pp. 77-91).

Within the *schizophrenic* position, this tenuous relationship with the other, particularly its symptomless form, manifests itself as a form of autism, characterised by a frail contact with the other rather than by a shunning of contact. The social connection is lacking or is minimal at best. This leads to a loss of self-evidence, a characterising trait of this condition. This point was discussed before, from the viewpoint of *intentionality*, with reference to a dysfunctional operative intentionality – a disorder of self-awareness accompanied by compensatory hyper-reflection. It was then elaborated using a *temporal* approach, the past, the 'having-been' being lost. Now, within the framework of the *inter-subjectivity* theme, it will again be explained, for the third time, conceiving this lack of self-evidence as a disturbed interpretation of human relationship as well as impaired practical knowledge (Stanghellini, 2007, p. 141). Obviously, a close mutual connection exists among these three levels.

Importantly, the relationship with the person's own body is impaired. Indeed, the body is the incarnation of subjectiveness, like the subjectiveness is corporeal. The dysfunctional relationship with the body as body proper corresponds to what has been described, in respect of the spatial relationship, as a state of deficiency of the central perspective, of the '*moi-ici*' (in Minskowski's sense). As mentioned before, this '*ipseity*' disorder and this concept of a weakened '*moi-ici*' may be considered to be equivalent to Lacan's concept of a deficient imaginary ego, a deficient '*moi*', as in the case of psychosis in Lacanian terms. This deficiency, phrased in different terms, leads to a fragmentation of the experienced unity of the body, resulting in haphazard actions, insofar as these actions require an intact relationship with corporeal subjectiveness (Soenen and Corveleyn, 2003). The body proper and its sphere define the boundaries with the outside world. In addition to a fragmentation of the body image, a blurring of the boundaries between body and outside world may result. This facilitates a kind of 'transitivism', a state in which the subject will actually feel what is happening in the outside world. Because there is no separation or distinction, the formative meaning of the sexual difference may also be lost. This may manifest itself in 'feminization' (with male patients) or a '*pousse à la femme*'.[21] This may be conceived as a perverse trait, here within the framework of a psychosis – which might equalized with perverse traits in neurosis (in line with the hysterical position, where

[21] Lacan (1966/2002, p. 472): "[...] unable to be the phallus the mother is missing, there remained the solution of being the woman that men are missing".

gender difference also plays a key role, obviously in a neurotic way). Essentially we see a non-operative or minimal function of the lack, which results in a loss of distance between the subject and his world, increasingly exposing the subject to a mentally unprocessed and non-symbolised reality.

Whenever difference and, consequently, the lack are absent, a special relationship with guilt will emerge. If there is no room for the lack to appear, it becomes non-existent and so the lack – in the form of a default – cannot be appropriated. In a sense, the subject is incapable of assuming responsibility and therefore cannot be held accountable, and so in all fairness we cannot attribute guilt for any behaviour, particularly felonies, when originating from a psychotic condition rooted in a schizophrenic position – in line with common legal practice in most countries.

Within the *melancholic* position the guilt theme also comes into play, be it differently. Indeed, the guilt theme becomes even predominant. The significance of the guilt can be explained most effectively on the basis of the time issue, as was demonstrated before. If the future is not accessible, then there is no way to return to the past from it. What has happened in the past, cannot be viewed in a different way and therefore cannot be revised. The guilt is fixed and unredeemable.

The guilt can also be approached from an intersubjective angle, the angle of desire. The subject's coming into being can be imagined, as previously discussed, as a renunciation of immediacy and immediate enjoyment, enabling a life characterised by distance between subject and other, and by a lack supporting the desire. It enables a life with the inherent pain of existence ('*douleur d'exister*'), imbued with melancholy, because of what 'was lost'. This 'bonne melancholie', this 'good melancholy' (Juranville, 2005, p. 17, 35) or 'capacité dépressive', 'depressive capacity' (Fédida, 2001, p. 16, 52, 73) suggests that through the mediation of symbolization a loss was suffered which, to a certain extent, will help shield the subject from the real losses that life will bring.

However, if this fundamental loss was *not* accepted, the subject will find it hard or even impossible to accept any loss (of a person, a person's love, or a function) – hard though that may turn out to be if there is a 'capacity for depression'. The impossibility to deal with this loss, in turn, will lead to a pain of existence in a pure state – '*douleur d'exister à l'état pur*' (Lacan, 1966/2002, p. 656) or a melancholy in its more specific meaning, to be distinguished from the '*douleur d'exister*' associated with life itself. Some evil had occurred to bring about this loss, with the melancholic person making a strategic choice by taking the blame: He himself is guilty, unworthy of life. Moreover, the unmediated enjoyment, part of which has been left unrenounced, is seated in the melancholic himself, following the same strategy. This destructive enjoyment will bring about aggression turned against the subject itself, leading to self-destruction and possibly even suicide, taking the form of extreme auto–sadism.

The *paranoid* position is often viewed as the very opposite of melancholy. The melancholic person will blame himself, while the paranoid person blames the other: 'the paranoid accuser and the melancholic self-accuser' (Soler, 1990, p. 37). The paranoid person will answer the same question as does the melancholic person (about the evil that brought about a loss), but their answers are opposed. The melancholic person will appropriate the mistake, but the paranoid person as a victim will point the finger at the other, the persecutor, the alleged source of his suffering. It reflects a masochistic trait in the field of psychosis.

And while the melancholy person appropriates the immediate enjoyment that causes him to pursue himself, the paranoid person will transfer this enjoyment to the other pursuing him. Thus melancholy and paranoia can in fact be opposed, while their opposite qualities can also be put into perspective. They share the non-acceptance or highly limited acceptance of an original lack or loss, because the connected symbolic function controlling separation and distinction is either ineffective or non-operative. This also constitutes a common foundation for the three types of psychosis, with the differences – seen from the present viewpoint – manifesting themselves in the way the guilt issue is dealt with: non-accountability (schizophrenic position), being overwhelmed by an unredeemable guilt (melancholic position) and transferring the – equally unredeemable – guilt to the other (paranoid position).

THE SYMBOLIC FUNCTION

The other presented himself to us as a person to be seduced, controlled or avoided, in the field of neurosis; as a person who should be broken, kept down or incorporated, in the field of personality disorder; or, finally, as a person who, from a psychotic position, simply cannot appear in a delimited form. This describes the three grades of separation, or the three grades of separation defining the relationship between the subject and the other.

Recapitulation. Speaking of grades of separation refers to the second, transcendental sphere – not that of the actual structure of a particular world (the empirical sphere) – of the neurosis, of the personality disorder or psychosis – but of the structuring principle to shape a world. The underlying thought would be that the symbolic function enables both separation and distinction, bringing a loss of a state of immediate presence and its associated enjoyment (*Jouissance*), related to (1) an immediate presence to external reality (the real outside man), (2) to the primordial other and (3) and to oneself, including the own body, the organism (the real inside man).The symbolic function serves to transform this triple immediacy into a time-space world, into intersubjectivity and into a body-subject that is not overwhelmed by *Jouissance* but is capable of intentional involvements, of reflection and desire as well as a limited level of (phallic) pleasure. Indeed, separation and symbolization go hand in hand. They result in an autonomous subject, a temporal-spatial world and subjective dividedness – enabling the subject to engage into a relationship with others, while distancing himself from himself, allowing both self-reflection and freedom to exist. Three themes require elaboration here.

Self. A particular type of distance involves the subject's state of autonomy. From the physiological body, made up of meaningless arousals, imbued with raw *Jouissance*, a body-subject emerges that is capable of engaging in intentional relationships, at reflexive but initially pre-reflexive level.

Time. Symbolization will also relate to the external environment – the second form of distance. The real is transformed into a temporal-spatial world that functions as the subject's object of focus, with the symbolic function ensuring (through the symbolic forms of space and time) sustained involvement of the subject with the world.

Reflection. Next to a separation between world and the real, a split occurs within the subject itself. Once a name and qualities have been attributed to the subject, it distinguishes itself from others receiving a different name and different qualities. Symbolisation, naming, brings separation between the subject and the other – the third form of distance. However, the subject does not actually become one with his symbolisations (identifications, interpretations). If he were to become one, fully coinciding with his symbolisations, the subject would become frozen, fixed, immutable. For the very reason that the subject fails to coincide with itself, it finds itself capable of reflection, which in turn allows it some degree of freedom of action.

How does this transcendental sphere relate to the empirical sphere? This question was addressed before, but may well be raised again. The fundamental symbolic function (including its elaborations in the fields of intentionality, world and reflection) is the effective carrier of actual symbolisations/separations. The symbolic function (of the transcendental sphere) enables the actual symbolisations, expressing itself in them (within the empirical sphere) as well as in deficient symbolisations resulting from a deficient symbolic function. Consequently, the symbolic function has a conditioning or 'transcendental' task to fulfil. Again, this should be taken functionally, not ontologically, as if dealing with an autonomous entity (see Chapter Six). It also explains why the reference to the transcendental sphere within the description (within the empirical sphere) was made before. A constant finding is that the two sphere may be distinct, but not separate.

This should not keep us from highlighting the (transcendental) sphere even more explicitly, a purpose to which the field of psychosis is eminently suited. We would do well to realise that transcendental issues are not limited exclusively to psychosis, and are in fact relevant to any psychopathological structure: What is it that enables normality, including the neurotic structure, what is it that enables the personality disorder, what is that enables a psychotic structure? The answer is: the symbolic function being operative, partially operative or predominantly non-operative. Yet, the psychotic disorder has a particularly clarifying role, because it essentially demonstrates the effects of the symbolic function, this function not being operative. With this disorder being inoperative to a major extent, we can tell *ex negativo* what the symbolic function effectuates 'behind our backs'. The question is *not* an empirical one – what is the precise cause of a psychosis? – but a 'transcendental' one. In what way does a psychosis represent a disruption of the conditions of possibility for being-in-the-world?

Two tours. When speaking of the predominantly inoperative state of the symbolic function in the case of psychosis, the psychotic person – to the degree that he is in fact psychotic – should *not* be seen as being removed from the symbolic or from the language sphere. Certainly not – the psychotic person has in fact entered the domain of the symbolic or the language and meaning, but to some extent remains caught in the exteriority of language, not being able to distance himself and to reflect. He has entered the 'Prison-House of Language' (Jameson, 1972), but he is not capable of making free use of language within the boundaries imposed by language. The second step, the second tour – free use of language – has been compromised, and prevents full free use of language within the range imposed by rules. Autonomization as an intentional subject, the capacity to construct a temporal-spatial world and to distance oneself in one's mind – the capacity to reflect – have been compromised. In Lacanian terms we might say that alienation e.g., with respect to access to language and meaning – the first tour – has occurred, but no separation – the second tour.

This scheme of 'two tours' or 'two moments' turns out to be a major figure in the stretch of symbolisation: a 'step in' followed by 'a step out', which brings separation and limitation. There are two tours in the constitution of space and time: entering (subjective and objective) space and time, followed by a limitation of these forms of space and time through acceptance of finiteness leading to symbolic, dimensional space and time. These two tours run parallel to 'entering' the symbolic, supported by imaginary means, and followed by 'distancing oneself' from the symbolic, supported by the establishment of a phantasm. Yet these 'two tours' should not be understood chronologically, but in a structural, or rather 'transcendental' way: it is what happens 'always', while living one's life as a divided subject – the psychotic subject failing in the second tour.[22]

Indeed, this 'distancing' in its both modalities will result in subjective dividedness and intentionality, in the acceptance of the finiteness of the world combined with dimensional space and time, and in the establishment of the intersubjective structure of desire, supported by a phantasm, combined with the possibility of reflection.

Psychosis Explained: the Self, Internal Time and Reflection

This inquiry into the conditions of possibility governing the constitution of the intentional subject (a self) of a temporal-spatial world and of reflection can be elaborated in a number of ways. In fact, this is what happened in anthropological psychopathology, where this theme is taken as a starting point for further development of this 'transcendental issue', more specifically to refine the inquiry into the condition of possibility for psychosis, in relation to schizophrenia, melancholy and paranoia. This

[22] These 'two tours' can be seen in the scheme of alienation/separation, but also, be it in a different way, in the 'graph of desire', to be reflected in its 'inferior' and 'superior line' (Lacan, 1966/2002, p. 692), and in the two moments of the paternal metaphor as well (Lacan, 1966/2002, p. 465).

points will be discussed briefly, in order to establish a connection with the symbolisation notion developed here (not aimed at fully describing the intent of each of these approaches).

The Self

The process of transformation of reality into a world creates a symbolising subject that is actively engaged in each single act of symbolisation. Indeed, symbolisation is both enabled and supported by an original symbolisation. Therefore, any synthesis of a thought, action or observation or social act is made possible by a supporting synthesis or 'natural self-evidence', which functions as a condition of possibility for any actual synthesis, preceding each specific engagement with others, things and oneself.[23]

This 'natural self-evidence' or 'primordial self' may be absent, however, which is exemplified particularly by the symptomless types of schizophrenia, as has been argued before, within the context of the three levels of the empirical sphere: *intentionality* (decay of operative intentionality, and the '*moi-ici*'), *time* (decay of having-been), *inter-subjectivity* (autism). Here, it will be discussed at a '*transcendental*' level.

In the case of a loss of 'natural self-evidence', this loss will have to be offset as part of each individual act: all syntheses (acts of thought, types of social action) normally carried out without thought now need to be reinvented. This leads to highly reflective type of schizophrenia, going back to the deficit or decay of the three moments of this 'primordial self'. What is lacking – an original 'knowing how', an 'original past' and an 'original being-with'– will have to compensated through hyper-reflection as part of each individual act. This may be interpreted in a transcendental way. This prompted Blankenburg to write the following: "Autism will manifest itself anywhere where the empirical I is about to step in, ready to take over the role of the transcendental I, to guarantee an 'autos', a Self".[24]

---

[23] Blankenburg (1971, p. 21): "Unter 'transcendentaler Organisation' verstehen wir [...] die Struktur der Bedingungen der Möglichkeit des jeweils fungierenden Selbst- und Weltverhältnisses".

[24] Blankenburg (1971, p. 104): "Der Autismus tritt überall dort ein, wo das empirische Ich sich anschickt, die Aufgabe des transzendentalen Ich zu übernehmen, einen 'autos', ein Selbst, zu gewährleisten." Negatively, this schizophrenic condition demonstrates the 'natural' effects of the transcendental function. See Blankenburg (1971, p. 103):

One might agree with this thesis that the symptomless type of schizophrenia does not meet three basic requirements, categories of human existence (ready-to-hand, having-been, and being-with) as articulated in this Heideggerian regional ontology of human existence. Yet, this thesis is in need of a completion. The remaining question is why these categories – offering a framework for symbolization – are not operative. The answer might be: because of a deficit of the symbolic function, which would have allowed the introduction of finiteness and establishment of intentional involvement, of dimensional time and of intersubjectivity. The symbolic function, being not-operative, brings the need for compensation – here in the form of hyper-reflection (being a 'supplementation' in a Lacanian sense). When, however, the compensation of a failing symbolisation fails in its turn, the subject will fall victim to an entirely non-mediated real, a quasi-linear time, and an all powerful Other. Schizophrenia characterised by so-called negative symptoms (the symptomless type of schizophrenia) will then develop into the positive-symptom type.

Internal Time Consciousness

Primarily, transforming the real into a world can also be interpreted based on the issue of time, with melancholy as a case in point. Melancholy can be interpreted as the loss of the dimension of the future within the dimensional, symbolic time, resulting in a disturbance of subjective time, of inner consciousness, which has become detached from objective time. Binswanger (1960), in the final years of his life, elaborated this point in his own unique way. Having put aside the task of providing descriptions of world designs (manic, schizophrenic) that marked his Daseins-analytical phase, he set out to define the way world formation or world constitution takes place from a transcendental consciousness (as defined by Husserl). Rather than analyse the cause, he tried to establish its origin, wholly inclined to concede that melancholy may well have a biological cause, representing a *experimentum naturae* (Binswanger, 1960, p. 15).

Instead of emphasising the decay of the dimension of future itself, he chooses to focus on the disruption of internal time consciousness as a whole (past, present, future). In the case of melancholy, the boundaries

---

"Die Konstitution von Selbst und Welt erweist sich nicht mehr als transcendental. Sie imponiert als eine physische Anstrengung".

between future expectation and past memories have become blurred, as a result of which the present becomes futile as well. The complaint ('if only I had/had not done this') is retrospective in nature, past-oriented, but is essentially prospective, while applying a future derived category (choice) on the past (as though it were the future). Then again, the future has become fixed (as though it were the past). Future possibilities are attributed to the past, whereas the future has become fixed and cannot be distinguished from the past. As a result, anything that would manifest itself in the present thus becomes irrelevant, effectively effacing the boundaries between present, past and future. At last, the unbolting of inner temporal awareness, of subjective time, also brings a fundamental disruption of objective time, of object constitution, allowing a melancholy delusion to develop. Then only loss, sheer loss ('*pure perte*') can be expected.

Once again one might agree with this thesis, while presupposing that it is also in need of completion. The question that presents itself is why this internal time consciousness has become unlimited, frantic, making it possible to interchange what cannot be interchanged. The answer might be the same as the one offered here: because of a deficit of the symbolic function. The introduction of subjective time (internal time consciousness) and its parallel objective, physical time, constitutes only a first step in symbolisation, which is in need of a second step. This second step, the introduction of dimensional, symbolic time, is curbing both, as a result of which the infinite internal time consciousness will be transformed into finite life-historical time, extending towards birth and death. The decay of the symbolic time causes objective time and subjective time to become disconnected, thereby unbolting internal, subjective time.

Reflection

There is yet another, third approach from which the 'transcendental' issue might be discussed, one that is based on the pool of inter-subjectivity and reflection. The subject is established through a process of symbolisation, of identifying with others, distancing oneself from a primordial other. Still, there is no full coalescence with one or more of his identifications. If it did coalesce, it would become fixed, immutable. Ricœur (1992) propounded his own view on this matter, arguing that human identity is characterised by two poles. This identity is shaped partly by actual behaviour and by daily interaction both with himself and with others, and consequently by the enduring character of a person. This quality of endurance will ensure that a person will remain himself in a variety of circumstances, while being recognisable as this person to others. This type of identity, referred to as 'identity as sameness' (*identity idem*), may be associated with a person's character or personality, which does make him 'the same' in his lifetime.

Next, a person's identity is shaped in part by the possibility to reflect on his actions, to what he commonly does or to the nature of his character itself. He may resolve to change his relationship to his past or character, and decide to do things in a different manner. This reflects his capacity to reach back beyond himself, to distance himself from what he is. This type of identity is referred to as 'identity as selfhood' (*identity ipse*) (Ricœur, 1992; Dastur, 2001). Commonly, these types of identity go together, because man cannot be equalised with his factuality nor with a capacity of pure reflection. He offers a combination in which factuality and reflection are alternately dominant. Man 'is what he is', while he also 'is not what he is'.

In the case of a psychotic disorder we could say that the dialectics of the two identity types is disturbed, and that the person has receded back into the sheer factuality of his character (behaviour and the sum of his experiences), from which he cannot distance himself. This is particularly true for the paranoia disorder. Assuming that mental health is characterised by 'a proper degree of melancholy' with an associated '*douleur d'exister*', likewise it is tied to 'a proper degree of distrust'. This distrust may have pathological dimensions, in which case, analogously to the '*Typus melancholicus*', we might speak of a '*Typus paranoïcus*', or a paranoid personality disorder. In the case of paranoia, the dialectics of the two identities is disturbed to such an extent that suspicion has become a dominant trait, without the capacity to distance oneself from what the person's character would present in the way of suspicion. Thus, the paranoid person finds himself overwhelmed by feelings of threat and persecution, not being able to distance himself from them reflectively.

Once again one might agree with this thesis, assuming that it still needs completion for a full transcendental discussion. The transcendental question is because of what the capacity to reflect could drop of. The answer might be the same as give up here: because of a deficit of the symbolic function, whose essence is allowing a subject to take distance towards his environment and his inner psychic world, allowing a subject to reflect, also on its own identity.

STANDARDS

It is obvious that standards are involved, for both the empirical and the transcendental sphere. In the transcendental sphere, the standard concerns the establishment of a well-formed world, being brought on by the workings of the symbolic function, which supports the process of symbolisation or separation. A criterion for measuring success would be the presence of the ability to maintain an adequate degree of distance. This will be reflected by the capacity of the subject to occupy an independent, supporting position, by the functioning of dimensional space and time, and by the dialectics of personal identity.

Next to it, there are the standards related to the thee levels of the empirical sphere: of intentionality, of the constituted world and of language and the lack, desire and reflection. Intentionalities may function differently in both its relevant fields (cognition and affectivity) and in its way of functioning (pre-predicatively and predicatively). Also, the intended world, in its structural moments, may diverge from normality with respect to the various psychopathological structures and positions, which in turn may be clarified by the various structures of desire. The normativity involved relates to the characterization of a complex whole – a subject position – in which both description and normativity are not separate but are intimately connected, as is always the case in psychopathology (Kenny, 1985, p. 52). This does not concern symptoms having their origin in a teleological discourse – the medical discourse – but is about meaningful phenomena abiding deontological rules (see Chapters Two and Five). More specifically, we need to investigate whether a specific normatively loaded description – under the heading of (non-)successful symbolization – will lead to the identification of a coherence occurring among phenomena occurring at the various levels. An example of the efficacy of the distinction between the three different positions within the neurotic structure may illustrate this point.

The hysteric position can be summarised as follows. In the field of intentionality, the affective prevails, more or less overshadowing the cognitive form; at the level of space, (ego)centricity is emphasised while at the level of time the emphasis is on the past. Intersubjectivity, on the other hand, is characterised by tempting the other to come closer. At the 'transcendental' level, the symbolic function (comprising the autonomy of the subject, dimensional time and personal identity) remain intact, but the aspect of separation is less prominent. Within the hysteric position, there is a tendency towards reducing the distance which, at each separate level, is expressed in a distinct but congruous manner.

The obsessive position is more or less its opposite. In the field of intentionality, the cognitive prevails, more or less overshadowing the affective form; at the level of space, the dimension of objectifiability, is predominant, while at the level of time the emphasis is on the future, characterised by anticipation and procrastination. Intersubjectivity, on the other hand, is characterised by keeping the other at bay. At the 'transcendental' level, the symbolic function (including its constituting moments) remains intact, but here the aspect of separation has become dominant. At all three levels distinguished within the obsessive position, we recognise a predisposition towards maximising the distance. Apparently, these separate levels are in fact congruous.

By contrast, the phobic position is characterised by a tendency towards cognitive and affective fleetingness in the field of intentionality, while at the level of space we see a preference for moving along the edge but within the boundaries, and the focus at the time level is on the present, as a result of constantly expecting impending danger. Intersubjectivity is characterised by observing a distance towards the other, who is watched closely and constantly. Again, at the 'transcendental' level, the symbolic function remains intact, but the distance towards the other is fragile and is rather critical: it should not be too close or too far.

A picture emerges of obsessive, hysteric and phobic positions as cohesive entities. The constellations of the various positions all seem to match at a particular level. Then again, they each express some degree of disproportion. The concept of proportion was introduced by Binswanger (1956, pp. 1-8), who spoke of 'anthropological proportion'. His focus was on the disproportion at the spatial level in a transcendental sense, more specifically with respect to the height-width polarity. Regardless whether this elaboration should be considered successful or not, we can say that the notion of proportion does have its value (Blankenburg, 1982). The examples offered (of the hysteric, obsessive and phobic positions) illustrate that we are dealing with highly complex entities, defined by some amount of disproportionality. Moreover, a lack of proportionality associated with a specific subject position, does not necessarily point to the presence of a significant inner or external conflict. For example, even a person with an obsessive position may be able to adapt and live a full life with little conflict. Conversely, proportionality is no guarantee for harmony. A person with both a obsessive and a hysteric repertoire will attain some degree of proportion, even if it leads to a life that lacks harmony, but is fulfilling nonetheless. In other words, mental health does not equal balance or harmony. Indeed, it can bring dividedness or even a sense of being torn. Consequently, the diagnosis of 'disorder' should not be made too hastily, whilst 'being not adapted to the environment' is not providing a decisive criterion. Passing judgment on a person's mental health therefore requires prudence, taking the form of an in-depth hermeneutical investigation into the person's world and the proportionality involved.

Any disproportions occurring in a person's world may have a unique origin. It is also the task of a hermeneutical diagnostics to establish how an individual's world emerged and took shape within his life history. This will be the central theme of the next chapter.

Eight

The Interpretation of a Life History

Just as the hermeneutical and structural diagnostics may be conceived as a description of a person's actual world, with its associated intentionalities and underlying symbolisations, so can we take this process a step further by exploring the process of genesis or historical development of this particular world. This will raise the question whether, in a person's life history, early stages of an identified world type can be traced and its structure be matched with a psychopathological structure. The implementation of this process is preceded by a theoretical question: what exactly is a life history? First of all a distinction should be made between an external type and an internal type of life history.

External Life History

The course of life or external life history can be interpreted as an external string of events that occurred in respect of a particular person, at a particular moment on a linear time axis, e.g., birth, child's diseases, going to school, etcetera. Bearing in mind the distinction between internal time and external time, the external life history can be placed on the axis of external time (see Chapter Seven). Yet, the concept of external life history brings a limitation in respect of the infinity of the external time, transforming it into calendar time: life history in an external sense is situated on the calendar time. Secondly, actions, experiences and events occur within the framework of the person's life, which is defined by the boundaries set by both birth and death. Thus, the real person's life is defined by external finiteness, by the limited lifespan stretching between birth and death, as well as by its being historically situated on the calendar time (into which the vast infinity of external time has been translated).

Can knowledge at all be inferred from a course of life or external life history, or from the past? This question is essential, as time and again doubt has been cast on the possibility of scientifically acceptable knowledge in respect of the past. Indeed, any branch of psychiatry dealing with such an issue exposes itself to being labelled as unscientific.

So what can we say about our knowledge of the past in general? The least we could say is that it refers to something that is no longer there. How then are we supposed to obtain knowledge of something that does not exist? The situation differs from that seen in most other empirical branches of science, where an 'object' is actually present (physical nature, human or animal organism, bodies of text, etcetera). Nevertheless, we might argue that the past – which undeniably does not exist anymore – manifests itself through the traces it left. Based on source studies and source criticism, we could prove rather convincingly that the emperor August lived in a particular historical period and that Jesus of Nazareth may or may not have existed. This concerns the level of historical research. Testing procedures may differ from those employed in natural scientific and social scientific models, but rigorous testing is certainly possible. Consequently, unless an extremely positivist stance is taken there is no reason to doubt the scientific quality of history as a scientific discipline. Still, the past (which no longer exists) can never be approached directly, only indirectly – a gap will remain between the 'lost reality of the past' and its description. There is no reason to dramatise this status by reducing the past to a mere construct, but we should point out that there is a distinction between the described reality of the past and the description itself (Mink, 1987).

A second level concerns the interpretation of what is offered by the description. Here, the historian makes a choice, adding structure and hierarchy to the overwhelming amount of descriptive data. For example, he will interpret the origins of the Golden Age, the characteristics of the Renaissance or the roots of the French Revolution. The multitude of descriptions is structured into a story that builds up to a conclusion, to a thesis. In doing so, he will use metaphor to shed new light on a particular time period or cultural movement. Alternatively, he may introduce a 'plot' into the course of events in order to summarise.[1] Therefore, a historical interpretation, as opposed to a historical description, is essentially creative. This aspect should not be misconstrued as resulting in lack of testability. Indeed, two testing options are available, viz.,

[1] The metaphoric nature of historical knowledge at this level is emphasised by H. White (1973). Ricœur also stresses the importance of using a metaphor at this level, highlighting the significance of structuring by the introduction of a 'plot' or 'intrigue' (also making reference to White). See Ricœur (1984). Another useful concept is the '*colligatory concept*' or overarching concept, introduced by W.H. Walsh (1974); see also Ankersmit (1995, p. 89).

internal or external testing. Internal testing focuses on the cohesion or integrative power of interpretation, on the coherent quality of interpretation. External testing does not focus on internal cohesion, but on the level of correspondence with the data produced by the description. Does interpretation reflect the multitude of data available, or were data used selectively? Also at this second level, testing procedures will differ from those employed in natural scientific and social scientific research, but they do exist, and there is no reason to doubt severely the scientific quality of a historical interpretation.

This will apply not only to historical investigation in general, but also to historical research focused on the life history. Based on findings contributed by others, historical research of this nature into the course or life or external life history may be called hetero-anamnestic. The biography is compiled from objective data, obtained from the registrar's office, from personal notes, etcetera. Based on these data, as a next step a 'plot' or clarifying metaphor may be presented to illustrate the life history of this person.

Internal Life History

The biography includes yet another aspect of the person's life, namely the fact that this person experienced it himself. If he is still alive, he can talk about it or be interviewed. This person will have a consciousness of past events, for example in the form of memories. This leads to auto-anamnestic analysis, which can supplement hetero-anamnestic analysis. It is called 'auto-anamnestic' because it proceeds from one's own memory, based on inner time consciousness.

There is also the issue of finiteness. The external life history has a beginning (birth) and will one day end (with death), thus taking its place in the generation chain, which makes it fundamentally historical – external time, stretching to the infinite, being transformed in finite calendar time. Like the external life history is defined by external time limits of birth and death, internal life history is bound by the relationship towards birth and death – internal time, stretching to the infinite as well, is being transformed into life historical time and its internal finiteness: resulting in an awareness of one's own finiteness. This will result in the idea of an internal life history, as a personal and changeable view of one's own history, which view in itself is also situated historically on the calendar time. The memory of an incident in early childhood can acquire the added meaning of "When I was young and life seemed endless".

External and internal finiteness are thus appropriated and integrated into a view expressing awareness of finiteness and awareness of being historical situated. It results in human existence being both historically situated and finite, in both senses: externally and internally. This conjunction expresses the dimensional (symbolic) time, the temporality of the subject itself (see Chapter Seven).

Within the framework of dimensional time a person is able to reach back to his past or to anticipate his future. The past is more than a past event to be remembered, and the future is more than just a future event waiting to occur. Indeed, the past is not complete but, within the mode of 'having been', is making its presence felt in the present time, while also shaping the anticipation of future events (Heidegger, 1927/ 1962, p. 376). Thus, man relates to and engages itself with past, present and future. Within the framework of inner consciousness, a person can have a memory of an early event – perhaps experienced as a toddler – the content of which has remained more or less intact over time. However this 'identical' event can be 'reviewed' and interpreted differently over time, modifying future perspectives.

Herein lies the focal point as well as the condition of possibility for any form of psychotherapy that aims to restore the connection between present and past. The past is never a historical fact per se but can always become part of the present, and a view of one's own past, of a past period in a person's life, can always be revised (Gadamer, 1960/1985, p. 265). Otherwise, psychotherapy in the sense indicated would be impossible and therefore pointless. A person's childhood is never a monolithic entity ("That is how it was"), but is open to interpretation and reinterpretation through the telling and retelling of life experiences. It creates the possibility for a large number of stories about a person's childhood to be told, some of which may be rejected by the person himself. It also highlights the connection with what psychoanalysis refers to as 'the unconscious'. This may be conceived as the whole body of stories that can be told or are being told by others (the Other) about a person, but which are rejected by the person himself although they may still find acceptance at some point in the future. Like the life history, the unconscious can be conceived as being narratively structured: "The unconscious is the Other's discourse", as an 'other discourse' (Lacan, 1966/2002, p. 316). Related to this concept of the unconscious, psychotherapy, aimed as it is on the life history as being a unified entity of past, present and future, may acquire yet another point of focus. The aim is not only to gain new insights into the past or to establish a new relationship with it, but also to accept – to the degree possible – the essence of life, which is found in its finite character, with life being delimited by both birth and death: limitation of life and enjoyment, the subjectification of death (Lacan, 1966/2002, p. 289).

External and Internal Life History Combined

Contrary to psychotherapy, psychodiagnostics cannot limit itself to a mere interpretation of the inner life history, and should instead aspire to integrate internal and external life histories. The description of the external course of life, it was shown, supplies us with testable data, based on which we can then arrive at a summarising interpretation, whose feasibility in turn can be put to the test. In a similar way, the description of the internal life history will yield testable components. The tenability of a person's actual memories can be assessed, and so can the – possibly – varying views of this past adopted by this person in the course of his lifetime. At any rate, both proposition types do not elude testing, as they together represent the building blocks that can become part of a comprehensive interpretation of the – in this case – life history as a whole. If the aim is to integrate external and internal life histories, as in the case of the life-historical psychodiagnostics, in practice both approaches will be used simultaneously and in tandem (Jaspers, 1913/1997, pp. 671-708).

Most likely, this will bring out marked differences among the various stories. There may be contradictions between the external and internal life histories (biography and autobiography), as well as between the various parts of the autobiography. For example, a person may disagree with others about the presence or significance of certain people in their own lives; or a person may at some point, or for a longer period of time, be in doubt about the specific nature of the past, holding different views of certain protagonists in their life at the same time. In such a case, man could be defined as possessing a multiple rather than a singular life history (Schafer, 1983, pp. 204-212). This sounds more dramatic than it actually is – all it means is that man can simultaneously hold a number of different views of himself or of significant others. A person may choose to either hate himself or not; likewise, he may admire or despise another person. Often, such views can be consolidated into one over-arching view. In their mutual differences, the stories acquire detail, can be qualified or modified. The story of a woman who hates her mother, and the story told by people around her who claim that she involves her mother in everything she does, can be unified into the thesis of a strong mutual symbiotic bond. Thus, various aspects of the life history, which at first glance may be strongly divergent, at closer inspection can sometimes reveal a well-defined underlying structure.

It is the interpretation of the life history – not to be confused with the description – that is supposed to bring out this underlying structure. This may result in an overall and integrating picture of the facts offered by the description. This may be done by way of a metaphor – “He is the scum of the family” – or by offering a ‘plot’ of the life history or life’s story: “Trust him to get hold of the short end of the stick”. A ‘plot’ brings unity (concordance) in the dispersed multitude of facts (discordance) (Ricœur, 1984).

Narrativisation of the life history turns a life history or life’s story into an interpretation of the past. It is a fallacy to think that at this level we might be able to actually reconstruct the past in its ‘true’ form (Spence, 1982). Facts from a course of life do offer indispensable building blocks for telling a life’s story, but that is all they do. Collecting external data constitutes the groundwork for the historical interpretation which, being narrative in nature, shapes the past by acknowledging an underlying structure. As was mentioned before, it holds the creative element that is part of any design, yet without precluding an assessment of its feasibility. To this end, the historian of the life history will refer to those facts that are supplied by the description of the course life to support his interpretation. He will also draw on the cohesive, integrative or binding power of the designed image or structure.

Interpretation and Prognosis

Even though a life history may include a multitude of stories, this does detract from the conception of life history as being a story. Remembering the past takes the form of a narrative of the past, as any attempt at structuring one’s own or someone else’s life in order to explain a life history will result in a narrative. The past is being told, and in the process a relationship between present and past is established.

How exactly are present, past and future related? Is this relationship causal, with the past causing the present first and then future? No, it is not, because there can never be an unequivocal causal relationship, as the past inevitably takes shape through interpretation and narration. The significance of interpretation and symbolization is also felt in the case of a traumatic past. Even a traumatic past will not be the outcome of a direct cause-effect chain. Indeed, any event will be traumatic insofar as interpretation or symbolization (i.e. mental processing) has failed, which again represents a reference to the factuality and possibility of interpretation or symbolization. Then again, extreme traumas may occur of such a grave nature that they elude symbolization, 'wandering around' wholly unprocessed in the mental space. Yet even in such extreme cases, reference to the psychic reality enabling – limited – interpretation or symbolization remains possible. In principle, any interpretation or symbolization constitutes an intermediate stage that allows the past to be processed and to perform its action. Next, it is very well conceivable that some interpretations or stories are profoundly unacceptable and therefore 'unconscious', bringing multiple concurrent stories into being, as was demonstrated before. However, because the past exercises its effect in an interpretative or narrative manner, life-historical explanations are also interpretative or narrative and can never be causal in nature. This does not imply that life historical events would be not effective: they most certainly are effective, be it in an internal and mediated (non-causal) way.

This does afford room for 'explanations' – an explanation does not mean that a given fact from a person's course of life included into a life's story is causal and therefore follows logically from the previous history, but merely has or acquires a degree of intelligibility when narratively structured. Typifying the relationship between present and past as non-causal opens up the possibility of considering whether freedom of action – reflection – actually existed when the event occurred. Indeed, this question cannot be posed within a deterministic context, where events by necessity lead to other events.

Next, a legitimate but limited prognosis can be offered of the future actions of a unique individual. These limitations are necessary because a non-deterministic view needs to take account of a degree of freedom and, consequently, of a certain amount of unpredictability. Still, a person's life story will bring out the interpretative schemes that drive both perception and action. As a result, any prognosis on future actions will not be based on extrapolation of past events, but on the 'interpretative schemes' that are most likely have been effective in the course of this subject's history, given the internal and external aspects of the life history. This approach makes an essential difference between hermeneutical prognosis and prediction of behaviour in an empiricist fashion, type HCR-20 – Historical Clinical Risk Assessment-20 (Webster et al., 1997).

Intrigue and Phantasm

In the above, the emphasis was on the variable nature of life stories, but the significance of this variety was also qualified. Often, a wide variety of stories can be consolidated into one single story, supported by an 'interpretative scheme' – most of the time anyway. For example, the story of a person who hates his father combined with the story that he still deeply loves him can be consolidated into the denominator of 'ambivalence'. The story of a person who claims only to love a person and not harbour any feelings of hatred, together with the story told by people around him who instead argue that this person does feel hatred for the other person, can be summed up as 'denial of feelings of hatred'. Thus, life stories that seemed discordant at first glance may in fact have a common underlying (concordant) structure or 'interpretative scheme' – an intrigue (Ricœur, 1984).

As a search model for revealing the structure of life stories, the structure of the original family situation is particularly significant. What exactly was the child's position within this family (Boszormenyi-Nagy and Spark, 1973)? Was the child supposed to give to the father or the mother what he or she supposedly lacked, to make up for the other's perceived lack, or to fill a void caused by one of the parents falling ill (parentification)? Did his birth signify the end of an ongoing struggle? Was the child supposed to serve as a whipping-boy or scapegoat for other problems occurring in the family (Girard, 1989)? Or was it expected to perform in a field where one of the parents had failed (delegation). And how did the parents respond if the child failed to fulfil the allocated role, to meet the demands of one or both parents, instead pursuing its own desires, for example by displaying unruly behaviour? Essentially, it is a variation on the theme phrased by Lacan, following Hegel: "*Le désir de l'homme, c'est le désir de l'Autre*". Man's desire finds its meaning in the other's desire, the desire is always a desire in relation to the Other's (the environment's) desire (Lacan, 1966/2002, p. 222). However, this does not rule out freedom of choice with regard to a subject position altogether: Freud's concept of *Neurosenwahl* is still valid (Freud, 1913/1958).

Moreover, the parents may have issues that originally brought them together – keeping them together or causing them to break up before long – which originate in the family structure from which they both came (Dolto, 1987, pp. 11-63). A life history may have origins that cause a fundamental issue to be carried from one generation to the next, from one family to the next. It seems to be dominated by an inert historical mass that cannot easily be escaped. Within this context, we may speak of a 'family gift' (Ortigues and Ortigues, 1988, pp. 51-72).

It does offer, however, a guide for identifying the structure of the life history, provided enough insight is available into a (possibly repeated) family structure. In fact, the course of events will be more cyclic in nature, with elements from the life stories pointing to a possible family structure, which allows ideas to be verified based on data presented by these life stories (see Chapter Five). Once again it turns out that the resulting interpretation of a life history in terms of an underlying structure represents a creative activity, whereas a factual and descriptive investigation into the course of life takes the form of 'data research'.

This leads us to inquire into the nature of the relationship between 'structure' and 'history'. If the structure is an invariant entity, this will render history irrelevant. If the life history merely expressed a unconscious basic phantasm (in the sense of Lacan) or an 'existential apriori' (following Binswanger), it would lose its autonomy.[2] The question is whether the relationship should rather be defined as one of mutual implication. A structure is not perceivable per se, but represents an abstraction of a factual and historically developed connection. Nor is the life history a disparate body of facts but, despite coincidences introduced by fate, is characterised by some degree of unity that makes a person's life uniquely recognisable. This unity may be cast into a construction that reflects its content, its 'plot' or 'intrigue' (Ricœur, 1984). The vastness (discordance) of historical facts is bound together by their structure (concordance). This unity may also be conceived in the construction of a phantasm, being the unconscious framework – in Lacan's sense – determining what can be desired and what produces a feeling of pleasure as well as defining what particular ties with the relational world are considered valid (see Chapter Seven).

---

[2] For the term 'existential apriori' in Binswanger's sense, see Needleman (1963/1975), pp. 70-72. Binswanger chose the term '*Daseinsgang*', on the one hand to do justice to the invariant and sustained character of an 'existential apriori', while on the other he wished to express the historicity of existence. He propounded and elaborated this issue in 'Der Fall Suzanne Urban'. See Binswanger (1957), pp. 359- 471.

Life History and Pathology

The variety seen among the different life stories is not necessarily cast in stone and may reflect a comparatively invariant structure. In some cases, this structure can be defined as pathological. Although a wide variety of life's stories may be found, there are in fact boundaries that any course of life will come up against.

In Chapter Seven we found that a person's world is characterised by a specific structure that includes structural moments, such as the relationship towards space and time, or to oneself and the other. What exactly defines the relationship towards others? Is a person capable of developing a personal bond, or does he experience the other merely as an object or as a means to an end? Next, is this person capable of facing his own finiteness and mortality, or does he essentially experience himself as eternal? Or is he perhaps preoccupied with his own death or another person's death, constantly exploring boundaries, limitations and impossibilities? In addition to the structural moments of a world, there are also intentionalities in the cognitive and affective sense indicated. As regards the cognitive form: allowing for some interpretative leeway, is a person prone to misrepresenting the common world? And with respect to desire: is a person capable of tolerating a particular lack, or is he instead reaching for something beyond his grasp which, once it has become attainable, loses its appeal, following a histrionic pattern? In each individual case, the structural moments mentioned can differ widely in their mutual relationships, but it is clear that boundaries may have been overstepped in a person's world.

Insofar as the world offers a cross-section of the life history, we may wonder if standards also apply in this domain. It may be presupposed that the life history meets or fails to meet a standard. In the latter case, the structure of the life history might well be defined as pathological. Children who used to be hit by their parents because these parents couldn't bear seeing their children unhappy when crying, will in turn become abusive parents. The parents or parent figures who look for in the child what they supposedly cannot offer each other, render another kind of contribution to a pathological life history. It allows this mechanism to repeat itself, with the child or later parent remaining captive of the parents' or educators' desires – the desire of the Other. The theme of a 'normative life history' thus presented has been elaborated as part of various specialties dealing with child development, including psychoanalysis, attachment theory and the theory of moral development.[3]

It also means that a number of types of normative life history may co-exist, which may actually engage in a relationship of mutual cohesion without necessarily being in conflict. We should start by mentioning Kohlberg's view who, in line with Piaget, has mapped moral development. He distinguished a preconventional stage in which the child is driven by entities such as fear of punishment, a conventional stage in which behaviour is authority-oriented, and a post-conventional stage where general consent or universality is pursued (Kohlberg, 1981). Another well-known theory is Freud's stage theory of sexual, libidinal development, involving the oral, anal and genital stages, respectively. According to Erikson, these stages are connected with the themes of trust and safety, of autonomy and control, and of complexity in sexual relationships, respectively (Erikson, 1967/1950). Significant is the concept of stage-adequate or stage-inadequate events, which holds that, depending on the stage, a 'similar' event will have either no impact or a major psychotraumatic impact. In addition to highlighting libidinal development, psychoanalysis employs the so-called object-relational approach, which focuses on relationships with other persons or 'objects' from a psychoanalytical perspective. Rather than conflict with the libido-theoretical approach, it might be considered to be complementary. These relationships may be imaginary in nature – as in the case of Melanie Klein's school (1977) – or relate to actual persons (Fairbairn, 1952; Greenberg and Mitchell, 1983). Lacan responded with his 'object' concept, in which the central theme is not the object as a person, but the lack of a 'partial object' sustaining the desire, the object little *a* that loses the subject in the course of separation, leaving a gap, ('*objet-trou*') that defines the outlines of what may give partial pleasure. Also noteworthy is the (normative) life history according to Kohut, who outlines the development of a narcissism needed to create a 'coherent and cohesive self'. Again, the notion of stage-inadequate events is seminal, more particularly, as stage-inadequate narcissistic injuries can disrupt early and necessary experiences of grandeur, which can have a major impact on the development of stable self-esteem (Kohut, 1971). We should also mention the scheme developed by Mahler, whose ideas on the

---

[3] The notion of a normative life history in a psychoanalytical context is discussed, but is rejected by Schafer (1983), pp. 237-239.

separation/individuation stage and the preceding autistic and symbiotic stages proved highly influential (Mahler, 1985).

Significant is the attachment theory which goes back to Bowlby (1969) and was elaborated in a less behaviour-centred manner by Fonagy, who introduced the concept of mentalisation (Fonagy and Target, 1996a and 1996b). Mentalisation refers to the capacity to attribute cognitions, affects and intentions to the other, in order to equip the child with a (at least rudimentary) 'theory of mind'. Its interiorisation will result in the child being able to understand both the other and itself in terms of affects and cognitions, and intentions that may be reflected upon, endowing it with a 'reflective function'.[4] First the child needs to be acknowledged by the other as a carrier of a 'mind', as a subject, in order to be able to mirror it. Primacy lies with its environment.

We also recognise a similarity with Lacan's views, who never failed to stress the significance of the environment (*l'Autre*) and of the mirroring process between parent and child (Verhaeghe, 2008, pp. 159-166). With Lacan, we see an emphasis on the distinction between mirrored or imaginary (dual) relations on the one hand, and symbolic (triangular) relations on the other. Their mutual connection is complex, with the child mirroring itself on an environment which, in its turn, on another, symbolic level, encompasses the child itself – by verifying the (imaginary) self-attributions of the child (Lacan, 1966/2002, p. 568). As the child later fully develops the symbolic function – again depending on its environment, on the Other and on Otherness – it will be able to distance itself from an immediate real, attributing a degree of autonomy to others and itself (having both a subject position, possessing both a '*mind*'). The distinction between imaginary and symbolic relations is not only meaningful within the context of development theory, but can also be applied in a structural fashion. What we are dealing with are not only historical periods – dominated by the imaginary and the symbolic, respectively – but rather permanent positions. In the former case, permanent dual or symbiotic 'one-on-one' relations predominate, while in the latter the relations are co-determined by a third term (rule or law).

This is not the place, however, to assess the internal coherence of the life history types or their relative value. It is pertinent, however, to draw the general conclusion that the concept of a normative life history will apply. Applying this notion, something that deviates from the life history

---

[4] This corresponds with the 'second tour' of the process of symbolization (See Chapter Seven).

can be seen as abnormal and pathological, or as a pathogen for subsequent chapters in life. Thus, the concept of pathology has been introduced, offering the possibility of rewriting a biography as a pathography, in which case the structure will be pathological – a specimen of a psychopathological structure.

In order to clarify and illustrate the thesis that the life history diagnostics represents a type of structural diagnostics, we will offer some examples of structures that may be distinguished and have been distinguished before, in Chapter Seven. We are referring to the distinction between the structure of a neurotic disorder, of a personality disorder and of a psychotic disorder. It offers the opportunity to run through the structural pathology in one final iteration. The emphasis will be on the register of intersubjectivity, that is, presenting an outline of the subject's relationships with itself as well as with the other. We should do well to realise that this outline is no more than an illustration of ideal-typical relationships not necessarily occurring in practice. With regard to an actual situation, the status would merely be that of search schemes that may or may not point the way towards understanding. Also in this case, the table in the Appendix outlining the psychopathological structures may be helpful.

Neurosis

The neurosis is not characterised by basic or fundamental disorders in the field of separation, i.e., between the subject and the other. The desire turns out the be intact, be it that the focus shifts depending on the subject position – hysteric, obsessive or phobic. As a reminder, we would like to stress the fact that, within the neurotic position, Lacan and most Lacanians take a different stance by only isolating the obsessive and hysteric neurosis, without attributing an independent status to phobia.

The fact of the desire being intact becomes evident first from the *hysteric* position, which is dominated by self-dramatization and theatrical behaviour of the subject, drawing the attention to itself. It reflects a focus on the other, causing the desire to assume a 'passive quality' in order to elicit the other's desire. The specific or 'neurotic' element is represented by the object supposed to offer satisfaction being rejected time and again for reasons of inadequacy – it fails to satisfy. In a sense, we see a search for perfection unfold (Israel, 1976). Perfection is looked for in the other but is also imposed on the subject itself, which results in a constant inner awareness of failing, of being imperfect. This awareness can be obscured by displaying a perfection that does not actually exist, by pretending. This hysteric mask, giving the impression of not being genuine, obscures a feeling of being imperfect rather than an awareness of an inner void.[5] This imperfection may be experienced in a number of ways, e.g., in the form of discontent with fate or with one's own gender, with social status or with a perceived lack of recognition. The person feels wronged, disillusioned, and is filled with resentment.

The life-historical background may be that the hysteric personality was confronted with a parent relationship defined by failure on the side of one of the parents in the eyes of the other parent, a failure that was measured unwittingly by the image of a superior figure (either male or female). This image had insinuated its way into the subject's imagination. A possible consequence may be that when choosing a partner, the subject expects the other to match this ideal type – a master – which never existed in reality. Thus, a partner will never turn out to be 'the one and only', and so the subject will reject the other in disappointment – he or she will never be able to live up to expectations. And so the search for an ideal partner, perfect job or full recognition continues, while setting oneself up for disappointment. As the search must continue, the underlying desire could be described as the desire for an unsatisfied desire.

As we have seen before, the *obsessive* position is more or less the opposite of the hysteric position. An obsessive or compulsive person has a strong tendency to control the people around him, while also keeping a tight rein on himself. In the case of a male obsessive person, we recognise something of a dichotomy: on the one hand, there is a tendency to acquiesce or submit to others, while on the other this person is suppressing feelings of protest. He will tread carefully when approaching women, displaying an aloof manner. He often finds himself in two minds, wondering whether he did the right thing, having to live up to the most rigid standards. Besides, he is reluctant to commit himself, always procrastinating. From the perspective of inner time, a time strategy is used that postpones rather than blocks the future.

---

[5] In this sense, it differs from the ingenuine behaviour seen in the borderline position, which essentially masks a 'void', which explains why dealing with a borderliner is so taxing for his or her environment. See also Kahn (1974). Also compare the 'As-if' personality in the sense of Helene Deutsch and the 'true/false-self' issue discussed by Winnicott. See Deutsch (1934); Winnicott (1965); Bollas (1987/1999, pp. 135-156).

The life history's background may – in an ideal-typical way – be one a family dominated by a degree of rigidity, while even an ostensibly tolerant family culture ('where everything is allowed') might still being experienced as enforced or dictated. Any conflict that may have arisen as a result was avoided rather than played out. This type of avoidance may be likened to the Master/Slave dialectic developed by Hegel: 'Lordship and Bondage'. Fearing death, the slave will avoid any struggle, submitting himself to the other and subsequently waiting for the other to die (the Master, the father, the elder).[6] A obsessive life pattern is often dominated by a preoccupation with life and death, because only death of the other will truly set the subject free. Essentially, an ancient but suppressed conflict seems to underlie the time strategy of procrastination (Leclaire, 1971, pp. 121-188; Lang, 2000a, pp. 131-152). As the obsessive neurotic person sees an opportunity, he will construct a deadlock or an impossible situation in order to perpetuate the 'waiting': "It cannot be done", or "It is not the proper thing to do". The desire is one for an impossible desire. Yet, a life history of this nature is bound to transgress borders. An essential aspect of a person's life is its finiteness – as life is defined by both a relationship to the future and an awareness of finiteness and death. This relationship may be denied, in the sense that the obsessive neurotic person may think he can endlessly continue postponing the future, but in doing so he makes a fundamental 'error of judgment'. In cases where human reality – its finite character – is actually denied, we may speak of a pathology.

The *phobic* position towards the other is characterised by a desire to escape this other, who is being experienced as dangerous, while at the same time the subject feels dependent upon this other. The subject is torn by an inner conflict, fearing loneliness and seeking contact with others, who in turn pose a perceived threat, causing the phobic person to retreat into his own safe and secluded world (Assoun, 2005, pp. 55-62). Whilst trying to escape loneliness he is also running away from the other.

The life-historical background may well reflect the loneliness that any child, or any human for that matter, is exposed to: being in a situation where man is at the mercy of others – Freud's helplessness (*Hilflosigkeit*) Heidegger's thrownness (*Geworfenheit*) or the Other's whims as defined

---

[6] The Master/Slave theme, taken from Hegel's *Phenomenology of the Spirit,* was frequently used by Lacan (1966/2002, e.g., pp. 98-99) and was associated more specifically with the obsessive neurosis (p. 258): "This sense is sustained by his subjective relation to the master insofar as it the master's death that he awaits".

by Lacan. For want of some measure of security, the child will bend to the desires of the Other, exhibiting docile and subservient behaviour. This 'choice for passiveness' also expresses fear of the other, who is given licence to do as he or she pleases. This, in turn, will lead to a fear of losing autonomy (of being 'devoured' by the other) or of losing one's reputation (as a result of being damaged by the other).[7] It will prompt the phobic person to resolve this fear (which can manifest itself in a variety of forms) by keeping his distance, once again bringing loneliness and associated fears to prominence. Thus, the strategy of desire is not one of seduction or action, or of control and postponement, but of acquiescence, compliance, and avoidance, of bowing to the inevitable.

Personality Disorder

The disturbance associated with the structure of the personality disorder (of perversion, of narcissism and the borderline position) runs appreciably deeper than in the case of a neurotic structure, as we have seen before. The process of separation and its dialectics of the inter-subjective relationships are patently disturbed, with most of the burden of subjectivity being put on the other's shoulders. We would do well to remember that Lacan and most Lacanians hold a different view in that they attribute sole autonomy to perversion and not to narcissism as position or the borderline position. Next, it is useful to remember the distinction made before between perverse, narcissistic and borderline traits on the one hand, and perverse, narcissistic, and borderline positions, which pervade the whole personality structure. If, for example, perverse traits become pervasive, we may speak of a perverse position. Likewise, this would apply to other traits and positions.

In the case of *perversion,* the other is involved in an action that transgresses boundaries, turning him by preference into an accomplice, whilst the boundary itself is ridiculed (Dor, 1997, pp. 31-71; Fink, 1977, pp. 165-202). Significant in this context is the theme of seeing and being seen, which is played out differently than in the case of the hysteric position. The hysteric wishes to be seen, while the pervert wishes to be seen and not to be seen (turning up only to disappear again), just like he

[7] Freud stresses the menacing role of the father. See the case of 'Little Hans' (Freud, 1909/1955a). Lacan, by contrast, highlights the threat posed by the mother. See Lacan (1994), p. 228: "[...] le term de la dévoration est toujours trouvable, par quelque coté, dans la structure de la phobie".

'knows' about the law he wishes to break without actually 'having knowledge' of it.[8] This type of duality, referred to as 'disavowal', is characteristic. To put it differently, the pervert will only see the alleged omnipotence of the Law (which does not exist) and not the impotence of the Law (which does exist). He simply lacks insight into the symbolic status of the Law, with the law being impotent in itself, becoming effective only if each and everyone submits to it. The Law will be presented as omnipotent only to be ridiculed for its impotence, upon which the pervert will leave the stage.

Ideal-typically, the life-historical background may be such that the child identifies with the other's lack, which is defined in terms of sexual difference. Lacan (1966/2002) writes (p. 462/3): "The whole problem of perversion consists in conceiving how the child, in its relationship with its mother [...] identifies with the imaginary object of her desire insofar as the mother herself symbolizes it in the phallus." From this sexualised – or rather 'phallicised' – bond with the mother, the figure of the 'third' will emerge (i.e., the other as a representative of the rule or the law prohibiting boundary-transgressing affective intimacy) as an impotent force. The child positions itself as the person who can be anything to the mother, as its imaginary phallus, whereas the father figure is virtually absent – a weak figure which only makes his presence felt through temper tantrums, which also betray his weakness. The pervert will repeat this basic scenario, positioning himself as an object ready to fill the lack in the other, with an immediacy and directness that will prompt a panic reaction with the other, who is expected to carry the full burden of subjectiveness. An immediate and unmitigated enjoyment is sought, which is connected rather with death and anxiety than with the gender difference (to put it differently: with aggression and fear). At the same time, the figure of the 'third' who is relegated to a background role becomes the object of mockery and derision – the cycle is complete and can begin anew. The awareness of the Law (embodied by the figure of the third) is present, but the Law itself is defied and scorned. [9]

The *narcissistic* position finds itself on a par with the level of psychic functioning. Again, most of the burden of subjectivity is put on the side of the other (the victim), positioning the perpetrator primarily as an

---

[8] Remember the title of the classic article by Octave Mannoni '*Je sais bien, mais quand-même ...*' See Mannoni (1969, pp. 9-33).

[9] To describe this aspect (the relationship with the powerful/powerless father), Lacan speaks of the '*père-version*' of the oedipal structure.

object or instrument. The disavowal of the lack is dominated not so much by phallicisation or the sexual difference as by a rejection of one's own insignificance. From an experienced sense of grandiosity, the own lack, in the sense of one's own insignificance and finiteness, is transferred to the other. The other is forced to do or submit to actions which he would never have engaged in voluntarily. While in the case of perversion some degree of cooperation on the part of the partner is expected to be sought, it is absent here. What we see here is intimidation or a form of brutal aggression, which we may refer to as 'desexualised sadism'.

Its life-historical background may be such that the gradual process of disillusionment which a child faces – *has* to face, from the perspective of a normative life history – was inadequate (Kohut, 1971). The gradual replacement of a mirroring and dual type of relationship – with the child being admired – by a more symbolic and triangular type of relationship, accepting one's own limitations by rules and laws, never came about fully. The reason may be that the child was a constant object of excessive admiration – leading to a type of narcissism dominated by feelings of excessive grandiosity, or to its psychopathic derivative. Then again, early (real or mental) traumatisation may have left the child strongly deprived in cases where it received little or no admiration, which leads to another type of narcissism with more antisocial characteristics or to its psychopathic derivative (see also Chapter Seven, psychopathy type 2 and 1, respectively). This antisocial type is probably the most well known variety, often involving a more or less violent father figure, not the figure of the so-called 'real father' that impotently refers to the symbolic law, but an imaginary and aggressive father (Verhaeghe and Willemsen, 2009). The Law is there, but only as a caricature in its violent pre-symbolic, imaginary form, leading to feelings of humiliations and shame. Yet the deep humiliation associated with it can be remedied in a compensatory way, leading to an illusional reinforcement of the feeling of grandiosity – the imaginary ideal-ego as opposed to the symbolic ego-ideals. However, its illusional character will make this grandiosity particularly vulnerable and open to injuries, which in turn may provoke narcissistic responses (in some cases leading the subject to commit more or less serious crimes).

Following the line of thought proposed here, the *borderline* position is found at the same level of psychic functioning, except that it involves the sphere of dependence (following on from the phobic position) rather than the sphere of provocation or enforcement. Where the phobic person submits to the other, transferring responsibility for his own existence (including all the risks involved), the borderline will put his fate into the other's hands. The lack is acknowledged insofar as the desire exists to fill the lack in the other. Yet at the same time the lack is denied, based on the belief that it can be filled completely. In other words, the lack is disavowed.

Its life-historical background may be that of a family situation with an overbearing parent claiming the child by saying: "You are everything to me". This type of overwhelming love is binding but not unconditional, because from it follows logically: "Without you I am nothing". This may prompt both partners to copy this by telling each other: "You are my everything, without you I am nothing", which effectively turns both into each other's prisoner. From a structural point of view, the opposite type of family may also exist, namely one of underinvolvement rather than overinvolvement: the child means little or nothing to the primary other. The child may attempt to attract attention by making itself explicitly available to the other, offering itself to remedy the lack in the other in an overinvolved ('hypermentalising', 'paranoid-sensitive') manner. The consequence of both constellations may be that the child will do anything to fill the lack with the other, which leads to a symbiotic and dual relational pattern.[10] In both cases, next to the primary (m)Other there is very little space for the secondary Other, the second parent, to express himself.

Psychosis

Compared to the two structures referred to in the above, the psychosis differs in the sense that it involves a fundamental disruption of intersubjectivity. Within the neurotic context, intersubjective relations are basically unaffected, as is the symbolic function, from the perspective of symbolization. In the case of the personality disorder, however, we see a profound disruption of intersubjective relations, with a symbolic function that is unable to bring full separation. This is reflected in the relations with both pleasure and the Law. In the case of the psychotic structure, however, structural relations are fundamentally disturbed, resulting from a thoroughly deficient symbolic function. 'Access to language' took place, but the 'encounter with the lack' (in respect to language and the Other) did not. As a result, the possibility of distancing

---

[10] An elaboration of the borderline states (not conceived as a position) from a Lacanian perspective is offered by Rassial (1999). See also Verhaeghe (2008, pp. 336-350).

oneself, which allows reflection, did not present itself either. To put it differently: there is alienation, but no separation. In the field of intentionalities, this leads potentially to a seriously impaired capacity for reality testing, although milder forms may also occur. The proximity of the other is overwhelming, who manifests himself in the form of inescapable hallucinations or as a single or multiple delusions in which the other is utterly powerful.

It is perfectly imaginable that such a profound defect of the symbolic function is constitutional in origin, going to back to inborn defects. From this perspective, the thesis of a non-operative symbolic function may well be in line with a biological rationale. It is equally conceivable that a proper development of the symbolic function is environment-dependent, and that any deficit is conditioned life-historically. A combination of the two conditions is also possible, with their mutual relations varying among cases (Lang, 2000b, pp. 296-309). The outcome would be that a fundamental disruption occurs (or has occurred) in the process of separation, which is normally characterised by the subject separating itself from the first other in the presence of 'a third', whilst leaving a remainder in this process of separation. The figure of 'the third' is a prerequisite for the process of separation between the two parties to be initiated, with this third serving as an instance to which both partners can relate.[11] The process of separation will be disturbed in the sense that there is no vacant chair or vacancy to be filled by a third (Mooij, 1993; 2003). Apparently, we are not dealing with a person, but with the performance of a function which, in one way or another, is perceived as 'tangible' (Nasio, 1987, pp. 120-126). That which is 'required' is nothing more than a reference to a vacant spot outside the twofoldness of the primary (m)Other and the child, regardless of how this takes shape. Whatever the case may be, at the very least it requires some kind of concretization of the lack in the (m)Other and some degree of openness on the part of the child which, based on its predisposition, needs to be able to perceive this vacancy and has some notion of how it should be filled.

---

[11] This refers to what Lacan describes as the 'foreclosure of the name-of-the-father', the '*forclusion du nom-du-père*', which underlies or is supposed to underlie the psychotic structure. The 'foreclosure of the name of the father' means that the father metaphor (*métaphore paternelle*), which represents the severing of the child's bonds with the mother's desire, is dysfunctional.

In the absence of such a vacancy or the possibility to perceive it, consistent 'agreements' or rules cannot be applied, which leads to permanent disruption of structured reality. Indeed, experiencing reality is also based on 'agreements' regarding this reality. In this case, reality testing is disturbed, paving the way for psychotic decompensation in the case of particularly stressful situations or sustained undermining to occur. The fact that such decompensation does not always occur may be put down to an adequate supplementation from the environment or effective protections built into the person's way of life to offset the lack, safeguarding this person against psychotic decompensation (Lacan, 1966/2002, p. 484; 1981/1993; 2005). It seems that a psychotic structure does not necessarily lead to full-blown psychotic symptoms (including hallucinations and/or delusions) while, by the same token, the presence of such symptoms does not always point to the supposed presence of such a structure (Maleval, 1981/1991; 2000).

Overall, the occurrence of episodes with a relapsing or chronic character will be associated with schizophrenic-like images where, depending on the seriousness of the disorder, the symbolic and separating function can be expected to be highly dysfunctional or even non-operative. They may also appear in the sphere of melancholy, in which case the process of separation will be 'focally' disturbed, with the subject identifying with the loss as a result of the process of symbolisation, which may result in a specific vulnerability for 'situations of loss' (Juranville, 2005, pp. 108-116).[12] Finally, paranoid episodes may occur in situations where disruption of separation specifically produces a loss of boundaries in the position of the perceived other, as 'common' dependence on the other will lead him to regard this other, in this particular case, as omnipotent. Within the context of a psychotic disorder, this may lead to a traditional type of delusion or paranoia.

This paragraph looked into ideal-typical connections between a pathological structure and a possible life-historical background, such in relation to a conception of a mental disorder in terms of a 'fundamental disturbance' – a defective symbolic function. This fundamental dis-

---

[12] Lambotte (1993/1999) distances herself from this conception, pp. 544-563, 'Ni névrose, ni psychose'. In the case of Lacan, the position of the melancholy is determined by a perfect identification with the lost object (object *a*), while the mania is determined by a non-functional object (to which he attributes its fleeting character). Lacan (2004, p. 388): "Dans la manie, […], c'est la non-fonction de a qui est en cause. Le sujet n'y est lesté par aucun a, ce qui le livre, quelque fois sans aucune possibilité de liberté, à la métonymie pure, infinite et ludique, de la chaîne signifiante".

turbance may manifest itself within the gamut of disorders comprising the neurosis, personality disorder and psychotic disorder, which reflect intact, partly disturbed and fundamentally disturbed intersubjective relationships, respectively. The intelligibility of these connections does not automatically justify conclusions being drawn on individual, factual cases, nor does it tell us anything about their role in the emergence and long-term presence of a psychotic structure. This limitation follows logically from the ideal-typical nature of the connection that refers only to an 'ideal' situation. It also follows from the condition that the environment does not causally determine the subject or the emerging subject, but that it merely offers the conditions to which it can and must relate. This implies a freedom in choosing a particular type of relation which, limited though it may be in individual cases, is always there. It makes one responsible in a sense for the subject position 'chosen' (Lacan, 1966/2002, p. 729). It also makes that any connection between a structure and life-historical background can only exist 'ideally', in a 'detached' form, which is why empirical-hermeneutical investigation into the real life history is needed. Man finding himself thrown into a particular situation will always have an option to define his relation towards it.

Psychiatry and Biography

As was pointed out before, the presumed significance of the life history for a psychic structure and a specific psychic disorder to emerge does not imply that it can be inferred in its entirety from the life history. This will prompt attempts to make sense of historical phenomena or, failing these attempts, to assume a fact of nature or natural law. Thus, assuming the presence of grades of intelligibility, we can descend the 'ladder of understanding', until we find ourselves at the level of events that can no longer be made sense of. This does impose limits on what can still be interpreted historically or (psycho)genetically: trauma, inborn errors, congenital defects, etcetera. Moreover, it is likely that psychic vulnerabilities that can be understood from a life-historical and structural perspective in turn are supported by a biological substrate – indeed, any action or experience is informed by mechanisms of the body and the central nervous system. Yet the focus is on the actual fortunes of the subject in relation to his situation of origin: the situation into which it is cast and to which it needs to relate. It is a fundamentally different approach from the one based on the notion that any psychic order has an underlying biological cause, ultimately leading to 'biography-less psychiatry'.

It makes that psychiatry focusing on the life history stands in a different relationship towards the 'criteria of scientific quality' than does the primarily natural-scientifically oriented brand of psychiatry. Among other things, it may look to the scientific discipline of history, to one of the humanities, as it also allows testing in the field of description and interpretation. That hermeneutical standards may also qualify as scientific does not alter the fact that there is a major divide between the natural-scientific and hermeneutical approaches. The natural-scientific or empirical-analytical approach is quantitative and measure-oriented, whereas the hermeneutical or empirical-hermeneutical approach is primarily qualitative and interpretative in nature.

This difference not only creates a potential division within psychiatry and a gap between the natural sciences and humanities, but also brings a more or less dualistic culture into being. Also here we find an uneasy relationship between a quality-focused mode of interpretation of understanding on the one hand, and an approach geared towards quantifying, measuring and controlling on the other. The ambiguous nature of this culture, which gave rise to the rift existing within psychiatry, will be discussed in the Epilogue.

Epilogue

This book distinguished between two types of psychiatry. The first type, focusing on the medical discourse, manifested itself as a natural, exact science. By extension, it addresses themes such as taxonomy, replicability, and effectiveness of interventions, while seeking to explain psychopathological phenomena in preferably biological terms. It is not particularly contemplative in nature, but rather empiricist and pragmatic, pursuing active intervention in favour of controlling aberrant behaviour.

Its orientation towards the humanities makes that the second type of psychiatry is not particularly focused on taxonomy or replicability, nor on identifying laws or statistical correlations. Instead, it aims to add a new dimension through description, establishing relationships of meaning, whilst seeking to address anthropological and existential issues associated with mental disorders. In doing so, it aims to express the psychic reality in all its dimensions. Adopting a practical but not a pragmatic approach, while being hermeneutical rather than empiricist in nature, it has a keen eye for the more tragic aspects of existence. This type of psychiatry has found itself exposed to criticism, with doubt being cast on its scientific quality as well as on its practical relevance. It is the classic and still ongoing battle on the legitimacy of the 'space of reasons' as being opposed to the 'realm of natural law'.

If psychiatry were to relegate the psychic reality to history, this would effectively put an end to the traditional manifestation of psychiatry as well as psychopathology, with its acknowledgement of a bipolarity recognizing the legitimacy of both perspectives. Psychiatry would then be virtually usurped by the medical discourse. If this were to occur, it would constitute a major departure from an established tradition, with the medical discourse creating a void left by the psychic reality to be filled by psychiatry.

Yet, regardless of the evolution of psychiatry as a medical specialty, the broad hermeneutical approach can continue to assert itself as a specialty in its own right in the field of mental disorders. It has been the major objective of this book to establish its viability in a philosophical and clinical sense. The distinction between the three levels of the psychic reality – experience, situation, structure – and its corresponding approaches – phenomenology, (narrowed-down) hermeneutics and a Lacanian analysis – having been validated may also define future developments. The same applies to the traditional distinction between neurosis, personality disorder and psychosis.

In the realm of experience, phenomenology, as a descriptive psychology, will remain indispensable. We might think of the description of psychic, intentional phenomena from the cognitive and affective spheres (e.g., anxiety, compulsive and impulsive behaviour associated with neurotic and personality disorders), but also of phenomena produced by disturbed pre-reflexive psychotic consciousness. The interpretative approach, e.g. the hermeneutics in a narrow-downed sense, is seminal to any in-depth description of specific modes of world constitution as well as its life-historical background in the fields of neurotic issues, personality disorders and psychotic disorders. Anthropological questions find expression in the structural perspective, as the concept of structure is tied to having a 'choice' to adopt a particular life design, regardless of the lack of freedom in having a choice. The Lacanian perspective adds an essential dimension to psychopathology, deepening it. Finally, the transcendental approach inquires into the conditions of possibility for normality and its disturbances. By highlighting the symbolic function of the human mind, it effectively forges a connection with traditional philosophical questions rooted in the transcendental tradition, while providing a disease criterion, being detached from any social standards.

It brings to light that in one sense a mental disorder cannot be compared to a physical disease: the former involves a person's individual subjectivity, with subjectivity itself being affected, fading or even imploding. This will raise a specific type of sense-giving's questions, which to some extent can be related to any particular disorder and subject position. A person suffering from anxiety provoked by a psychotrauma will do so as a result of a particular event, while also potentially suffering from the human condition itself, which is vulnerable and fragile, exposed to infringements from both within and outside. It turns a mental disorder tied to a subject position into more than just the expression of a disturbed experience, a life-historically defined conflict, of a specific psychopathological structure or a brain function disorder. Indeed, it is also an expression of the essentially fragile nature of human existence and of individual subjectivity, which a decaying of its basic conditions of possibility – the symbolic function – can cause to dissolve, fade or even implode.

Ultimately, the future of the hermeneutical perspective, conceived in a broad sense, hinges on the notion of experience. The natural-scientific approach limits the experience to what is repeatable, measurable and possibly calculable within an impersonal framework. It presupposes a generic 'Bewusstsein überhaupt'. The concept of the hermeneutical experience, in its most generalised context, is much broader, while also implying a contribution of a person's subjectivity as well as a sense of awareness of this contribution, purifying it. Where the natural-scientific experience strives to eliminate subjectivity, the hermeneutical experience proceeds from the notion that no insight into actual experience, background and underlying structure can be gained unless this aspect is taken into account. This is the tenet of the humanities and any of the various human sciences gravitating around it, as well as the hermeneutical philosophy as such.

Where our approach to reality in modernity creates a divide between a natural-scientific and a hermeneutical view, this will effectively reduce the world by half, as it recognises only the natural-scientific approach as legitimate. And yet, making a choice is not that dramatic in itself: rather than either/or, it is a matter of and/and. Moreover, the two psychiatric views outlined here do not exist in isolation, but each corresponds to generic approaches to reality that transcends the boundaries of the psychiatric field itself. Indeed, psychiatry will step beyond its reach because both brands of psychiatry reflect a type of culture or a line of thought that in its turn is suited to psychiatric interpretation. Depending on which line of thought prevails, either a natural-scientific and pragmatic view *or* a hermeneutical and more tragic view is dominant. A pragmatic view within psychiatry as well as in culture at large highlights what is measurable, geared towards short-term interventions in favour of controlling behaviour whose effect is easily identifiable. A hermeneutical view, by contrast, is sceptical of the requirement of countability, measurability and controllabilty , instead pleading the case of a scientific approach that accommodates prudential interpretation, whilst emphasising that any process of change, if possible at all, is likely to take time.

These two lines of thought are not likely to find common ground any time soon, if ever, considering that the barriers to be overcome are fundamentally not empirical but conceptual in nature. Thus neither approach should win out, as both cultures represent a dimension of human existence that must never be obscured. Again, it is not a matter of 'or/or', but of 'and/and', involving a comprehensive integration of both perspectives that is *not* supposed to be forthcoming yet. This, however, should not be taken as an excuse to favour the natural-scientific approach at the expense of hermeneutics. Besides, whenever activism and pragmatism is the dominant culture, the case for the hermeneutical and tragic dimension should be made even more strongly. Therefore, in the field of psychiatry, the empiricist and pragmatic approach has become firmly established. But if psychiatry, psychopathology deals with psychic reality – through experience, conflict and loss, life history and psychopathological structure – hermeneutics would be the path to follow. A psychiatry or psychopathology that is truly open to the psychic reality in all its manifestations will hold greater promise for the future. Only then will psychiatry become a truly human science.

Simultaneously, psychiatry will contribute to a more balanced culture, one that takes both perspectives into account, the realm of law as well as the space of reason, the way of controlling behaviour or understanding its meaning. More than that, it may deepen the philosophical conception of man, while recognising man's psychic reality – his openness to experience, his being situated, and the language-dependent mode of his existence, all supported by his ability to interpret and symbolise the real, outside or within himself. Ultimately, psychopathology may put flesh and bones on this conceptual scheme, by referring to the various ways people live their unique individual lives: in a more or less (neurotic) normal or in a more or less disturbed way (personality disorder and psychosis). This will lead to a broadening of the horizon of understanding of the rich spectrum of the human mind.

In doing so, psychiatry, or psychopathology conceived as a human science, may contribute to the further development of a philosophical anthropology, or at least to its concretization. Indeed, philosophical anthropology without empirical content is essentially empty, while a human science without a philosophical scheme is more or less blind, the scheme itself having to be rooted in experience. In conclusion, psychiatry as a human science offers a philosophical anthropology made concrete, adding qualification to the one-sidedness of both modern psychiatry and modern culture.

Appendix

Table Outlining Psychopathological Structures

Neurotic structure			
POSITION	*hysteric*	*obsessive*	*phobic*
Time dimension	past +	future +	present +
Space dimension	centre +	height +	boundary +
Desire (lack recognized)	unsatisfied	impossible	inevitable
Personality disorder structure			
POSITION	*perverse*	*narcissistic*	*borderline*
Time dimension	past –	future –	present –
Space dimension	centre –	height –	boundary –
Disavowal (lack acknowledged and not-acknowledged)	sexual difference	one's own insignificance	the other's lack
Psychotic structure			
POSITION	*schizophrenic*	*melancholic*	*paranoid*
Time dimension, decay of	past 0	future 0	present 0
Space dimension, decay of	centre 0	height 0	boundary 0
Lack not acknowledged	incapability of guilt	identification with guilt	identifying the other with guilt

Explanation of symbols used:
+ means: emphasis on the dimension concerned
– means: weakening of the dimension concerned
0 means: imploding of the dimension concerned

Bibliography

Alexander, F. (1950). *Psychosomatic Medicine.* New York: Norton.

American Psychiatric Association (2000). *Diagnostic and Statistical Manual of Mental Disorders* (IV-TR). Washington, DC.

André, S. (1993). *L'Imposture Perverse.* Paris: Seuil.

Andreasen, N. (1984). *The Broken Brain. The Biological Revolution in Psychiatry.* New York: Harpar and Row.

Andreasen, N. (2001). *Brave New Brain: Conquering Mental Illness in the Era of the Genome.* Oxford: Oxford University Press.

Andreasen, N. (2007). DSM and the death of phenomenology in America: An example of unintended consequences. *Schizophrenia Bulletin, 33*, 108-112.

Ankersmit, F.R. (1995). De activiteit van de historicus. In *Hermeneutiek en Cultuur. Interpretatie in de Kunst- en Cultuurwetenschappen*, F.R. Ankersmit, M. van Nierop & H. Pott (Eds.), 70-97. Amsterdam: Boom.

Anscombe, G.E.M. (1963). *Intention.* Oxford: Basil Blackwell. (Original work published 1957)

Apel, K.-O. (1979). *Die Erklären-Verstehen-Kontroverse in Transzendental-Pragmatischer Sicht.* Frankfurt a.M.: Suhrkamp.

Aristotle (1984). *The Complete Works of Aristotle.* The revised Oxford translation. Editor J. Barnes. Princeton, NJ: Princeton University Press.

Arnold, M.B. (1960). *Emotion and Personality*, Part I: Psychological Aspects. New York: Columbia University Press.

Assoun, P.-L. (2005). *Les Phobies.* Paris: Anthropos.

Atwood, G.E., & Stolorow, R.D. (1984). *Structures of Subjectitivity: Explorations in Psychoanalytic Phenomenology.* Northvale, NJ: Jason Aronson.

Audi, R. (1993). *Action, Intention and Reason.* Ithaca and London: Cornell University Press.

Austin, J.L. (1970). Three ways of spilling ink. In *Philosophical Papers*, 272-288. London/Oxford: Oxford University Press. (Original work published 1961)

Austin, J.L. (1971). *How to Do Things with Words.* London: Oxford University Press. (Original work published 1962)

Baas, B. (1992). *Le désir pur. Parcours philosophiques dans les parages de J. Lacan.* Louvain: Peeters.

Bailly, L. (2009). *Lacan.* London: Oneworld.

Balmès, F. (1999). *Ce que Lacan dit de l'être.* Paris: Presses Universitaires de France.

Bechtel, W. (2001). Representations: From neural systems to cognitive systems. In *Philosophy and the Neurosciences. A Reader*, W. Bechtel, P. Mandik, J. Mundale & R.S. Sufflebeam (Eds.), 332-349. Oxford/Malden, MA: Blackwell Publishers.

Bennet, M.R., & Hacker, P.M.S. (2003). *Philosophical Foundations of Neuroscience*. Oxford: Basil Blackwell.

Benoist, J. (2007). Two (or three) conceptions of intentionality. *Tijdschrift voor Filosofie, 69*, 79-105.

Bercherie, P. (1980). *Les Fondements de la Clinique: Histoire et Structure du Savoir Psychiatrique*. Paris: Navarin.

Berg, J.H. van den (1965). *Het Menselijk Lichaam,* Part 1: Het geopende lichaam. Nijkerk: Callenbach. (Original work published 1959)

Bermúdez, J.L. (2005). The phenomenology of body awareness. In *Phenomenology and the Philosophy of Mind,* D. Woodruff Smith & L. Thomassen (Eds.), 295-317. Oxford: Clarendon Press.

Bernard, Cl. (1865). *Introduction à l'Étude de la Médecine Expérimentale.* Paris: Baillière.

Bernet, R. (2004). Husserl's transcendentalism revisited. *New Yearbook for Phenomenology and Phenomenological Philosophy, 4*, 1-20.

Betti, E. (1988). *Zur Grundlegung einer Allgemeinen Auslegungslehre.* Tübingen: Mohr.

Binswanger, L. (1931-1932). Über Ideenflucht. *Schweizer Archiv Für Neurologie Und Psychiatrie, Teil XXVII-XXX.*

Binswanger, L. (1947). *Ausgewählte Vorträge und Aufsätze*, Part I: Zur phänomenologischen Antropologie. Bern: Francke.

Binswanger, L. (1953). *Grundformen und Erkenntnis Menschlichen Daseins.* Zürich: Max Niehans. (Original work published 1942)

Binswanger, L. (1955). *Ausgewählte Vorträge und Aufsätze*, Part II: Zur Problematik der psychiatrischen Forschung und zum Problem der Psychiatrie. Bern: Francke.

Binswanger, L. (1956). *Drei Formen Missglückten Daseins: Verstiegenheit Verschrobenheit Manieriertheit.* Tübingen: Niemeyer.

Binswanger, L. (1957). *Schizophrenie.* Pfullingen: Neske.

Binswanger, L. (1960). *Melancholie und Manie: Phänomenologische Studien.* Pfullingen: Neske.

Binswanger, L. (1965a). *Einführung in die Probleme der Algemeinen Psychologie.* Amsterdam: Bonset. (Original work published 1922)

Binswanger, L. (1965b). *Wahn: Beiträge zu einer Phänomenologischen und daseinsanalytischen Erforschung.* Pfullingen: Neske.

Binswanger, L. (1998). *Le Problème de l'Espace en Psychopathologie.* Toulouse: Presses Universitaires Mirail.

Binswanger, L. (2000). *Sur la Fuites des Idées* (Trans. of *Über Ideenflucht*). Grenoble: Millon. (Original work published 1931-32)

Bion, W.R. (1986). *Attention and Interpretation*. London: Karnac Books. (Original work published 1970)

Black, M. (1962). *Models and Metaphors*. Ithaca, NY: Cornell University Press.

Blankenburg, W. (1971). *Der Verlust der Natürlichen Selbstverständlichkeit: Ein Beitrag zur Psychopathologie Symptomarmer Schizophrenien*. Stuttgart: Enke.

Blankenburg, W. (1980). Ein Beitrag zur Normproblem. In *Medizinisch-psychologische Anthropologie*, W. Bräutigam (Ed.), 273-290. Darmstadt: Wissenschaftliche Buchgesellschaft.

Blankenburg, W. (1982). A dialectical conception of anthropological proportion. In *Phenomenology and Psychiatry*, A.J.J. de Koning & F.A. Jenner (Eds.), 35-50. London/Toronto/Sydney/New York: Academic Press/ Grune and Stratton.

Blom, J.D. (2004). *Deconstructing Schizophrenia*. Amsterdam: Boom.

Boer, Th. de (1978). *The Development of Husserl's Thought*. The Hague: Nijhoff.

Bollas, B. (1999). *The Shadow of the Object*. London: Free Association Books. (Original work published 1987)

Bollnow, O.F. (1943). *Das Wesen der Stimmungen*. Frankfurt a.M.: Klostermann.

Bonnet, G. (1981). *Voire et Être Vu*, Part I: Études cliniques sur l'exhibitionisme. Paris: PUF.

Bonnet, G. (1993). *Les Perversions Sexuelles*. Paris: PUF. (Original work published 1983)

Boss, M. (1954). *Einführung in die Psychosomatische Medizin*. Stuttgart: Huber.

Bowlby, J. (1969). *Attachment and Loss*, Volume I: Attachment. London: Hogarth Press and the Institute of Psycho-Analysis.

Boszormeyi-Nagy, I & Spark, G.M. (1973). *Invisible Loyalities*. New York: Harper and Row.

Bracken, P., & Thomas, P. (2005). *Postpsychiatry: Mental Health in a Postmodern Environment*. Oxford: Oxford University Press.

Brandon, R.B. (2001). *Articulating Reasons. An Introduction to Referentialism*. Cambridge, MA/London: Harvard University Press.

Braunstein, N. (2003). Desire and jouissance in the teachings of Lacan. In *The Cambridge Companion to Lacan*, J.-M. Rabaté (Ed.), 102-116. Cambridge: Cambridge University Press.

Brenner, C. (1980). *An Elementary Textbook of Psychoanalysis*. New York: International Universities Press.

Brentano, F. (1973). *Psychology from an Empirical Standpoint*. London: Routlege and Kegan Paul. (Original work published 1874)

Buytendijk, F.J.J. (1965). *Prolegomena van een Antropologische Fysiologie*. Utrecht/Antwerpen: Spectrum.

Cartwright, N. (1983). *How the Laws of Physics Lie*. Oxford: Clarendon Press.

Cartwright, N. (1999). *The Dappled World. A Study on the Boundaries of Science*. Cambridge: Cambridge University Press.

Cassell, E.J. (2004). *The Nature of Suffering and the Goals of Medicine*. Oxford/New York: Oxford University Press. (Original work published 1991)

Cassirer, E. (1943). The place of Vesalius in the culture of the Renaissance. *Yale Journal of Biology and Medicine, 16* (December), 109-119. Quoted in Krois 2004, 293.

Cassirer, E. (1953). *Language and Myth* (S.L. Langer, Trans.). New York: Dover. (Work original published 1946)

Cassirer, E. (1953-1957). *The Philosophy of the Symbolic Forms*, Volume 1-3 (R. Manheim, Trans.). New Haven: Yale University Press.

Cassirer, E. (1966). *An Essay on Man: An Introduction to a Philosophy of Human Culture*. New Haven/London: Yale University Press. (Work orginal published 1944)

Cassirer, E. (1969). *Wesen und Wirkung des Symbolbegriffs*. Darmstadt: Wissenschaftliche Buchgesellschaft. (Work original published 1956)

Cassirer, E. (1971). *Idee und Gestalt. Goethe, Schiller, Hölderlin, Kleist*. Darmstadt: Wissenschafliche Buchgesellschaft.

Cassirer, E. (1994a). *Philosophie der Symbolischen Formen,* Part I: Die Sprache. Darmstadt: Wissenschaftliche Buchgesellschaft. (Work original published 1923)

Cassirer, E. (1994b). *Philosophie der Symbolischen Formen,* Part III: Phänomenologie der Erkenntnis. Darmstadt: Wissenschaftliche Buchgesellschaft. (Work original published 1929)

Cassirer, E. (2000). *Substanzbegriff und Funktionsbegriff. Untersuchungen über die Grundfragen der Erkenntniskritik. Gesammelte Werke: Hamburger Ausgabe*, edited by B. Recki, Volume 6, edited by R. Schmücker. Darmstadt: Wissenschaftliche Buchgesellschaft. (Original work published 1910).

Cassirer, E., Cohen, H., & Natorp, P. (1998). *L'École de Marburg*. Paris: Éditions du Cerf.

Castanet, H. (Ed.) (1990). *Le Sujet dans la Psychose: Paranoïa et Mélancolie*. Nice: Z'éditions.

Chalmers, D.J. (1996). *The Conscious Mind: In Search of a Fundamental Theory*. Oxford: Oxford University Press.

Chamond, J. (Ed.) (2004). *Les Directions de Sens: Phénoménologie et Psychopathologie de l'Espace Vécu*. Paris: Cercle Herméneutique.

Changeux, J.P., & Ricoeur, P. (1998). *Ce Qui Nous Fait Penser: La Nature et la Règle*, Paris: Odile Jacob.

Charbonneau, G. (2004). L'être en deçà de soi ou la hantise de l'outrepassement. In *Les Directions de Sens: Phénoménologie et Psycho-*

pathologie de l'Espace Vécu, J. Chamond (Ed.), 117-131. Paris: Cercle Hermeneutique.

Charbonneau, G. (2010). *Introduction à la Psychopathologie Phénoménologique*, Part II, 177-215. Paris: MJW Fédition.

Chiesa, L. (2007). *Subjectivity and Otherness. A Philsophical Reading of Lacan.* Cambridge, MA: MIT Press.

Church, J. (2004). Social constructionist models: making order out of disorder – On the social construction of madness. In *The Philosophy of Psychiatry: A Companion*, J. Radden (Ed.), 393-406. Oxford: Oxford University Press.

Churchland, P. (1984). *Matter and Consciousness: A Contemporary Introduction to the Philosophy of Mind.* Cambridge, MA: MIT Press.

Clark, A. (1997). *Being There: Putting Brain, Body and World Together.* Cambridge, MA/London: MIT Press.

Clark, A. (2008). *Supersizing the Mind: Embodiment, Action and Cognitive Extension.* Oxford: Oxford University Press.

Clavreul, J. (1978). *L'Ordre Médical.* Paris: Seuil.

Clavreul, J. (1980). The perverse couple. In *Returning to Freud: Clinical Psychoanalysis in the School of Lacan,* S. Schneiderman (Ed.), 214-234. New Haven/London: Yale University Press.

Cleckley, H. (1976). *The Mask of Sanity.* St Louis, MO: Mosby.

Collingwood, R.G. (1978). *An Autobiography.* Oxford: Oxford University Press.

Conrad, K. (1959). Gestaltanalyse und Daseinsanalytik. *Der Nervenarzt, 30,* 405-410.

Conrad, K. (1987). *Die Beginnende Schizophrenie: Versuch einer Gestaltanalyse des Wahns.* Stuttgart: Thieme. (Work orginal published 1958)

Courtine, J.-F. (Ed.), (1992). *Figures de la Subjectivité.* Paris: CNRS.

Damasio, A.R. (1994). *Descartes' Error: Emotion, Reason and the Human Brain.* New York: Avon Books.

Damasio, A.R. (2003). *Looking for Spinoza: Joy, Sorrow and the Feeling Brain.* Orlando, FL: Harcourt.

Dastur, F. (2001). Autobiographie et narrativité. In *Phénoménologie de l'Identité Humaine et Schizophrénie,* D. Pringey & F.S. Kohl (Eds.), 43-50. Paris: Cercle Herméneutique.

Davidson, D. (1980). *Action and Events.* Oxford: Clarendon Press.

Depraz, N. (2001). Pratiquer l' épochè: Pertinence de l'épochè schizophrénique comme phénomène-limite. In *Phénoménologie de l'Identité Humaine et Schizophrénie*, D. Pringey & F.S. Kohl (Eds.), 134-144. Paris: Cercle Herméneutique.

Derrida, J. (1982). *Margins of Philosophy* (A. Bass, Trans.). Chicago: University of Chicago Press. (Work original published 1972)

Descartes, R. (1988). *Les Passions de l'Âme.* Parijs: Gallimard.

Deutsch, H. (1934) Über einen Typus der Pseudoaffektivität ('Als Ob'). *Internationale Zeitschrift für Psychoanalyse, 20,* 323-335.

Dijksterhuis, E.J. (1986). *The Mechanization of the World Picture*. Princeton, NJ: Princeton University Press.

Dillmann, R. (1990). *Alzheimer's Disease: The Concept of Disease and the Construction of Medical Knowledge*. Amsterdam: Thesis.

Dilthey, W. (1961). Der Aufbau der geschichtlichen Welt in den Geisteswissenschaften. In *Die Philosophie des Lebens*. (Selected by H. Nohl), 131-230. Stuttgart/Göttingen: Teubner/Vandenhoeck & Ruprecht. (Original work published 1910)

Dolto, F. (1987). *Dialogues Québécois*. Paris: Seuil.

Dor, J. (1997). *The Clinical Lacan*. Northvale, NJ/London: Jason Aronson Inc.

Dreyfus, H.L. (2007). The return of the myth of the mental. *Inquiry: An Interdisciplinairy Journal of Philosophy*, *50*, 352-365.

Ebtinger, R. (1986). Modèles phénoménologiques et psychiatriques en psychiatrie. In *Phénoménologie Psychiatrie Psychanalyse*, P. Fédida (Ed.), 79-123. Paris: Echo-Centurion.

Ehrenberg, A. (2009). *The Weariness of the Self: Diagnosing the History of Depression in the Contemporary Age* (D. Homel, Trans.) Montreal: McGill-Queen's University Press.

Ellenberger, H. (1970). *The Discovery of the Unconscious: The History and Evolution of Dynamic Psychiatry*. London: Allen Lane/The Penguin Press.

Engel, G.L. (1980). The clinical application of the biopsychosocial model. *American Journal of Psychiatry*, *137*, 129-136.

Engelhardt, D. von, & Schipperges, H. (1980). *Die Inneren Verbindungen zwischen Philosophie und Medizin im 20. Jahrhundert*. Darmstadt: Wissenschaftliche Buchgesellschaft.

Erikson, E.H. (1967). *Childhood and Society*. New York/London: Norton. (Original work published 1950)

Ey, H. (1954). *Études Psychiatriques*, Part III: Structure des psychoses aigues et déstructuration de la conscience. Paris: Desclée de Brouwer.

Fairbairn, W.R.D. (1952). *Psycho-analytic Studies of the Personality*. London: Tavistock.

Fédida, P. (2001). *Des Bienfaits de la Dépression: Éloge de la Psychothérapie*. Paris: Odile Jacob.

Fédida, P., & Villa, F. (Eds.) (1999). *Le Cas en Controverse*. Paris: PUF.

Feigl, H. (1958). The 'Mental' and the 'Physical'. In *Minnesota Studies in the Philosophy of Science*, Part II, H. Feigl, G. Maxwell, & M. Scriven (Eds.), 370-497. Minneapolis: University of Minnesota Press.

Fenichel, O. (1945). *The Psychoanalytic Theory of Neurosis*. New York: Norton.

Fink, B. (1995). *The Lacanian Subject: Between Language and Jouissance*. Princeton, NJ: Princeton University Press.

Fink, B. (1997). *A Clinical Introduction to Lacanian Psychoanalysis: Theory and Technique*. Cambridge, MA/London: Harvard University Press.

Fink, B. (2007). *Fundamentals of Psychoanalytic Technique: A Lacanian Approach for Practioners*. New York: Norton.

First, M.B., Gibbon, M., Spitzer, R.L., Williams, J.B.W., & Benjamin, L. (1997). *Structured Clinical Interview for DSM-IV Axis II Personality Disorders* (SCID-II). New York: Biometric Research Department, New York State Psychiatric Institute.

First, M.B., Spitzer, R.L., Gibbon, M, & Williams, J.B.W. (1996). *Structured Clinical Interview for DSM-IV Axis I Disorders* (SCID-I). New York: Biometric Research Department, New York State Psychiatric Institute.

Fodor, J. (2000). *The Mind Doesn't Work that Way: The Scope and Limits of Computational Psychology*. Cambridge, MA/London: MIT Press.

Fonagy, P. (2001). *Attachment Theory and Psychoanalysis*. New York: Other Press.

Fonagy, P., Gergely, G., Jurist, E., & Target, M. (2002). *Affect Regulations, Mentalization and Development of the Self*. New York: Other Press.

Fonagy, P., & Target, M. (1996a). Playing with reality: I. Theory of the mind and the normal development of psychic reality. *International Journal of Psychoanalysis*, *77*, 217-233.

Fonagy, P., & Target, M. (1996b). Playing with reality: II. The development of psychic reality from a theoretical perspective. *International Journal of Psychoanalysis*, *77*, 459-479.

Foucault, M. (1971). *L'Ordre du Discours*. Paris: Gallimard.

Foucault, M. (1989). *The Archeology of Knowledge* (A. M. Sheridan Smith, Trans.) London: Routledge. (Work original published 1969)

Foucault, M. (1994). *The Birth of the Clinic: An Archeology of Medical Perception*. New York: Vintage Books. (Work original publisehed 1963)

Fraassen, B. van (1980). *The Sientific Image*. Oxford: Oxford University Press.

Frances, A., First, M.B., & Pincus, H.A. (1995). *DSM-IV Guidebook*. Washington: American Psychiatric Association.

Frank, M. (1997). *The Subject and the Text: Essays on Literary Theory and Philosophy* (Edited, with an introduction by Andrew Bowie). Cambridge: Cambridge University Press.

Frankena, W.F. (1973). *Ethics*. Englewood Cliffs, NJ: Prentice Hall.

Freud, S. (1953a). The interpretation of dreams. In *The Standard Edition of the Complete Psychological Works of Sigmund Freud*, J. Strachey (Ed.), Volume 4 & 5. London: The Hogarth Press & The Institute of Psycho-Analysis. (Original work published 1900)

Freud, S. (1953b). Three essays on the theory of sexuality. In *The Standard Edition of the Complete Psychological Works of Sigmund Freud*, J. Strachey (Ed.), Volume 7, 130-243. London: The Hogarth Press & The Institute of Psycho-Analysis. (Original work published 1905)

Freud, S. (1955a). Analysis of a phobia in a five-year-old boy. In *The Standard Edition of the Complete Psychological Works of Sigmund Freud*, J.

Strachey (Ed.), Volume 10, 5-149. London: The Hogarth Press & The Institute of Psycho-Analysis. (Original work published 1909)

Freud, S. (1955b). Notes upon a case of obsessional neurosis. In *The Standard Edition of the Complete Psychological Works of Sigmund Freud*, J. Strachey (Ed.), Volume 10, 155-249. London: The Hogarth Press & The Institute of Psycho-Analysis. (Original work published 1909)

Freud, S. (1957). Some character-types met with in psycho-analytic work. In *The Standard Edition of the Complete Psychological Works of Sigmund Freud*, J. Strachey (Ed.), Volume 14, 311-333. London: The Hogarth Press & The Institute of Psycho-Analysis. (Original work published 1916)

Freud, S. (1958). The disposition to obsessional neurosis: a contribution to the problem of choice of neurosis. In *The Standard Edition of the Complete Psychological Works of Sigmund Freud*, J. Strachey (Ed.), Volume 12, 317-326. London: The Hogarth Press & The Institute of Psycho-Analysis. (Original work published 1913)

Freud, S. (1966). The originins of psychoanalysis. In In *The Standard Edition of the Complete Psychological Works of Sigmund Freud*, J. Strachey (Ed.), Volume 1, 177-387. London: The Hogarth Press & The Institute of Psycho-Analysis. (Original work published 1950

Freud, H.C. (1991). *Freud, Proust, Perversion and Love*. Amsterdam: Swets & Zeitlinger.

Frie, R. (2003). Language and subjectivity: From Binswanger through Lacan. In *Understanding Experience: Psychotherapy and Postmodernism*, R. Frie (Ed.), 137-160. Hove: Routledge.

Friedman, M. (2000). *A Parting of the Ways: Carnap, Cassirer, and Heidegger*. Chicago/La Salle, IL: Open Court.

Frijda, N.H. (1986). *The Emotions*. Cambridge: Cambridge University Press.

Fulford, K.W.M. (2001). Losing sight of insight. In *Phénoménologie de l'Identité Humaine en Schizophrénie*, D. Pringuey en F.S. Kohl (Eds.), 26-34. Paris: Cercle Herméneutique.

Fulford, K.W.M. (2004). Fact/values: ten principles of values based medicine. In *The Philosophy of Psychiatry: A Companion*, J. Radden (Ed.), 205-234. Oxford: Oxford University Press.

Fulford, K.W.M., Morris, K, Sadler, J.Z., & Stanghellini, G. (Eds.), (2003). *Nature and Narrative: An Introduction to the New Philosophy of Psychiatry*. Oxford: Oxford University Press.

Gadamer, H.-G. (1985). *Truth and Method* (G. Barden & J. Cumming, Trans.). New York: Crossroad.

Gallagher, S. (2005). *How the Body Shapes the Mind*. Oxford: Clarendon Press.

Gebsattel, V.E. von (1954). *Prolegomena einer Medizinischen Anthropologie*. Berlin/Göttingen/Heidelberg: Springer.

Geertz, Cl. (1973). *The Interpretation of Culture*. New York: Basic Books.

Gehlen, A. (1966). *Der Mensch: Seine Natur und Stellung in der Welt.* Frankfurt a. M./Bonn: Atheneum.

Gill, M.M. (1983). The point of view of psychoanalysis: Energy discharge or person? *Psychoanalysis and Contemporary Thought, 6*, 523-551.

Girard, R. (1986). *The Scapegoat* (Y. Freccero, Trans.). Baltimore: Johns Hopkins University Press.

Giudicelli, S. (1990). La dépressivité humaine. In *Le Sujet dans la Psychose; Paranoïa et Mélancolie,* H. Castanet (Ed.), 17-35. Nice: Z'éditions.

Giudicelli, S. (1996). *Journal de Bord d'un Thérapeute.* Paris: Seuil.

Glas, G. (2003). Anxiety: Animal reactions and the embodiment of meaning. In *Nature and Narrative. An Introduction to the New Philosophy of Psychiatry*, B. Fulford, K. Morris, J. Sadler, & G. Stanghellini (Eds.), 231-249. Oxford: Oxford University Press.

Goldstein, K. (1934). *Der Aufbau des Organismus: Einführung in die Biologie unter Besonderer Berücksichtigung der Erfahrungen am Kranken Menschen.* Den Haag: Nijhoff.

Goodman, N. (1978). *Ways of Worldmaking.* Indianapolis: Hackett Publishing Company.

Gordon, P.E. (2010). *Continental Divide. Heidegger, Cassirer, Davos.* Cambridge MA: Harvard University Press.

Granger, G.-G. (1967). *Pensée Formelle et Sciences de l'Homme.* Paris: Aubier-Montaigne.

Green, A. (1973). *Le Discours Vivant: La Conception Psychoanalytique de l'Affect.* Paris: Presses Universitaires de France.

Greenberg, J.R., & Mitchell, S.A. (1983). *Object Relations in Psychoanalytic Theory.* Cambridge, MA/London: Harvard University Press.

Griesinger, W. (1964). *Die Pathologie und Therapie der Psychischen Krankheiten für Arzte und Studirende.* Amsterdam: Bonset. (Original work published 1845)

Grondin, J. (1994). *Der Sinn für Hermeneutik.* Darmstadt: Wissenschaftliche Buchgesellschaft.

Grondin, J. (2001). *Einführung in die philosophische Hermeneutik.* Darmstadt: Wissenschaftliche Buchgesellschaft.

Grondin, J. (2002). Gadamer's basic understandings of understanding. In *The Cambridge Companion to Gadamer*, R.J. Dostal (Ed.), 36-51. Cambridge: Cambridge University Press.

Grondin. J. (2003). *Le Tournant Herméneutique de la Phénoménologie.* Paris: Presses Universitaires de France.

Guir, J. (1983). *Psychosomatique et cancer.* Paris: Point Hors Ligne.

Guze, S.B. (1989). Biological psychiatry: is there any other kind? *Psychological medicine, 19*, 315-323.

Habermas, J. (1988). *Der Philosophische Diskurs der Moderne.* Frankfurt a.M.: Suhrkamp.

Habermas, J. (2008). *Between Naturalism and Religion: Philosophical Essays* (C. Cronin, Trans.). Cambridge: Cambridge University Press.

Hacking, I. (1999). *The Social Construction of What?* Cambridge/London: Harvard University Press.

Häfner, H. (1961). *Psychopathen: Daseinsanalytische Untersuchungen zur Struktur und Verlaufsgestalt von Psychopathien.* Berlin/Göttingen/Heidelberg: Springer Verlag.

Hanson, M.J., & Callahan, D. (Eds.) (1999). *The Goals of Medicine: The Forgotten Issues in Health Care Reform.* Washington, DC: Georgetown University Press.

Hanson, N.R. (1958). *Patterns of Discovery.* Cambridge: Cambridge University Press.

Hare, R.D. (1991). *Manual for the Hare Psychopathy Checklist Revised.* Toronto: Multi Health Systems.

Hart, H.L.A. (1948-1949). The ascription of responsibility and rights. *Aristotelian Society Proceedings, 49*, 171-194.

Hartmann, H. (1964). *Essays on Ego Psychology.* New York: International Universities Press.

Hegel, G.W.F. (1979). *Hegel's Phenomenology of the Spirit* (A.V. Miller, Trans.). Oxford: Clarendon Press. (Original work published 1807)

Heidegger, M. (1962). *Being and Time* (J. Macquarrie & E. Robinson, Trans.). London/New York: Harper and Row. (Original work published 1927)

Heidegger, M. (1973). *Kant und das Problem der Metaphysik.* Franfurt a.M.: Vittorio Klostermann (Original work published 1929)

Heidegger, M. (1987). *Zollikoner Seminare* (Medard Boss, Ed.). Frankfurt a.M.: Klostermann.

Heinroth, J.C.A. (1823). *Lehrbuch der Seelengesundheitskunde*, Part I. Leipzig: Vogel.

Hell, D. (1993). *Schizophrenien: Verständnisgrundlagen und Orientierungshilfen.* Berlin/Heidelberg/New York: Springer. (Original work published 1988)

Hell, D. (2002). *Welchen Sinn macht Depression? Ein Integrativer Ansatz.* Hamburg: Rohwolt. (Original work published 1994)

Hell, D. (2003). *Seelenhunger. Der Fühlende Mensch und die Wissenschaften vom Leben.* Bern/Göttingen/Toronto: Huber Verlag.

Hempel, C.G. (1965). Fundamentals of taxonomy. In *Aspects of Scientific Explanation and other Essays in the Philosophy of Science*, 137- 154. New York: Free Press.

Hempel, C.G. (1966). *Philosophy of Natural Science.* Englewood Cliffs, NJ: Prentice Hall.

Henry, J.M. (2001). La passivité hallucinatoire. In *Introduction à la Phénoménologie des Hallucinations*, G. Charbonneau (Ed.), 79-89. Paris: Cercle Herméneutique.

Holzhey-Kunz, A. (1994). *Leiden am Dasein: Die Daseinsanalyse und die Aufgabe einer Hermeneutik Psychopathologischer Phänomenen.* Vienna: Passagen.

Homer, S. (2005). *Jacques Lacan.* London and New York: Routledge.

Hume, D. (1966). *A Treatise of Human Nature,* Book II: Of the Passions, 3-165. London/New York: Everymans Library. (Original work published 1739-1740)

Husserl, E. (1964). *Phenomenology of Internal Time-Consciousness* (J.S. Churchill, Trans.). The Hague: Nijhoff. (Original work published 1928)

Husserl, E. (1970a). *Cartesian Meditations: An Introduction to Phenomenology* (D. Cairns, Trans.). The Hague: Nijhoff. (Orignal work published 1950)

Husserl, E. (1970b). *The Crisis of the European Sciences and the Transcendental Phenomenology* (D. Carr, Trans.). Evanston: North Western University Press. (Orignal work published 1953)

Husserl, E. (1983). *Ideas Pertaining to a Pure Phenomenology and a Phenomenological Philosophy,* Book 1: General Introduction to a Pure Phenomenology (F. Kersten, Trans.). The Hague: Nijhoff. (Orignal work published 1913)

Husserl, E. (1989). *Ideas Pertaining to a Pure Phenomenology and a Phenomenological Philosophy,* Book 2: Studies in the Phenomenology of Constitution (R. Rojcewicz & A. Schuwer, Trans.). Dordrecht: Kluwer. (Orignal work published 1952)

Husserl, E. (1964). *Phenomenology of Internal Time-Consciousness* (J.S. Churchill, Trans.). The Hague: Nijhoff. (Original work published 1928)

Hyppolite, J. (1957). Phénoménologie de Hegel et psychanalyse. *Psychanalyse, 3,* 1-16.

Ineichen, H. (1991). *Philosophische Hermeneutik.* München: Karl Aber.

Israël, L. (2001). *L'Hystérique, le Sexe et le Médecin.* Paris: Masson. (Original work published 1976)

Israël, L. (1984). *Initiation à la Psychiatrie.* Paris: Masson.

Jameson, F. (1972). *The Prinson-House of Language. A Critical Account of Structuralism and Russion Formalism.* Princeton, NJ: Princeton University Press.

Jaspers, K. (1997). *General Psychopathology,* Vol. I and II (J. Hoenig & M. Hamilton, Trans.). Baltimore/London: Johns Hopkins University Press. (Original work published 1913; translation of the extended seventh edition 1959)

Jones, E. (1981). *The Life and Work of Sigmund Freud.* Harmondsworth: Penguin Books. (Original work published 1953)

Julien, Ph. (2000). *Psychose, Perversion, Psychose. La lecture de Jacques Lacan.* Toulouse: Érès.

Juranville, A. (2005). *La Mélancolie et ses Destins.* Paris: Éditions in Press.

Kandel, E.R. (1999). Biology and the future of psychoanalysis: A new intellectual framework for psychiatry revisited. *American Journal of Psychiatry*, *156*, 505-524.

Kant. I. (1965). *Critique of Pure Reason* (N. Kemp Smith, Trans.). New York: St Martin's Press (original work published 1781)

Kant. I. (2002). *Prolegomena to Any Future Metaphysics* (J.W. Ellington, Trans.). Indianapolis: Hackett (Original work published 1783)

Kendler, K.S. (2005). Towards a philosophical structure for psychiatry. *American Journal of Psychiatry*, *162*, 433-440.

Kendler, K.S., & Zachar, P. (2008). The incredible insecurity of psychiatric nosology. In *Philosophical Issues in Psychiatry: Explanation, Phenomenology and Nosology*, K.S. Kendler & J. Parnas (Eds.), 368-382. Baltimore: Johns Hopkins University Press.

Kenny, A. (1963). *Action, Emotion and Will.* London/Henley: Routledge and Kegan Paul.

Kenny, A. (1969). Mental health in Plato's 'Republic'. *Proceedings of the British Academy*, *55*, 229-253.

Kenny, A. (1985). *The Ivory tower: Essays in Philosophy and Public Policy.* Oxford: Basil Blackwell.

Kernberg, O. (1984). *Severe Personality Disorders: Psychotherapeutic Strategies.* New Haven/London: Yale University Press.

Kernberg, O. (2006). Perversion, perversity and normality. In *Perversion*, D. Nobus and L Downing (Eds.), 19-40. London: Karnac Books.

Kimura, B. (1982). The phenomenology of the between: on the problem of the basic disturbance in schizophrenia. In *Phenomenology and Psychiatry*, A.J.J. de Koning & F.A. Jenner (Eds.), 173-185. London/Toronto/Sydney/ New York: Academic Press/Grune and Stratton.

Klein. G.S. (1976). *Psychoanalytic Theory: An Exploration of Essentials*. New York: International Universities Press.

Klein, M., Heiman, P., & Money-Kyrle, R.E. (1977). *New Directions in Psycho-analysis.* London: Maresfield. (Original work published 1955)

Kockelmans, J.J. (1987). Husserl's original view on phenomenological psychology. In *Phenomenological Psychology: The Dutch School*, 1-19. Dordrecht: Nijhoff.

Kohlberg, L. (1984). *Essays on Moral Development*, II: The psychology of moral development. San Francisco: Harper and Row.

Kohut, H. (1971). *The Analysis of the Self: A Systematic Approach to the Psychoanalytic Treatment of Narcissistic Personality Disorders.* New York: International Universities Press.

Koning, A.J.J. de, & Jenner, F.A. (Eds.) (1982). *Phenomenology and Psychiatry.* London/Toronto/Sydney/NewYork: Academic Press/Grune and Stratton.

Koyré, A. (1957). *From the Closed World to the Infinite Universe.* Baltimore: John Hopkins Press

Kraft, V. (1960). *Erkenntnislehre.* Vienna: Springer.

Kräpelin, E. (1909). *Psychiatrie: Ein Lehrbuch für Studierende und Ärzte*, Part I (8th rev. ed.). Leipzig: Barth.

Kraus, A. (2007). Schizophrenic delusion and hallucination as the expression and consequence of an alteration of the existential a prioris. In *Reconceiving Schizophrenia*, M.C. Chung, K.W.M. Fulford, & G. Graham (Eds.), 97-113. Oxford: Oxford University Press.

Kreis, G. (2010). *Cassirer und die Formen des Geistes.* Frankfurt a.M.: Suhrkamp.

Kretschmer, E. (1950). *Der Sensitive Beziehungswahn.* Berlin/Göttingen/ Heidelberg: Springer. (Original work published 1927)

Krois, J.M. (1987). *Cassirer: Symbolic Forms and History.* London/New Haven: Yale University Press.

Krois, J.M. (2004). Ernst Cassirer's philosophy of biology. *Sign Systems Studies*, *32* (1/2), 277-295.

Kronfeld, A. (1920). *Das Wesen der Psychiatrischen Erkenntnis.* Berlin: Springer.

Kuhn, T.S. (1970). *The Structure of Scientific Revolutions* (2nd enlarged ed.). Chicago: University of Chicago Press. (Original work published 1962)

Kulenkampff, C. (1956). Erblicken und Erblickt-werden: Das Für-Andere-Sein (J.-P. Sartre) in seiner Bedeutung für die Anthropologie der paranoiden Psychosen. *Der Nervenarzt*, *27*, 2-12.

Kulenkampff, C. (1963). Entbergung, Entgrenzung, Überwältigung als Weisen des Standverlustes: Zur Anthropologie der paranoiden Psychosen. *Der Nervenarzt*, *26*, 89-95.

Kupfer, D.J., First, M.B., & Regier, D.A. (Eds.) (2002). Introduction. In *A Research Agenda for DSM-V*, xv-xxiii. Washington: American Psychiatric Association.

Kusters, W. (2004). *Pure Waanzin: Een Zoektocht naar de Psychotische Ervaring.* Amsterdam: Nieuwezijds.

Lacan, J. (1961-1962). *Le Séminaire de Jacques Lacan: L'Identification*, session of 20 December 1961. Unedited.

Lacan, J. (1973). *Télévision.* Paris: Seuil.

Lacan, J. (1975). *De la Psychose Paranoïaque dans ses Rapport avec la Personnalité.* Paris: Seuil. (Original work published 1932)

Lacan, J. (1977). *Écrits. A selection* (A. Sheridan, Trans.). London: Tavistock & Routledge (Work original published 1966).

Lacan, J. (1986). *The Seminar of Jacques Lacan,* Book XI: The four fundamental concepts of psycho-analysis, 1965 (J.A. Miller, Ed. & A. Sheridan, Trans.). (Original work published 1973)

Lacan, J. (1992). *The Seminar of Jacques Lacan,* Book VII: The ethics of psychoanalysis, 1959-1960 (J.A. Miller, Ed. & D. Porter, Trans.). New York: Norton (Orginal work published 1986)

Lacan, J. (1993). *The Seminar of Jacques Lacan*, Book III: The psychoses, 1955-56 (J.A. Miller, Ed. & R. Grigg, Trans.), session of 8 February 1956. New York: Norton. (Original work published 1981)

Lacan, J. (1994). *Le Séminaire de Jacques Lacan*, Livre IV: La relation d'objet, 1956-1957 (J.A. Miller, Ed.). Paris: Seuil.

Lacan, J. (1998). *Le Séminaire de Jacques Lacan*, Livre V: Les formations de l'inconscient, 1957-1958 (J.A. Miller, Ed.). Paris: Seuil.

Lacan, J. (2001). *Autres Écrits*. Paris: Seuil.

Lacan, J. (2002). *Écrits: The First Complete Edition in English* (B. Fink, Trans.). New York/London: Norton. (Original work published in 1966)

Lacan, J. (2004). *Le Séminaire de Jacques Lacan*, Livre X: L'angoisse, 1962-1963 (J.A. Miller, Ed.). Paris: Seuil.

Lacan, J. (2005). *Le Séminaire de Jacques Lacan*, Livre XXIII: Le sinthome, 1975-1976 (J.A. Miller, Ed.). Paris: Seuil.

Lacan, J. (2006). *Le Séminaire de Jacques Lacan*, Livre XVI: D'un Autre à l'autret, 1968-1969 (J.A. Miller, Ed.). Paris: Seuil.

Lacan, J. (2007). *The Seminar of Jacques Lacan*, Book XVII: The other side of psychoanalysis, 1969-1970 (J.A. Miller, Ed. & R. Grigg, Trans.). New York: Norton. (Orignal work published 1991)

Lain-Entralgo, P. (1970). *The Therapy of the Word in Classical Antiquity*. New Haven: Yale University Press.

Lambotte, M.-C. (1999). *Le Discours Mélancolique: De la Phénoménologie à la Métapsychologie*. Paris: Anthropos. (Original work published 1993)

Lang, H. (2000a). *Das Gespräch als Therapie*. Frankfurt a.M.: Suhrkamp.

Lang, H. (2000b). *Strukturale Psychoanalyse*. Frankfurt a.M.: Suhrkamp.

Lantéri-Laura, G. (2003). Introduction historique et critique à la notion de dépression en psychiatrie. In *Phénoménologie des Sentiments Corporels*, B. Granger & G. Charbonneau (Eds.), Part I, 89-103. Paris: Cercle Herméneutique.

Latour, B. (1987). *Science in Action: How to Follow Scientists and Engineers through Society*. Harvard: Harvard University Press.

Leclaire, S. (1968). *Psychanalyser: Essai sur l'Ordre de l'Inconscient et la Pratique de la Lettre*. Paris: Seuil.

Leclaire, S. (1971). *Démasquer le Réel: Un Essai sur l'Objet en Psychanalyse*. Paris: Seuil.

LeDoux, J. (1998). *The Emotional Brain*. New York: Touchstone Books. (Original work published 1996)

Lefort, R. & Lefort, R. (1988). *Les Structures de la Psychose: L'Enfant au Loup et le Président*. Paris: Seuil.

Le Gaufey, G. (1997). *Le Lasso Spéculaire*: *Une Étude Traversière de l'Unité Imaginaire*. Paris: E.P.E.L.

Leguil, C. (2012). *Sartre avec Lacan: Corrélation Antinomique, Liaison Dangereuse*. Paris: Navarin/Le Champ freudien.

Lemoine-Luccioni, E. (1976). *Partages de Femmes*. Paris: Seuil.

Levinas, E. (1969). *Totality and Infinity: An Essay on Exteriority* (A. Lingis, Trans.). Pittsburgh: Duquesne University Press. (Original work published 1961)

Levine, S.Z. (2008). *Lacan Reframed.* London: Tauris.

Libbrecht, K. (2001). *Les Délires de l'Hystérique: Une Approche Historique.* Toulouse: Érès.

Linschoten, J. (1964). *Idolen van de Psycholoog.* Utrecht: Bijleveld.

Lofts, S.G. (1994). L'ordre symbolique de Jacques Lacan à la lumière du symbolique d'Ernst Cassirer. In *La Pensée de Jacques Lacan*, S. Lofts & P. Moyaert (Eds.), 83-107. Leuven/Paris: Peeters.

Lofts, S.G. (1997). *Ernst Cassirer: La Vie de l'Esprit.* Paris/Leuven: Peeters-Vrin.

Lovejoy, A.O. (1973). *The Great Chain of Being.* Cambridge, MA: Harvard University Press. (Original work published 1934)

Mackie, J.L. (1980). *The Cement of the Universe. A Study of Causation.* Oxford: Clarendon Press

MacLean, P.D. (1980). Sensual and perceptual factors in emotional functioning in the triune brain. In *Explaining Emotions*, A. Oksenburg Rorty (Ed.), 9-36. Berkeley/Los Angeles/London: University of California Press.

Magner, L.N. (2005). *A History of Medicine.* London/New York/Singapore: Taylor and Francis.

Mahler, M., Pine, F., & Berman, A. (1985). *The Psychological Birth of the Human Infant: Symbiosis and Individuation.* London: Hutchinson. (Original work published 1975)

Maldiney, H. (1961). Comprendre. *Revue de Métaphysique et de Morale, 66,* 35-89.

Maldiney, H. (1991). *Penser l'Homme et la Folie. A la Lumière de l'Analyse Existentielle et de l'Analyse du Destin.* Grenoble: Millon.

Maleval, J.-C. (1991). *Folies Hystériques et Psychoses Dissociatives.* Paris: Payot. (Original work published 1981)

Maleval, J.-C. (2000). *Logique du Délire.* Paris: Masson.

Mannoni, O. (1969). *Clefs Pour l'Imaginaire ou l'Autre Scène.* Paris: Seuil.

Mansfeld, J. (1973). *Theorie en Empirie: Filosofie en Geneeskunde in de Voorsocratische Periode.* Assen: Van Gorcum.

Marty, P., M'Uzan, M. de, & David, C. (1963). *L'Investigation Psycho-somatique.* Paris: PUF.

Matthews, E. (2003). How can a mind be sick? In *Nature and Narrative: An Introduction to the New Philosophy of Psychiatry*, B. Fulford, K. Morris, J. Sadler, & G. Stanghellini (Eds.), 73-92. Oxford: Oxford University Press.

Matthews, E. (2006). *Merleau-Ponty: A Guide for the Perplexed.* London/New York: Continuum Publishing Group.

McDowell, J. (1994). *Mind and World.* Cambridge, MA: Cambridge University Press.

McGinn, C. (1999). *The Mysterious Flame: Conscious Minds in a Material World*. New York: Basic Books.

Merleau-Ponty, M. (1962). *Phenomenology of Perception* (C. Smith, Trans.). London: Routlege and Kegan Paul. (Original work published 1945)

Miller, J.-A.. (2007). Jacques Lacan and the voice. In *The Later Lacan. An Introduction*, V. Voruz and B. Wolf (Eds.), 137-146. New York: SUNY.

Miller, M.J. (2011). *Lacanian Psychoanalysis: Theory and Practical Applications*. New York/London: Routledge.

Millon, T. (1981). *Disorders of Personality, DSM-III: Axis II*. New York/ Chichester: John Wiley.

Mills, J. (2000). Dialectical psychoanalysis: Towards process psychology. *Psychoanalysis and Contemporary Thought, 23* (3), 20-54.

Mills, J. (2002). *The Unconsciuous Abyss: Hegel's Anticipation of Psychoanalysis*. New York: SUNY.

Mills, J. (2005). Process psychology. In *Relational and Intersubjective Perspectives in Psychoanalysis: A Critique*, J. Mills (Ed.), 279-308. Northvale, NJ: Aronson/ Rowman & Littlefield.

Mink, L.O. (1987). *Historical Understanding*. Ithaca: Cornell University Press.

Minkowski, E. (1997). *La Schizophrénie*. Paris: Payot. (Original work published 1927)

Mishara, A.L. (1997). On Wolfgang Blankenburg, common sense and schizophrenia. *Philosophy, Psychiatry and Psychology, 8*, 317-322.

Mitscherlich, A. (1967). *Krankheit und Konflikt: Studien zur Psychosomatischen Medizin*. Frankfurt a.M.: Suhrkamp.

Mooij, A.W.M. (1991). *Psychoanalyis and the Concept of a Rule: An Essay in the Philosophy of Psychoanalysis* (S. Firth, Trans.) Berlin/Heidelberg/New York: Springer.

Mooij, A.W.M. (1993). The symbolic father. In *The Dutch Annual of Psychoanalysis*, H. Groen-Prakken & A. Ladan (Eds.), 161-168. Amsterdam/Lisse: Swets & Zeitlinger.

Mooij, A.W.M. (1995). Towards an anthropological psychiatry. *Theoretical Medicine, 16*, 73-91.

Mooij, A.W.M. (2001). *Taal en Verlangen: Lacans Theorie van de Psychoanalyse*. Meppel/Amsterdam: Boom. (Original work published 1975)

Mooij, A.W.M. (2003). Die Bedeuting des Vaters in der Psychosenbehandlung. Überlegungen zur Theorie und Technik. *RISS: Zeitschrift für Psychoanalyse; Freud-Lacan, 18* (no. 56), 81-93.

Mooij, A.W.M. (2008). Deux rencontres avec Lacan. *La Cause freudienne. Nouvelle revue de psychanalyse, no. 69*, 200-203.

Mooij, A.W.M. (2010). *Intentionality, Desire, Responsibility: A Study in Phenomenology, Psychoanalysis and Law*. Leiden/Boston: Brill.

Morel, G. (2008). *La Loi de la Mère: Essai sur le Sinthome Sexuel*. Paris: Anthropos.

Mul, J. de (2004). *The Tragedy of Finitude. Dilthey's Hermeneutics of Life* (T. Burrett, Trans.). New Haven/London: Yale University Press.

Nagel, E. (1971). *The Structure of Science*. London: Routledge and Kegan Paul. (Original work published 1961)

Nagel, Th. (1974). What is it like to be a bat? *Philosophical Review, 83*, 435-450.

Nagel, Th. (1986). *The View from Nowhere*. Oxford: Oxford University Press.

Nasio, J.-D. (1987). *Les Yeux de Laure: Le Concept de l'Object a dans la Théorie de J. Lacan*. Paris: Aubier.

Nasio, J.-D. (1995). *L'Hystérie ou l'Enfant Magique de la Psychanalyse*. Paris: Payot.

Nasio, J.-D. (2005). *L'Œdipe: Le Concept le Plus Crucial de la Psychanalyse*. Paris: Payot.

Nasio, J.-D. (2007). *Mon Corps et ses Images*. Paris: Payot.

Needleman, J. (Trans. & Ed. & critical introduction) (1975). *Being-in-the-World: Selected Papers of Ludwig Binswanger*. London: Souvenir Press. (Original work published 1963)

Nobus, D. (1998). Life and Death in the Glass. A New Look at the Mirror Stage. In *Key Concepts of Lacanian Psychoanalysis*, D. Nobus (Ed.), 101-139. London: Rebus Press.

Noë, A. (2009). *Out of Our Heads: Why You Are Not Your Brain, and Other Lessons from the Biology of Consciousness*. New York: Hill and Wang.

Northoff, G. (2011). *Neuropsychoanalysis in Practice: Brain, Self and Objects*. Oxford: Oxford University Press.

Nussbaum, M.C. (1986). *The Fragility of Goodness: Luck and Ethics in Greek Tragedy and Philosophy*. Cambridge/New York: Cambridge University Press.

Orth, E.W. (2004). *Von der Erkenntnistheorie zur Kulturphilosophie*. Würzburg: Königshausen & Neuman.

Ortigues, M.C., Ortigues, E. (1988). *Comment Se Décide une Psychothérapie d'Enfant*. Paris: Denoël.

Owen, J.R. (2006). *Psychotherapy and Phenomenology: On Freud, Husserl and Heidegger*. New York: Universe.

Panksepp, J. (1998). *Affective Neuroscience: The Foundations of Human and Animal emotions*. New York/Oxford: Oxford University Press.

Pascal, B. (1964). *Pensées*. Paris: Garnier. (Original work published 1667)

Pellegrino, E.D., & Thomasma, D.C. (1981). *A Philosophical Basis of Medical Practice: Towards a Philosophy and Ethics of the Healing Professions*. New York/Oxford: Oxford University Press.

Phillips, J. (2004). Understanding/explanation. In *The Philosophy of Psychiatry: A Companion*, J. Radden (Ed.), 180-190. Oxford: Oxford University Press.

Plato (2004). *Republic* (C.D.C. Reeves, Trans.). Indianapolis: Hackett.

Plügge, H. (1962). *Wohlbefinden und Missbefinden*. Tübingen: Niemeyer.

Pluth, E. (2007). *Signifiers and Acts: Freedom in Lacan's Theory of the Subject*. Albany: State University of New York Press.

Pommier, G. (2004). *Comment les Neurosciences Démontrent la Psychanalyse.* Paris: Flammarion.

Popper, K.R. (1968). *The Logic of Scientific Discovery.* London: Hutchinson. (Original work published 1959)

Popper, K.R. (1969). Back to the presocratics. In *Conjectures and Refutations.* London: Routledge and Kegan Paul.

Popper, K.R. (1972). *Objective Knowledge: An Evolutionary Approach.* Oxford: Clarendon Press.

Popper, K.R., & Eccles, J.C. (1977). *The Self and Its Brain.* Berlin/New York/ London: Springer.

Porter, R. (1996). What is disease? In *The Cambridge Illustrated History of Medicine,* R. Porter (Ed.), 82-117. Cambridge/New York: Cambridge University Press.

Postal, R.J. (Ed.) (2002). *The Cambridge Companion to Gadamer*. Cambridge: Cambridge University Press.

Putnam, H. (1974). The 'corroboration' of theories. In *The Philosophy of Karl Popper*, P. Schilpp (Ed.), 221-240. La Salle: Open Court (Library of Living Philosophers).

Putnam, H. (1975). The meaning of 'meaning'. In *Mind, Language and Reality*, 215-271. Cambridge: Cambridge University Press.

Quine, W.V.O. (1961). *From a Logical Point of View: Logico-philosophical Essays.* New York: Harper Torch Books. (Original work published 1953)

Rabinovitch, S. (1998). *La forclusion: Enfermés dehors*. Ramonville: Érès.

Radden, J. (2007). Defining persecutory paranoia. In *Reconceiving Schizophrenia*, M.C. Chung, K.W.M. Fulford & G. Graham (Eds.), 255-275. Oxford: Oxford University Press.

Renik, O. (1998). The analyst's subjectivity and the analyst's objectivity. *The International Journal of Psychoanalysis*, *79*, 487-499.

Rentsch, Th. (1980). Leib-Seele-Verhältnis. In *Historisches Wörterbuch der Philosophie,* J. Ritter & K. Grunder (Eds.), Part 5, 185-206. Darmstadt: Wissenschaftliche Buchgesellschaft.

Reynaert, P. (2002). Qualia en het subjectieve beleven. In *Het bewustzijn in de Fysische Wereld: Filosofische Essays over Materialisme en Fenomenaal Bewustzijn*, J. Leilich, P. Reynaert & J. Veldeman (Eds.), 271-292. Leuven: Peeters.

Richardson, W.J. (1983). Psychoanalysis and the Being-question. In *Interpreting Lacan*, J.H. Smith and W. Kerrigan (Eds.), 139-160. New Haven/ London: Yale University Press.

Rickert, H. (1921). *Die Grenzen der Naturwissenschaftlichen Begrifsbildung: Eine Logische Einleitung in die Historischen Wissenschaften.* Tübingen: Mohr. (Original work published 1902)

Ricœur, P. (1970). *Freud and Philosophy* (D. Savage, Trans.). New Haven: Yale University Press.

Ricœur, P. (1975). *La Métaphore Vive*. Paris: Seuil.

Ricœur, P. (1984). *Time and Narrative 1* (K. McLaughin & D. Pellauer, Trans.). Chicago, IL: University of Chicago Press.

Ricœur, P. (1992). *Oneself as an Other* (K. Blamey, Trans.). Chicago, IL: University of Chicago Press.

Ricœur, P. (2001). *Hermeneutics and the Human Sciences* (J.B. Thompson, Ed.). Cambridge: Cambridge University Press. (Original work published 1981)

Rorty, R. (1979). *Philisophy and the Mirror of Nature*. Princeton NJ: Princeton University Press.

Rosenberg, Ch. (2007). *Our Present Complaint: American Medicine, Then and Now*. Baltimore: Johns Hopkins University Press.

Rosolato, G. (1985). *Éléments de l'Interprétation*. Paris: Gallimard.

Ross, W.D. (1961). *Aristotle: De Anima*. Oxford: Clarendon Press.

Ryle, G. (1963). *The Concept of Mind*. Harmondsworth: Penguin. (Original work published 1949)

Sackett, D.L., Strauss, S.E., Richardson, W.S., Rosenberg, W., Haynes, R.B. (2000). *Evidence-Based Medicine: How to Practice and Teach EBM*. Edinburgh: Churchill Livingstone.

Sadler, J.Z. (1992). Eidetic and empirical research: A hermeneutic complementarity. In *Phenomenology, Language and Schizophrenia*, M. Spitzer, F. Uehlein, M.A. Schwarz, C.H. Mundt (Eds.), 103-114. New York: Springer.

Sadler, J.Z. (2005). *Values and Psychiatric Diagnosis*. Oxford: Oxford University Press.

Sadler, J.Z., Wiggens, O.P., & Schwartz, M.A. (Eds.) (1994). *Philosophical Perspectives on Psychiatric Diagnostic Classification*. Baltimore: Johns Hopkins University Press.

Safouan, M. (1974). *Etudes sur l'Oedipe*. Paris: Seuil.

Sartre, J.-P. (1939) *Esquisse d'une Théorie des Émotions*. Paris: Hermann.

Sass, L.A. (1994). *The Paradoxes of Delusion: Wittgenstein, Schreber and the Schizophrenic Mind*. Ithaca/London: Cornell University Press.

Sass, L.A. (2001). Culture, schizophrenia and the self. On the so called 'Negative Symptoms'. In *Phénoménologie de l'Identité Humaine et Schizophrénie*, D. Pringey & F.S. Kohl (Eds.), 112-121. Paris: Cercle herméneutique.

Sass, L.A., & Parnas, J. (2001). Phenomenology of self-disturbances in schizophrenia: some research findings and directions. *Philosophy, Psychiatry and Psychology, 8*, 347-356.

Saussure, F. de (1986). *Course in General Linguistics*. (R. Harris, Trans.). Chicago: Open Court. (Original work published 1916)

Schafer, R. (1976). *A New Language for Psychoanalysis.* New Haven/London: Yale University Press.

Schafer, R. (1983). *The Analytic Attitude.* London: Hogarth Press.

Schaffner, K.F. (2008). Etiological Models in Psychiatry: Reductive and Non-reductive Approaches. In *Philosophical Issues in Psychiatry: Explanation, Phenomenology and Nosology*, K.S. Kendler & J. Parnas (Eds.), 48-89. Baltimore: Johns Hopkins University Press.

Scheler, M. (1948). *Wesen und Formen der Sympathie: Phänomenologie und Theorie der Sympathiegefühle.* Frankfurt a.M.: Schulte-Bulmke. (Original work published 1912)

Schneider, K. (1980). *Clinical Psychopathology.* Stuttgart/York: Thieme. (Original work published 1959)

Schokker, J., & Schokker, T. (2000). *Extimiteit: Jacques Lacans Terugkeer naar Freud.* Amsterdam: Boom.

Schwarz, A.L., & Wiggins, O.P. (2004). Phenomenological and Hermeneutical Models: Understanding and Interpretation in Psychiatry. In *The Philosophy of Psychiatry: A Companion*, J. Radden (Ed.), 251-363. Oxford: Oxford University Press.

Schwemmer, O. (1997). *Ernst Cassirer: Ein Philosoph der Europäischen Moderne.* Berlin: Academie Verlag.

Searle, J.R. (1974). *Speech Acts: An Essay in the Philosophy of Language.* Cambridge: Cambridge University Press. (Original work published 1969)

Searle, J.R. (2002). *Consciousness and Language.* Cambridge/New York: Cambridge University Press.

Searle, J.R. (2007). *Freedom and Neurobiology: Reflections on Free Will, Language, and Political Power.* New York: Columbia University Press.

Sellars, W. (1963). Philosophy and the Scientific Image of Man. In *Science, Perception and Reality*, 1-40. London/New York: Routledge & Kegan Paul/Humanities Press.

Sellars, W. (1997). *Empiricism and the Philosophy of Mind.* Cambridge, MA: Harvard University Press. (Original work published 1956)

Shaffer, J. (1972). Mind-body problem. In *The Encyclopedia of Philosophy*, P. Edwards (Ed.), Part V, 336-347. London/New York: Macmillan. (Original work published 1967)

Shaffer, J. (1975). Roundtable discussion. In *Evaluation and Explanation in the Biomedical Sciences*, H.T. Engelhardt en S.F. Spickers (Eds.), 215-255. Dordrecht/ Boston/London: Reidel.

Sifneos, P.E. (1973). The prevalence of alexithymic characteristics in psychosomatic patients. *Psychotherapy and Psychosomatics*, *26*, 270-285.

Slade, M., Priebe, S. (2001). Are randomised controlled trials the only gold that glitters? (Editorial). *British Journal of Psychiatry*, *179*, 286-288.

Smart, J.J.C. (1963). *Philosophy and Scientific Realism.* London: Routledge and Kegan Paul.

Socarides, C.W. (2004). A psychoanalytical classification of paedophilias: Two clinical illustrations. In *The Mind of the Paedophile: Psychoanalytic Perspectives*, C.W Socarides & L.R. Loeb (Eds.), 7-62. London: Karnac Books.

Soenen, S., Corveleyn, J. (2003). The vicissitudes of corporeality in schizophrenia: A psychoanalytic approach. In *Psychosis: Phenomenological and Psychoanalytical Approaches,* J. Corveleyn & P. Moyaert (Eds.), 27-41. Leuven: Leuven University Press.

Soler, C. (1990). Paranoïa et mélancolie. In *Le Sujet dans la Psychose: Paranoïa et Mélancolie,* H. Castanet (Ed.), 35-45. Nice: Z'éditions.

Soler, C. (1996). Hysteria and obsession. In *Reading Seminars I and II: Lacan's Return to Freud,* R. Feldstein, B. Fink & M. Jaanus (Eds.), 248-283. Albany: State University of New York Press.

Soler, C. (2011). *Les Affects Lacaniens.* Paris: Presses Universitaires de France.

Sousa, R. de (1980). The rationality of emotions. In *Explaining Emotions*, A. Oksenberg Rorty (Ed.), 127-153. Berkeley/Los Angeles/London: University of California Press.

Spence, D.P. (1982). *Narrative Truth and Historical Truth.* New York/London: Norton.

Spiegelberg, H. (1972). *Phenomenology in Psychology and Psychiatry.* Evanston: Northwestern University Press.

Spitzer, M. (1988). Psychiatry, philosophy and the problem of description. In *Psychopathology and Philosophy*, M. Spitzer, F.A. Uehlein & G. Oepen (Ed.), 3-18. Berlin/Heidelberg/New York: Springer.

Spitzer, M. (1990). Why philosophy? In *Philosophy and Psychopathology*, M. Spitzer & B.A. Mahrer (Ed.), 3-19. New York/Heidelberg/Berlin: Springer.

Stanghellini, G. (2004). *Disembodied Spirits and Deanimated Bodies: The Psychopathology of Common Sense.* Oxford: Oxford University Press.

Stanghellini, G. (2007). Schizophrenia and the sixth sense. In *Reconceiving Schizophrenia*, M.C. Chung, K.W.M. Fulford & G. Graham (Eds.), 129-150. Oxford: Oxford University Press.

Stolorow, R.D., Atwood, G.E., & Orange, D.M. (2002). *World of Experience: Interwaving Philosophical and Clinical Dimensions in Psychoanalysis.* New York: Basic Books.

Strasser, S. (1956). *Das Gemüt: Grundgedanken zu einer Phänomenologischen Philosophie und Theorie des Menschlichen Gefühlslebens.* Utrecht/Antwerpen/Freiburg: Spectrum/Herder.

Strasser, S. (1985). *Understanding and Explanation: Basic Ideas Concerning the Humanity of the Human Sciences.* Pittsburg, PA: Duquesne University Press.

Straus, E. (1935). *Vom Sinn der Sinne: Ein Beitrag zur Grundlegung der Psychologie.* Berlin/Göttingen/Heidelberg: Springer.

Straus, E. (1963). Das Zeiterleben in der endogenen Depression und in der psychopathischen Verstimmung. In *Die Wahnwelten (Endogene Psychosen)*, E. Straus en J. Zutt (Eds.), 337-351. Frankfurt a.M.: Akademische Verlagsgesellschaft. (Original work published 1928)

Straus, E., & Zutt, J. (Eds.) (1963). *Die Wahnwelten (Endogene Psychosen).* Frankfurt a.M.: Akademische Verlagsgesellschaft.

Strawson, P.F. (1964). Freedom and resentment. In *Freedom and Resentment and Other Essays*, 1-25. London: Methuen.

Sullivan, H.S. (1953). *Conceptions of Modern Psychiatry*. New York: Norton.

Szasz, T.S. (1961). *The Myth of Mental Illness: Foundations of a Theory of Personal Conduct*. New York: Dell.

Tatossian, A. (1992). La subjectivité melancolique. In *Figures de la Subjectivité*, J.-F. Courtine (Ed.), 103-109. Paris: CNRS.

Tatossian, A. (1997). *Phénoménologie des Psychoses*. Paris: L'Art du comprendre. (Original work published 1979)

Taylor, Ch. (1964). *The Explanation of Behaviour*. London: Routledge and Kegan Paul.

Taylor, Ch. (1985a). *Human Agency and Language: Philosophical Papers 1.* Cambridge/New York; Cambridge University Press.

Taylor, Ch. (1985b). *Philosophy and the Human Sciences: Philosophical Papers 2*. Cambridge/New York: Cambridge University Press.

Tellenbach, H. (1956). Die Räumlichkeit der Melancholischen. I. Über Veränderungen des Raumerlebens in der endogenen Melancholie; II. Analyse der Räumlichkeit melancholischen Daseins. *Der Nervenarzt*, *27*, 12-18; 289-298.

Tellenbach, H. (1983). *Melancholie: Problemgeschichte Endogenität Typologie Pathogenese Klinik*. Berlin/Heidelberg/New York: Springer. (Original work published 1961)

Theunissen, M. (1984). *The Oher: Studies in the Social Ontology in Husserl, Heidegger, Sartre and Buber* (Ch. Macann, Trans.). Cambridge, MA: MIT Press.

Theunissen, M. (1991). Melancholisches Leiden unter der Herrschaft der Zeit. In *Negative Theologie der Zeit*, 218-285. Frankfurt a.M.: Suhrkamp.

Thibierge, S. (1999). *L'image et le Double. La Function Spéculaire en Pathologie*. Ramonville: Érès.

Thompson, M.G. (2005). Phenomenology of intersubjectivity: A historical overview of the concept and its clinical implications. In *Relational and Intersubjective Perspectives in Psychoanalysis*, J. Mills (Ed.), 35-70. Northvale, NJ: Jason Aronson.

Thornton, T. (2002). Reliability and validity in psychiatric classification: Values and neo-humeanism. *Philosophy, Psychiatry and Psychology*, *9*, 229-235.

Thornton, T. (2004). Reductionism/Antireductionism. In *The Philosophy of Psychiatry: A Companion*, J. Radden (Ed.), 191-204. Oxford: Oxford University Press.

Ueling, T.E. Jr (1996). *Wahrnehmungsurteile* und *Erfahrungsurteile* Reconsidered. In *Immanuel Kant's Prolegomena to Any Future Metaphysics in Focus*, B. Logan (Ed.), 165-175. London: Routledge.

Uexkull, Th. von (1963). *Grundfragen der Psychosomatischen Medizin.* Hamburg: Rowohlt.

Van Haute, Ph. (2001). *Against Adaptation: Lacan's Subversion of the Subject.* New York: Other Press.

Van Heule, S. (2011). *The Subject of Psychosis: A Lacanian Perspective.* Basingstoke: Palgrave Macmillan.

Varela, F. (2002). The consciousness in neurosciences. *Journal of European Psychoanalysis*, *14*, 109-123.

Veldeman, J. (2002). Inleiding: Materialisme en fenomenaal bewustzijn. In *Het Bewustzijn in de Fysische Wereld: Filosofische Essays over Materialisme en Fenomenaal Bewustzijn*, J. Leilich, P. Reynaert & J. Veldeman (Eds.), 1-47. Leuven: Peeters.

Ver Eecke, W. (2006). *Denial, Negation and the Forces of the Negative. Freud, Hegel, Lacan, Spitz, and Sophocles.* New York: SUNY Press.

Vergote, A. (1980). *Bekentenis en Begeerte in de Religie: Psychoanalytische Verkenning.* Antwerpen/Amsterdam: Nederlandse Boekhandel.

Verhaeghe, P. (1998). *Does the Woman Exist? From Freud's Hysteric to Lacan's Feminine.* New York: Other Press.

Verhaeghe, P. (2001). *Beyond Gender. From Subject to Drive.* New York: The Other Press.

Verhaeghe, P. (2008). *On Being Normal and Other Disorders: A Manual for Clinical Psychodiagnostics.* (S. Jottkandt, Trans.). London: Karnac.

Verhaeghe, P. (2009). *New Studies of Old Villains: A Radical Reconsideration of the Oedipus Complex.* New York: Other Press.

Verhaeghe, P. & Willemsen, J. (2009). When psychoanalysis meets law and evil: perversion and psychopathy in the forensic clinic. In *Law and Evil: Philosophy, Politics, Psychoanalysis*, A. Hirvonen & J. Porttikivi (Eds.), 237-259. Abingdon/New York: Routledge.

Verwey, G. (1980). *Psychiatrie tussen Antropologie en Natuurwetenschap: Een Historische Studie over het Zelfbegrip van de Duitse Psychiatrie van ca. 1820 tot ca. 1870.* Meppel: Krips Repro.

Verwey, G. (2004). *Wilhelm Griesinger: Psychiatrie als Ärztlicher Humanismus.* Nijmegen: Arts en Boeve.

Wakefield, J.C. (1992). Disorder as harmful dysfunction: a conceptual critique of DSM-III-R's definition of mental disorder. *Psychological Review*, *99*, 232-247.

Waldenfels. B. (1985). *In den Netzen der Lebenswelt.* Frankfurt a.M.: Suhrkamp.

Waldenfels. B. (2000). *Das leibliche Selbst. Vorlesungen zur Phänomenologie des Leibes*. Frankfurt a.M.: Suhrkamp.

Waldenfels, B. (2004). *Phänomenologie der Aufmerksamkeit.* Frankfurt a.M.: Suhrkamp.

Walker, C. (1994). Karl Jaspers and Edmund Husserl: II, The divergence. *Philosophy, Psychiatry, and Psychology*, *1*, 245-266.

Walker, C. (1995). Karl Jaspers and Edmund Husserl: III, Jaspers as a Kantian phenomenologist. *Philosophy, Psychiatry, and Psychology*, *2*, 65-82.

Walsh, W.H. (1974). Colligatory concepts in history. In *The Philosophy of History*, P. Gardiner (Ed.), 127-144. Oxford; Oxford University Press.

Webster, C.D., Douglas, K.S., Eaves, D., & Hart, S.D. (1997). *HCR-20: Assessing Risk for Violence, Version 2.* Burnaby, British Columbia: Simon Frazer University.

Wegner, D.M. (2002). *The Illusion of Conscious Will.* Cambridge MA: MIT Press.

Weizsäcker, V. von (1973). *Der Gestaltkreis: Theorie der Einheit von Wahrnehmen und Bewegen.* Frankfurt a.M.: Suhrkamp. (Original work published 1940)

Welton, D. (2000). *The Other Husserl: The Horizons of Transcendental Phenomenology.* Bloomington/Indianapolis: Indiana University Press.

White, H. (1973). *Metahistory: The Historical Imagination in Nineteenth-Century Europe.* Baltimore/London: Johns Hopkins University Press.

White, P. (Ed.) (2004). *Biopsychosocial Medicine: An Integrating Approach to Understanding Illness.* Oxford/London: Oxford University Press.

Widmer, P. (2006). *Die Metamorphosen des Signifikanten. Zur Bedeutung des Körperbilds für die Realität des Subjekts.* Bielefeld: Transcript Verlag.

Wiggins, O.P., & Schwartz, M.A. (2007). Schizophrenia: a phenomenological-anthropological approach. In *Reconceiving Schizophrenia*, M.C. Chung, K.W.M. Fulford, & G. Graham (Eds.), 113-129. Oxford: Oxford University Press.

Williams, D.D.R., & Garner, J. (2002). The case against 'the evidence': A different perspective on evidence-based medicine. *British Journal of Psychiatry*, *180*, 8-12.

Winch, P. (1976). *The Idea of a Social Science and Its Relation to Philosophy.* London: Routledge and Kegan Paul. (Original work published 1958)

Windelband, W. (1904). *Geschichte und Naturwissenschaft.* Strasbourg: Heitz. (Original work published 1894)

Wing, J.K., Cooper, J.E., & Sartorius, N. (1974). *The Measurement and Classification of Psychiatric Symptoms.* Cambridge: Cambridge University Press.

Winnicott, D.W. (1965). Ego distortion in terms of true and false self. In *The Maturational Processes and the Facilitating Environment*, 140-152. London: Hogarth Press.

Winnicott, (1980). *Playing and Reality*. Harmondsworth: Penguin. (Original work published 1971)

Wittgenstein, L. (1963). *Philosophical Investigations*. Oxford: Basil Blackwell. (Original work published 1958)

Wright, G.H. von (1971). *Explanation and Understanding*. London: Routledge and Kegan Paul.

Wyrsch, J. (1956). *Zur Geschichte und Deutung der Endogenen Psychosen*. Stuttgart: Thieme.

Wyss, D. (1987). *Neue Wege in der Psychosomatischen Medizin*, Part 3: Der psychosomatisch Kranke. Göttingen: Vandenhoeck & Ruprecht.

Zacher, P. (2000). Psychiatric disorders are not natural kinds. *Philosophy, Psychiatry, Psychology*, *7*, 167-182.

Zacher, P., & Kendler, K. (2007). Psychiatric disorders: a conceptual taxonomy. *American Journal of Psychiatry*, *164*, 557-565.

Zahavi, D. (2003). *Husserl's Phenomenology*. Stanford: Stanford University Press.

Zarifian, E. (1998). *Des Paradis Plein la Tête*. Paris: Odile Jacob. (Original work published 1994)

Zarifian, E. (2005). *Le Goût de Vivre: Retrouver la Parole Perdue*. Paris: Odile Jacob.

Žižik, S. (2008). *Enjoy Your Symptom. Jacques Lacan in Hollywood and Out*. New York and London: Routledge (Work original published 1992)

Zutt, J. (1957). Blick und Stimme: Beitrag zur Grundlegung einer verstehenden Anthropologie. *Der Nervenarzt*, *28*, 350-355.

Zutt, J. (1963a). Über den tragenden Leib: Über den werdenden, wachsenden, blühenden, welkenden und vergehenden Leib. In *Die Wahnwelten (Endogene Psychosen)*, E. Straus & J. Zutt (Eds.), 384-399. Frankfurt a.M.: Akademische Verlagsgesellschaft. (Work original published 1938)

Zutt, J. (1963b). Über Daseinsordnungen. Ihre Bedeutung für die Psychiatrie. In *Die Wahnwelten (Endogene Psychosen)*, E. Straus & J. Zutt (Eds.), 169-192. Frankfurt a.M.: Akademische Verlagsgesellschaft. (Work original published 1953)

Zutt, J. (1963c). Vom ästhetischen im Unterschied zum affektiven Erlebnisbereich. In *Die Wahnwelten*, E. Straus en J. Zutt (Eds.), 155-168. Frankfurt a.M.: Akademische Verlagsgesellschaft. (Work original publised 1955)

Zwart, H. (1998). Medicine, symbolization and the 'real' body: Lacan's understanding of medical science. *Journal of Medicine, Healthcare and Philosophy*, *1*, 107-117.

Name Index

Subject Index

Printed in the United States
By Bookmasters